THE HANDBOOK OF
CANCER
IMMUNOLOGY

THE HANDBOOK OF CANCER IMMUNOLOGY

Volume 4
Immune Status in Cancer Treatment and Prognosis —Part B

THE HANDBOOK OF CANCER IMMUNOLOGY

Edited by
Harold Waters
Smithsonian Science Information Exchange

Garland STPM Press
New York & London

15   14   13   12   11   10   9   8   7   6   5   4   3   2   1

Library of Congress Cataloging in Publication Data
Main entry under title:

Immune status in cancer treatment and prognosis.

  (The Handbook of cancer immunology; v. 3–4)
  Includes bibliographies and index.
    1.   Cancer—Immunological aspects.   2.   Brain—
Tumors—Immunological aspects.   3.   Immunotherapy.
4.   Tumor antigens.   I.   Waters, Harold, 1942–
II.   Series.   [DNLM: 1.   Neoplasms—Immunology.
QZ200 H235 v. 3 etc.]
RC268.3.H35   vol. 3, etc.   616.9'94'07908s [616.9'94'079]

  ISBN 0–8240–7003–8   77–18079

Printed in the United States of America

CONTENTS

PREFACE

Detailed information about the strengths and weaknesses of the immune system at and before diagnosis of cancer may soon be essential in helping determine courses of treatment. A patient with a powerfully well-developed immune system and with a resectable tumor, promising to leave little residual burden, might be in line for more supportive types of therapy and less of the aggressive immunosuppressive approaches, whereas one presenting with details of a devastated immune system might be a candidate for an all-out therapeutic effort employing commonly used tumor and immune destructive agents.

More immediately, immune status determinations are becoming crucial for monitoring the progression of cancer and in helping document the durations of remissions and cures.

What we need more of now is to find out specifically what these tests of immunity mean. Exactly how do they relate to immune competence? Exactly what base lines have to be superimposed over cancer patient data? What are the effects of age, sex, diurnal rhythms, and acute and chronic stress? How can we expect the lymphocytes of a 47-year-old woman to perform when they are collected one hour or one day after she has been told that she has breast cancer?

There are many spaces left blank in this puzzle. The fact is, we have not even pieced together all of the edges and corners yet. And as Professor Sigel succinctly says of cancer-related immunology, "It can do good or it can make mischief." In these two volumes, 34 contributors attempt to relate immune status to cancer treatment and prognosis: they contribute to the separation of the good from the mischief.

Harold Waters
Washington, D.C.
March, 1978

CHAPTER 1

IMMUNOLOGIC ASPECTS OF HODGKIN'S DISEASE

Richard I. Fisher
and Robert C. Young

The Medicine Branch
National Cancer Institute
Bethesda, Maryland 20014

Untreated patients with Hodgkin's disease have decreased delayed hypersensitivity skin tests, E rosette formation, and mitogen-induced lymphocyte proliferation. Serum inhibitors may account for some of these observations. Abnormalities in the humoral immune system have not been convincingly demonstrated. Immunologic studies suggest that Reed-Sternberg cells are derived from monocytes and not lymphocytes. Hodgkin's disease may result from an autoimmune reaction against a virus-infected T cell. Radiotherapeutic treatment for Hodgkin's disease causes prolonged immunosuppression. The effects of combination chemotherapy on the immune system of patients with Hodgkin's disease have not been adequately analyzed. Controlled trials are needed to determine whether immunotherapy has any therapeutic efficacy.

Introduction

During the twentieth century significant progress had been made both in understanding the natural history of Hodgkin's disease and in developing effective treatment. However, the pathogenesis of Hodgkin's disease remains undeciphered. Confusion over the true nature of Hodgkin's disease, that is, whether it was an inflammatory disease or lymphoreticular malignancy, hindered early research. The association of Hodgkin's disease with tuberculosis had led to the suggestion that Hodgkin's disease was an infectious process with an inflammatory or immunologic reaction like that seen in tuberculosis (82). In 1902 Reed finally established that tuberculosis and Hodgkin's disease were separate entities (75).

Several aspects of the pathology and natural history of Hodgkin's disease still suggest that immunologic abnormalities are an integral part of this lymphoreticular malignancy. Unlike many carcinomas, the microscopic appearance of Hodgkin's disease is not composed of a uniform population of malignant cells. The cellular infiltrate consists of microscopically normal lymphocytes, eosinophils, and plasma cells plus the characteristic Reed-Sternberg cells. Reactive follicular hyperplasia can be found in many lymph nodes surrounding the actual tumor. In addition, Lukes and Collins have cited the common mediastinal presentation of nodular sclerosing Hodgkin's disease and the tendency to find early focal involvement in the paracortical region of lymph nodes as evidence that Hodgkin's disease may develop selectively in those areas of lymphoid tissue that are normally populated by thymus-derived lymphocytes (66). Peripheral blood lymphocyte counts are decreased in patients with Hodgkin's disease, particularly those with advanced-stage, constitutional symptoms and mixed cellularity or lymphocyte-depleted histologies (3, 15, 44, 84, 91). There is clearly an association between certain infections and Hodgkin's disease. In addition to tuberculosis, increased susceptibility to fungal infections and Herpes zoster has been documented by many authors (4, 16, 61). These infections are often associated with failure of normal immunologic responses. The observations by Parker et al. and Steiner, that even during the course of active tuberculosis patients with Hodgkin's disease frequently have negative tuberculin reactions, suggest that the increased susceptibility to tuberculosis might be caused by a defect of cellular immunity (72, 81). Other studies also suggest defects in cellular immunity. Kelly et al. studied patients with Hodgkin's disease who were not receiving any chemotherapy, including steroids; thirteen of seventeen patients either had no evidence of or a significant delay in rejection of an allogeneic skin graft (55).

More sophisticated techniques in immunology have provided better understanding of human immunologic mechanisms and an increased ability to measure various aspects of the immune response. The application of these techniques to patients with Hodgkin's disease now permits a more complete definition of the immunologic abnormalities associated with that illness. This review will summarize our current understanding of the *in vivo* and *in vitro* abnormalities of the immune response in patients with Hodgkin's disease; these data provide clues to understanding the pathogenesis of Hodgkin's disease as well as suggesting new methods of effective treatment.

In Vivo Abnormalities of the Non-specific Immune Response

The normal immune response involves a complex series of events, including antigen uptake and processing, antigen recognition by precursor cells with subsequent blastogenesis and proliferation, and finally antibody production or specific cell-mediated reactions. A patient's *in vivo* generation of a primary delayed hypersensitivity skin test or specific antibody formation requires that all events in the sequence of the immune response be functional.

DELAYED HYPERSENSITIVITY. Extensive skin testing of patients with Hodgkin's disease has been conducted since the 1950s, yet the degree of impairment of delayed hypersensitivity remains controversial. Much of the confusion in the literature relates to both the clinical status of the patients being analyzed and the techniques employed. The status of a patient's cell-mediated immune response has been studied *in vivo* by determining the patient's ability either to react to recall skin test antigens or to form a primary delayed hypersensitivity skin test reaction to a new antigen. In the latter case, the patient may be sensitized with a new antigen and one to two weeks later rechallenged with that antigen.

Many of the early studies suggested an impairment of delayed hypersensitivity in patients with Hodgkin's disease. In 1954, Schier *et al.* studied 43 patients (4). Only 23% had delayed hypersensitivity reactions to purified tuberculoprotein, 14% to mumps skin test antigen, 19% to *Candida albicans*, and 16% to *Trichophyton gypseum*. Positive reactions among 79 controls were observed in 71%, 90%, 92%, and 68%, respectively. The patients' stage, constitutional symptoms, and treatment were not specified.

Lamb *et al.* reported that 53% of patients with Hodgkin's disease who were "in good condition" did not react to diphtheria toxoid, streptokinase-streptodornase (SK-SD), mumps, Trichophyton, or Candida (57). Anergy to that battery of skin test antigens was observed in 1.4% of their normal control population. None of their patients had received chemotherapy within four weeks of study, but information regarding stage or other therapy was not presented.

In 1964 Aisenberg attempted to sensitize 37 patients with Hodgkin's disease to a new antigen 2,4-Dinitrochlorobenzene (DNCB) (2). He reported that all patients with active disease, even if it was localized, failed to develop a delayed hypersensitivity reaction. However, patients whose disease was inactive for over two years did have a normal response. All these studies suggested an impairment in delayed hypersensitivity but the heterogeneity of patients studied precluded definite conclusions.

The results of delayed hypersensitivity skin testing in untreated patients with Hodgkin's disease are summarized in Table 1. Young et al. in 1972 reported the first prospective study of delayed hypersensitivity in untreated Hodgkin's disease (91). The 103 patients had clinical staging and skin tests performed at the National Cancer Institute (NCI) between November 1965 and November 1967. The battery of skin test antigens included mumps, Candida, histoplasmin, coccidiodin, and intermediate-strength purified protein derivative (I-PPD). In addition, patients were sensitized with 2000-μg DNCB and rechallenged in 14 days with 50 and 100 μg of DNCB. The skin test reactivity of patients was less than controls for each antigen, and 34% of all patients did not react to any of the recall skin tests. However, when the above data were combined with the percent of patients capable of responding to DNCB, only 11.7% of patients were considered anergic. The incidence of anergy increased with stage so that none of the Stage I patients, but 26.6% of Stage IV patients, were anergic. Anergy was more common in patients with mixed cellularity or lymphocyte-depleted histologies, with profound lymphopenia, and with constitutional symptoms.

Because previous studies had suggested that the ability to develop a delayed hypersensitivity response might be a fundamental characteristic of the Hodgkin's patients who had long survival (79), Young et al. also analyzed skin test reactivity as an independent prognostic variable. All patients had been followed for at least 40 months after initial evaluation and therapy. No relationship could be determined between initial skin test reactivity and duration of remission, frequency of relapse, or survival. The authors concluded that anergy was less common in untreated Hodgkin's disease than had been previously suggested and was not a useful prognostic sign.

The experience at Stanford University was summarized by Eltring-

Table 1. Delayed hypersensitivity skin tests in untreated patients with Hodgkin's disease

Series	% Responding	
	Recall Antigens	DNCB
Young, (NCI)	66	67
Eltringham (Stanford University)	34	45
Winkelstein (University of Pittsburgh)	59	—
Chung (Rosewell Park Memorial Institute)	53	—
Case (Memorial Sloan-Kettering Institute)	66	52

ham and Kaplan in 1973 (26). One hundred fifty four untreated patients were studied. The recall skin test antigens utilized were identical to those used in the NCI study with the addition of blastomycin; however, the per cent of patients responding to each intradermal test was approximately one-half that reported by Young et al. (92). When patients were sensitized to DNCB with a 2000-μg dose, 45% of the Stanford patients responded. A greater percentage of unresponsive patients had advanced stages of disease. This did not differ statistically from the NCI report. However, if one analyzed the five recall antigens and the 2000-μg DNCB dose used in both studies, the incidence of anergy to the above tests was 25% at Stanford and 11% at the NCI. Since both series had approximately equal ratios of localized/advanced disease patients, the differences in results are difficult to explain. The discrepancy cannot be explained by the 75% incidence of nodular sclerosis in the Stanford series, which was approximately twice that of the NCI study. As previously noted, Young et al. demonstrated that skin test reactivity was highest in patients with nodular sclerosis or lymphocyte-depleted histologies (91).

Several additional groups have now reported skin test data from smaller numbers of untreated patients. Winkelstein et al. (90) studied the delayed hypersensitivity response of 27 untreated patients to mumps, Candida, Trichophyton, and SK-SD. Fifty-nine percent of patients responded to one or more of the antigens and the response rate did decrease with advanced stages. Chang et al. studied 55 patients who had minimal or no prior therapy (17). Patients who had completed one course of single-agent chemotherapy or radiotherapy to no more than two anatomic regions were defined as having minimal therapy. Using I-PPD, mumps, SK-SD (10 U), Candida, and Trichophyton, 53% of patients had at least one positive test. Furthermore, in agreement with data of Young et al., the response rate, duration of remission, and survival did not differ statistically between anergic and non-anergic patients. The experience at Memorial Sloan-Kettering Cancer Center with 52 untreated patients was reported by Case et al. (15). The skin tests utilized included I-PPD, mumps, Candida, and SK-SD. DNCB was utilized to test the capacity for primary sensitization. Overall, 34% of the patients were anergic to recall antigens: 65% of Stages III and IV and 12% of Stages I and II patients. Fifty-two percent of patients responded to DNCB sensitization.

None of the above studies addressed the possible existence of subclinical disturbances in delayed hypersensitivity, especially in patients with localized Hodgkin's disease. Eltringham and Kaplan concluded that many patients with localized disease had abnormalities in delayed hypersensitivity when tested with suboptimal doses of antigen (26). If a 500-μg dose of DNCB was used to sensitize the patients, only 25% of patients responded. This lack of response to the lower dose of DNCB occurred as frequently in patients with localized disease as those with advanced disease. Studies with SK-SD also revealed that the percentage of unresponsive patients was higher if a lower dose of antigen was used. Only 10.3% of patients with Hodgkin's disease responded to a dose (5 U) that produced positive skin tests in 60–100% of controls. If those patients who did not respond to 5 U SK-SD were rechallenged with 50 U, an additional 27.6% developed a positive test.

In summary, early studies suggested that most patients with Hodgkin's disease had profound abnormalities of delayed hypersensitivity. These results must be interpreted with the knowledge that many of the patients studied were undergoing radiotherapy or chemotherapy. As we will discuss later, both of these modalities can severely depress cell-mediated immunity. Recent studies of untreated patients (Table 1) also reveal impaired delayed hypersensitivity responses in patients with advanced stages of Hodgkin's disease. Moreover, when lower doses of antigens such as SK-SD or DNCB are utilized, a significant number of patients with Stage I or Stage II Hodgkin's are also found to have abnormal skin tests, indicating a subtle defect in cell-mediated immunity. However, available data suggest that a patient's ability to develop a delayed hypersensitivity response does not have prognostic significance in Hodgkin's disease. This is in contrast to the results found in many solid tumors, such as melanoma or sarcoma, where anergy is a poor prognostic factor regardless of stage. This difference could be attributed to the fact that highly successful therapeutic programs are now available for all stages of Hodgkin's disease—a situation not present in the treatment of melanoma or sarcoma. These successful treatment programs may overwhelm any prognostic effect of delayed hypersensitivity reactivity.

HUMORAL IMMUNITY.   Historically most patients with Hodgkin's disease have been thought to have normal humoral immunity.
An assessment of a patient's ability to form antibodies can be obtained by
measuring levels of circulating immunoglobulins, naturally occurring antibodies, or specific antibody production following immunization with a
new antigen. Results have varied somewhat, depending on the nature of
the assay and the treatment status of the patient.

Goldman and Hobbs studied the serum immunoglobulin levels of 50
radiotherapy treated patients with all stages of Hodgkin's disease (37).
They reported that IgG was increased, IgA was low normal, and IgM was
decreased, especially in advanced stages. These results were not supported by Case et al., who studied the immunoglobulin levels of 52 untreated patients (15). Most patients had normal levels of all immunoglobulins but 10–20% of patients in each stage had low immunoglobulins. No
author has reported a significant number of hypogammaglobulinemic patients (4).

Studies of the ability of patients with Hodgkin's disease to form antibodies to new antigens have given conflicting results. Previously treated
patients generally had abnormal humoral responses. Dubin originally observed that no anti-brucella antibody could be detected in 14 patients
with Hodgkin's disease who had clinically documented brucellosis (25).
Barr and Fairley noted that only 4 of 10 Hodgkin's patients developed
significant antibody titers to tetanus toxoid after primary sensitization
while the majority had normal titers after secondary immunization (9).
Saslaw et al. reported that only 40.5% of patients had positive titers to
tularemia determined 3 to 6 weeks after immunization (77). In contrast,
Aisenberg and Leskowitz immunized 19 patients with pneumococcal
polysaccharide. The only patients not producing significant antibody titers were 4 "terminal patients" (1). They also observed that although peak
titers were normal, the duration of the antibody response was shorter than
that seen in controls. Hoffman and Rottino found 81% of patients develop
a normal antibody response to typhoid-paratyphoid immunization (46).
Stage and prior radiotherapy of patients were not described.

The preceding studies all analyzed the humoral immune response in
patients undergoing treatment for their disease. Two groups have studied
untreated patients and in both cases normal antibody titers are described.
Brown et al. studied 50 untreated cases of Hodgkin's disease (14). All
patients were immunized with tularemia vaccine and antibody levels
were assayed 2 weeks later. Median titers in patients and controls were
identical; only three failed to develop a significant response. DeGast et al.
evaluated 30 untreated patients for their response to the hemocyanin protein of Helix-pomatia (αHPH) (21). IgM antibody was determined and was
normal in 24 Stage I–III patients but abnormal in two of 6 Stage IV pa-

tients. Thus most untreated patients can develop a normal humoral response to new antigens; if there are any defects in antibody production, they may occur only in the most advanced patients. Prior treatment may explain some of the early reports suggesting abnormal antibody production.

In Vitro Abnormalities
of Nonspecific Immune Response

Since the in vivo tests of the immune response have suggested an abnormality of delayed hypersensitivity, recent in vitro investigations have attempted to define the precise cause of the immune defect. Potentially, this lack of skin test reactivity could be caused by a decrease either in the number or function of effector cells.

CIRCULATING T AND B CELLS. Peripheral blood lymphocytes of man have been shown to be composed of two major subpopulations. Humoral immune responses are mediated by lymphocytes, which have easily detectable immunoglobulin on their cell surface. They are called B cells from the first letter of the bursa of Fabricius, from which they are derived, in experimental animals. Cell-mediated immunity is a function of the thymus-derived (T) lymphocytes. These cells lack easily detectable surface immunoglobulin. They are identified by their ability to form spontaneous rosettes with sheep erythrocytes (E rosette assay) or to be killed by an anti-T cell antiserum. The precise numbers of B and T cells determined will vary with the assay conditions. Therefore all results must be compared to those with controls studies in the same manner. Several groups have now attempted to determine the number of T and B cells in the peripheral blood of patients with Hodgkin's disease.

Early studies were performed on small numbers of patients undergoing various treatment programs and gave conflicting results. The population studied by Chin et al. was composed of 20 Hodgkin's disease patients, the majority having Stage III or IV disease and undergoing chemotherapy (18). Using antihuman T cell and antihuman immunoglobulin antisera, the authors reported that most patients had normal levels of T cells (mean 75%) and of B cells (mean 22%). A few patients had B cell proportions as high as 60%. In contrast Aiuti and Wigzell, using a rabbit anti-human T cell antibody, found low levels of T cells in 7 patients (mean 24% vs 50% in normals) (6). No details regarding the stage or previous treatment of the patients were provided. Cohnen et al. studied 10 patients with Hodgkin's disease; most had advanced stage and some were undergoing treatment (19). They reported low E rosettes (< 45%). B cells were low in untreated patients and high in treated patients (normal range 15–40%). Engeset et al. confirmed a normal percentage of B cells (< 20%) in 16 untreated patients, mostly Stage III or IV (27). Seven previously irradiated patients had much higher B cell levels (mean 34%). Andersen reported the results of the E rosette assay for 32 patients (19 previously untreated) (7). When compared to their controls, the untreated patients had a statistically significant decrease in E rosettes (mean 35% vs 49%). Thus some patients with Hodgkin's disease appeared to have low E rosettes and normal B cell numbers. Following radiotherapy, B cell percentages appeared to increase. However, the small numbers of patients studied and the diversity of stages and prior treatments included in these studies make any definitive conclusions impossible.

Gajl-Peczalska et al. reported the first large series of untreated patients who had simultaneous determination of B and T cells (35). Eighty-nine percent were Stage I–IIIA. They concluded that only 17% of patients had low B cells (< 11%) and 8% had low T cells determined by the E rosette assay (< 44%). They could not correlate the abnormal tests with stage, histology, or age. After radiotherapy 7 of 9 patients had increased B cells (> 34%). Swain and Trounce measured E rosettes in 32 untreated patients (83). Patients with Stage I, II, or III had normal levels of E rosettes. Those patients with Stage IV Hodgkin's disease had significantly decreased E rosettes (< 46%). Holm et al. produced a comprehensive analysis of nonspecific immune function in 38 untreated patients (47). Fifty percent of patients had levels of E rosettes below the normal range while mean B cell levels were normal. When the results were analyzed according to the patient's stage, 65% of patients with Stage III or IV were below the normal range of E rosettes while 40% of Stage I or II were low.

Bobrove et al. studied T and B cells in 42 untreated patients with Hodgkin's disease referred to Stanford University (12). Peripheral blood T cells were quantitated both by an anti-T cell antiserum and by E rosette formation. The percentage of T cells determined by the cytotoxicity assay was identical to that of a normal control population but there was a statistically significant decrease in the percent of E rosettes (mean, < 53%). No difference in the decreased E rosettes was found between patients with early or advanced stages. The percentage of B cells did not differ from that of the control population.

The apparent reduction in E rosettes in Hodgkin's disease could be caused by a true decrease in the number of T cells, an abnormal sheep erythrocyte receptor on the cells, or a serum factor interfering with the binding of sheep red cells to T cells. The finding of normal T cells by anti-T cell antibody assays with reduced T cells by the E rosette technique suggested that the actual number of T cells might be normal. The discrepancy between the two techniques for determining T cells has been investigated further by Fuks *et al.* (31). Overnight incubation of peripheral blood lymphocytes from untreated Hodgkin's patients in 20% fetal calf serum restored the percentage of E rosettes to normal. Reincubation with 20% Hodgkin's disease serum again reduced the percentage of E rosettes. This reduction in E rosettes, caused by serum from Hodgkin's disease, appeared specific for lymphocytes from patients with Hodgkin's disease. The serum factor was reported to be a low-density lipoprotein and not an immunoglobulin. This represents the first convincing demonstration that a factor present in the serum of patients with Hodgkin's disease might interact directly with T cells and could perhaps account for some of the observed defects in cellular immunity.

Thus, any determination of circulating T and B cells in Hodgkin's disease must consider the stage and treatment status of the patient as well as the technique utilized. Most determinations of T cells by anti-T cell antisera suggest a normal percent. While E rosettes are usually decreased in advance stages, some patients with limited disease also have depressed levels of E rosettes. Preliminary evidence suggests that the decrease in E rosettes may be caused by a serum inhibitor. B cell levels in untreated patients are normal or slightly decreased, while B cell levels appear to increase following treatment.

LYMPHOCYTE PROLIFERATION INDUCED BY MITOGENS, ANTIGENS, AND ALLOGENEIC CELLS.

Even though circulating T cells may be reduced in patients with Hodgkin's disease, T cell determinations are rarely less than 50% of normal levels. Whether the reduced level of T cells can account for the *in vivo* abnormalities of cell mediated immunity is unknown; however, the functional capacity of the residual lymphocytes may be just as important in determining *in vivo* immune defects.

An essential process in the formulation of an immune response is the ability of lymphocytes to proliferate following an immunologic stimulus. The capacity to proliferate can be assessed *in vitro* by incubation of lymphocytes with mitogens, antigens, or allogeneic cells. Plant lectins or mitogens can be selected to stimulate different subpopulations of lymphocytes. Under the usual experimental conditions, phytohemagglutinin (PHA) and concanavalin (Con A) stimulate T cells while pokeweed mitogen (PWM) stimulates both T and B cells to proliferate. While there is some controversy whether T or B cells stimulate a mixed leukocyte culture (MLC), incubation of lymphocytes with allogeneic cells definitely leads to a proliferation of T cells.

In 1965 Hersh and Oppenheim reported the initial studies of PHA-induced lymphocyte transformation in patients with Hodgkin's disease (45). Twenty-three patients were studied and eleven had no prior therapy.

Eighty-seven percent had responses less than that of the lowest control patient. Anergic patients had the lowest stimulations. Han and Sokal found a normal median response to PHA stimulation in 11 untreated patients with advanced stage although several patients had low stimulations (39). Jackson et al. studied 32 patients prior to radiotherapy. They suggested that PHA-induced proliferation was not significantly depressed in patients with localized disease but was decreased in patients with advanced stage or constitutional symptoms (49). The conclusion that PHA stimulation was abnormal only in patients with advanced disease was also supported by Winkelstein (90).

Forty-three patients were studied at the NCI prior to therapy and then followed to determine the prognostic significance of PHA stimulation (92). Mean PHA-induced lymphocyte transformation for the entire group was significantly lower than that of normal controls. However, when analyzed according to stage of disease, only Stage IIIB or IV patients had a significantly depressed response. Furthermore, life table analysis revealed that there was no correlation between pretreatment PHA-induced transformation and remission duration, frequency of relapse, or survival. Again one can question whether the effectiveness of treatment for Hodgkin's disease is not the dominant factor determining survival and therefore the prognostic significance of immune function tests can no longer be detected.

Most assays of mitogen stimulation determine the percentage of blast cells in the culture by direct visualization or measure tritiated thymidine incorporation into dividing cells. Levy and Kaplan measured protein synthesis in PHA-stimulated cells (63). They determined a dose response curve for various concentrations of PHA. At conventional doses of PHA only Stage III or IV patients had a suppressed response but, at lower concentrations of PHA, patients with Stage I and II disease had a response statistically lower than controls.

Faguet used the standard thymidine incorporation assay for PHA stimulation and tested 35 untreated patients with Hodgkin's disease (29). Instead of using a single PHA concentration, he constructed a dose response curve for PHA-induced stimulation over a wide range of PHA concentrations. He demonstrated that 74% of patients had abnormal PHA stimulations detected by this method although only 17% would have been detected by the usual single concentration tests. Furthermore these abnormalities were independent of stage.

Another approach to PHA stimulation assays was utilized by Matchett (67). He studied 25 untreated patients with Hodgkin's disease by calculating the kinetics of PHA stimulation. The PHA response was determined daily for 7 days at a single concentration of PHA. Under these conditions, all patients had abnormal responses. Furthermore, Matchett found that stimulation with PWM was normal; thus he suggested a selective T cell defect in Hodgkin's disease.

The well-studied series of patients reported by Holm et al. analyzed mitogen stimulation at several concentrations following PHA, Con A, and PWM, as well as antigen stimulation with PPD (47). Patient studies were considered abnormal if the stimulations fell below the range established by the authors for normal controls. PHA responses were decreased in 50% of Stage III and IV and 20% of Stage I and II. Con A response was decreased in 63% of Stage III and IV and 33% of Stage I and II. PPD stimulation was abnormal in 55% with advanced disease and 47% with localized disease. The only test involving B cell stimulation used PWM. Responses were abnormal in 55% of Stage II or IV but only 7% of Stage I or II.

Several investigators have attempted to determine whether the reduced mitogen stimulation they observed was caused by a serum inhibitor. In the initial study of mitogen stimulation by Hersh and Oppenheim, plasma from patients with Hodgkin's disease did not inhibit the proliferation of normal lymphocytes (45). In contrast, Trubowitz et al. suggested the existence of a plasma inhibitor (86). They reported that the response of patients' lymphocytes did improve when cultured with normal plasma although the difference was not statistically significant. In addition, they reported that the proliferation of control lymphocytes was less in patient's plasma than it was in autologous plasma. Unfortunately, PHA stimulations performed in autologous plasma may exceed assays performed in allogeneic plasma. There was no attempt to demonstrate a serum inhibitor by comparing the stimulation of normal lymphocytes in patients' plasma with that obtained in normal allogeneic plasma. For the above reasons, this study does not provide conclusive evidence for a plasma inhibitor of PHA stimulation. Han and Sokal noted that plasma from patients with Hodgkin's disease did not inhibit the proliferation of normal lymphocytes (39). Likewise when Matchett replaced autologous plasma with fetal calf serum in his system, no consistent change in stimulation was noted (67). However, the Stanford group has recently reported that the depressed response of patients' lymphocytes to PHA can be reversed by incubation of the cells in fetal calf serum (33). Further studies are needed to confirm the observation, but the analogy to the serum inhibitor of the E-rosette assay proposed by the same authors is obvious.

Lymphocyte transformation with the antigens Toxoplasma and SK-SD was analyzed by Gaines et al. in 23 untreated patients with Hodgkin's disease (34). Only 1 out of 23 Hodgkin's disease patients, in contrast to 13 of 14 normal controls, responded. Plasma for Hodgkin's patients inhibited transformation of normal cells and in fact patient's lymphocytes transformed normally in the presence of normal plasma.

The mixed lymphocyte culture (MLC) also measures the ability of a lymphocyte to proliferate. However, in contrast to the nonspecific mitogen-induced proliferation, the MLC proliferation is in response to a foreign antigen present on a cell membrane. A strong MLC response correlates with the ability of the donor animal to reject a graft from the stimulatory animal. Therefore the proliferation induced in an MLC might be more clearly analogous to a patient's potential response to his own tumor cells.

Bjorkholm studied the MLC response of 39 untreated patients with Hodgkin's disease (11). The mean response to randomly chosen allogeneic, mitomycin-treated, normal lymphocytes was not diminished. The 10 patients who did have a lower response could not be predicted by any clinical parameter. In contrast, the stimulatory capacity of patient's lymphocytes was markedly reduced. This conclusion was consistent with the report of Lang et al. in 1972 (58). They studied 11 untreated patients with Hodgkin's disease and found that 9 patients had normal responses to allogeneic lymphocytes.

Ruhl et al. had reached an opposite conclusion (76). They analyzed lymphocytes from 30 patients with Hodgkin's disease. Most had active advanced disease but the extent of prior treatment was unknown. They found the responding capacity of the patients' lymphocytes reduced, while the stimulatory capacity was normal. In addition they studied the kinetics of the MLC, and found that the patients had a normal peak response at 144 – 168 hours.

Kasakura performed a similar assay on lymphocytes from 10 untreated patients (53). The patients who had limited disease could both respond to allogeneic cells and also stimulate them in a normal manner. In patients with advanced disease, both stimulating and responding capacity were reduced.

In 1975, Twomey et al. analyzed the ability of lymphocytes from 30 patients with Hodgkin's disease to stimulate normal lymphocytes in an MLC (87). Subnormal stimulation was found in 15 of 22 Stage III or IV and 1 of 8 Stage I or II patients. Subnormal stimulation was also more common in patients with constitutional symptoms and mixed cellularity or lymphocyte depleted histologies. This decreased stimulation of allogeneic cells by patient mononuclear leukocytes was attributed to excessive suppressor lymphocytes since removal of adherent cells from the patient mononuclear leukocytes or inhibition of protein synthesis by those cells restored a normal stimulatory capacity. Removal of phagocytic cells did not alter the stimulatory capability. Unfortunately experiments where patient adherent cells were mixed with normal stimulatory leukocytes were not reported. The latter experiment would have determined whether the suppressor lymphocytes could suppress normal MLC response as well as the MLC of patients with Hodgkin's disease.

Table 2.   Mean PHA stimulations in untreated patients with Hodgkin's disease

Author (Technique)	Stage I–II	Stage III–IV
Jackson (maximal PHA conc.)	Normal	Decreased
Winkelstein (maximal PHA conc.)	Normal	Decreased
Young (maximal PHA conc.)	Normal	Decreased
Holm (maximal PHA conc.)	Normal	Decreased
Levy (maximal PHA conc.)	Normal	Decreased
(suboptimal PHA conc.)	Decreased	Decreased
Faquet (PHA dose response curve)	Decreased	Decreased
Matchett (suboptimal lymph conc. with kinetic analysis)	Decreased	Decreased

In summary, patients with untreated Hodgkin's disease have abnormal proliferation of their lymphocytes in response to PHA, as summarized in Table 2. At high concentration of PHA, the defect is detected only in patients with advanced stages. However, patients with localized disease also have abnormal proliferation if a dose response curve or kinetic analysis of PHA stimulation is calculated. To date there is no conclusive evidence supporting the existence of a plasma inhibitor of PHA induced proliferation. The ability of lymphocytes to stimulate or respond in the MLC is subnormal in some patients with advanced stages of Hodgkin's disease. Studies of patients with early stages of disease have produced conflicting results. Some of the discrepancies may relate to methods of performing the MLC. One investigator has presented evidence which suggests that a suppressor lymphocyte may inhibit the stimulatory capacity of lymphocytes from patients with Hodgkin's disease.

Immunologic Clues to Etiology of Hodgkin's Disease

The preceding data have dealt with the status of the immune system in patients with Hodgkin's disease. Since Hodgkin's disease is a malignancy of lymphoid tissue, investigators have also attempted to determine the origin of the cellular infiltrates in involved tissues. Such information might provide clues to the etiology or pathogenesis of this disease.

ORIGIN OF CELLULAR INFILTRATES.   Fairley *et al.* first described the presence of an abnormal population of lymphoid cells in the peripheral blood of patients with Hodgkin's disease (30). These circulating cells were larger than 15 μ in diameter, had abundant pale-staining cytoplasm, and showed monocytoid or lymphoblast-like nuclei. They resembled the circulating cells seen in infectious mononucleosis. The cells also had increased DNA synthesis, determined by thymidine incorporation. This abnormal population was related to the activity of disease but could not be correlated with stage, histology, or prognosis. Huber et al. performed simultaneous DNA incorporation and E rosette assays on these cells (48). The majority of cells formed E rosettes. Schiffer et al. were able to visualize similar cells in 8 patients with viral upper respiratory infections as well as 33 patients with Hodgkin's disease (78). They could not correlate the presence of these cells with histology, stage, splenic involvement, or response to therapy and concluded that the cells were probably "reactive," that is, did not represent circulating tumor cells.

Several investigators have attempted to analyze the cellular infiltrate in lymphoid tissues. Kaur et al. studied the mononuclear cells obtained from 7 spleens from patients with all stages of nodular sclerosis Hodgkin's disease (54). The number of immunoglobulin-bearing cells was reduced compared to that found in nonmalignant spleens. In addition 67% of cells from spleens infiltrated with Hodgkin's disease responded to PHA while 28% of cells from uninvolved spleens underwent PHA-induced transformation, suggesting an increased T cell population in involved nodes. Braylan et al. confirmed an increase in T cells in suspensions made from the spleens or lymph nodes of 5 patients with Hodgkin's disease (13). E rosettes were detected in 73.6% of patients versus 36.2% of normals, while surface immunoglobulin positive cells were found in 20.6% of patients and 30.6% of normals. Aisenberg and Long did not find such dramatic differences in a series of patients when 5 normal and 13 inflammatory nodes were used as controls (5). The authors used an anti-T cell antiserum and E rosettes to detect T cells and a fluoresceinated anti-Ig to detect B cells. All but one nonmalignant node had greater than 60% of cells reacting with the anti-T cell antiserum and most had greater than 80% T cells by this test. The E rosette assay consistently yielded lower results (34% mean in normal nodes and 44% in hyperplastic nodes). Fourteen patients with Hodgkin's disease had similar results with the anti-T cell antiserum (73% mean) but higher results by E rosette assay (57% mean). No monoclonal populations of B cells were seen in nodes from patients with either Hodgkin's disease or nonmalignant conditions. Gajl-Peczalska studied the lymph nodes from 10 patients with Hodgkin's disease using the E rosette assay and found that 80% had normal percentages of T cells while the other 20% had increased percentages (35).

The cell most characteristic of Hodgkin's disease is the Reed-Sternberg cell. Several investigators have attempted to determine the origin of these cells. Peckham and Cooper studied short-term in vitro cultures derived from the involved lymph nodes of patients with Hodgkin's disease (73). They were unable to demonstrate any labeling of Reed-Sternberg cells and concluded that they were a nonproliferative cell. In long-term cultures, Kaden and Asburg reached a different conclusion (50). Multinecleated Hodgkin's cells showed evidence of DNA synthesis and nuclear division. Kaden et al. later reported that Hodgkin's cells (the mononuclear variant of Reed-Sternberg cells) from fresh splenic or lymph node preparations had intracytoplasmic IgG by immunofluorescence but did not form E rosettes or react with an antithymocyte antiserum (51). This observation was confirmed by Leech and Garvin et al. (36, 60). Taylor used an anti-light chain antibody followed by an immunoperoxidase labeled anti-Ig on sections from nodes of 20 patients with Hodgkin's disease (85). The number of stained Reed-Sternberg cells within a given case was highly variable, suggesting that not all Reed-Sternberg cells contain cytoplasmic immunoglobulin. In contrast, Boecker et al. obtained cells from the pleural effusions of two patients with Hodgkin's disease and placed them in short-term culture. Approximately 80% of the Hodgkin cells and Reed-Sternberg cells had detectable cell surface immunoglobulin while neither cell formed E rosettes.

Kaplan has reported preliminary results of his immunologic characterization of short term cultures from Hodgkin's disease tissue (52). The cells appeared morphologically similar to macrophages, adhered to plastic, and phagocytized India ink particles. They formed IgG-EA rosettes indicating the presence of an F_c receptor. They also formed IgM-EAC rosettes when the C_{3b} component of complement was used but not when the C_{3d} component was tested. This later test suggests that the complement receptor on these cells resembles the complement receptor on monocytes and not B cells. Finally, the cells lacked surface IgM, which cannot adhere to cell membranes via the F_c receptor. Therefore Kaplan concluded that all evidence derived from his in vitro cultures suggests that cultured Hodgkin's cells are derived from monocytes and not lymphocytes.

Thus there is no convincing evidence that the lymphocytic infiltrate in spleens or lymph nodes of patients with Hodgkin's disease represents a monoclonal proliferation of B or T cells. The peripheral blood of patients with active disease does contain some atypical lymphoblastoid cells which are probably "reactive" cells and not tumor cells. The characteristic Reed-Sternberg cell probably contains intracytoplasmic immunoglobulin, an F_c receptor, and a complement receptor, all suggesting that the cell is derived from monocytes and not lymphocytes.

EVIDENCE FOR TUMOR-ASSOCIATED ANTIGENS. Tumor-associated antigens have been described in numerous animal and human malignancies. In animal models, carcinogen-induced tumors appear to have unique antigenic determinants for each tumor while viral-induced tumors share some common antigens when caused by the same virus. Thus characterization of a tumor associated antigen might provide some clues to the etiology of Hodgkin's disease. In addition, detection of tumor-associated antigens might assist in separating the true malignant manifestations of Hodgkin's disease from the reactive process that occurs in response to the tumor.

Order, Porter, and Hellman provided the first evidence of a tumor associated antigen in Hodgkin's disease (68). They obtained suspensions of involved nodes and spleens from 2 patients with Hodgkin's disease. These cells were used to immunize rabbits and the resulting antisera were absorbed with autologous normal spleen cells. Using indirect immuno-fluorescence, they demonstrated that the antisera stained tumor nodules and not normal spleen. Common antigenicity was also demonstrated between the two tumors. The same results were later demonstrated in 18 Hodgkin's involved spleens (70). A homogenized tumor yielded a crude antigen preparation that could be analyzed by gel diffusion and im-munoelectrophoresis. Results indicated that three distinct antigens were being detected by the antisera: a fast migrating band (F-antigen), a slowly migrating band (S-antigen), and a band present in the lysates of peripheral lymphocytes (PL-antigen) (71). In addition to being present in Hodgkin's disease, the F-antigen could be found only in thymus, fetal tissue, and Burkitt lymphoma cell cultures. It has now been characterized as being identical to ferritin (28). It is of interest that Bieber et al. detected ferritin by counterelectrophoresis in the serum of 68% of Stage III or IV and 32% of Stage I or II patients but not in normal serum (10). Serum ferritin was also elevated in 28% of non-Hodgkin's lymphomas, 60% of patients with hepatitis, and a few patients with metastatic carcinoma. The S-antigen and PL-antigen reacted with normal serum components which had been absorbed to or constitute part of the lymphocyte membrane.

Long, Aisenberg, and Zamecnik used material obtained from the supernatants of monolayer cultures of spleens involved by Hodgkin's disease to immunize rabbits (64). The resulting antibody reacted strongly with the cell surface of the Hodgkin's spleen cells in culture but not with non-cultured Hodgkin's spleen cells. Since there was some cross-reactivity with normal spleen, the antigen was called tumor-associated and not tumor-specific. The exact nature of the antigen was not charac-terized further.

Longmire et al. demonstrated that in vitro splenic IgG synthesis was increased in Hodgkin's disease (65). Synthesis was greatest in uninvolved or slightly involved spleens. Massively involved spleens produced less IgG, although IgG production was still above normal controls. The IgG produced was shown to react strongly with autologous peripheral blood lymphocytes, suggesting that the antibody might be directed against a tumor-associated antigen.

The leukocyte migration inhibition (LMI) assay has also suggested the presence of tumor associated immunity in Hodgkin's disease (42, 43). A factor was obtained from the homogenate of a spleen from one patient with Hodgkin's disease. This factor inhibited leukocyte migration in 56% of 77 untreated patients but only 4% of normal controls. There was no correlation between LMI and stage or histology. Patients entering complete remission did have higher LMI than those with partial or no response to therapy. At the time of relapse, most patients lost evidence of LMI.

If a virus infection was the initial step in the pathogenesis of Hodgkin's disease, one might expect to find viral antigens in the tumor. Likewise, if the host could generate an immune response against the tumor, antiviral antibodies might be present. Therefore several authors have attempted to detect antiviral antibodies instead of focusing on the detection of tumor-associated antigens. In 1971, Levine et al. reported elevated antibody titers to Epstein-Barr virus (EBV) in Hodgkin's disease (62). Antibodies to four other Herpes viruses did not differ between patients and controls. The authors could not distinguish between an etiologic role for EBV and that of a passenger virus. However, Goldman and Aisenberg did not detect a difference in EBV titers between patients and age-matched controls (38). Furthermore, Langenhuysen et al. reported elevated antibody titers to both EBV and cytomegalovirus in patients with Hodgkin's disease (59). Thus, there is no conclusive data suggesting that either EBV infection is more common in patients with Hodgkin's or has an etiologic role.

The preceding immunologic data have led to several theories regarding the development of Hodgkin's disease. Order and Hellman postulated that initially some T cells were selectively infected by a virus (69). The infected T cells underwent an antigenic alteration of their surface membranes which led normal T cells to develop a chronic autoimmune reaction against them. This immune reaction resembled a graft-versus-host reaction and led to a malignant reticulum cell line and lymphocyte depletion with anergy. In contrast, DeVita stressed the significance of Longmire's report of increased IgG capable of reacting with autologous lymphocytes (24). He postulated that it was a B cell that created the autoimmune reaction against a virus-infected, antigenically altered T cell. The B cell production of autoantibodies led to reactive hyperplasia, circulating lymphoblast cells, and progressive loss of T cell function with advancing stage. It is obvious that both theories stress very similar occurrences in the pathogenesis of Hodgkin's disease. The major discrepancy involves the question of whether the initial reaction against a viral-infected T cell is a humoral or cell-mediated reaction. This latter question will probably remain unresolved until a tumor-associated antigen can be easily detected on a viral-infected T cell; then assays can be designed to determine whether the reaction to that antigen is mediated by T or B cells.

Alterations in Immune Response Following Staging and Therapy

EXPLORATORY LAPAROTOMY AND SPLENECTOMY. Exploratory laparotomy with splenectomy has been utilized as a routine staging procedure in many institutions. This procedure has provided immunologists an opportunity to determine what effects the removal of a major lymphoid organ would have on the various immune alterations that accompany Hodgkin's disease. In addition, young children undergoing splenectomy are known to have an increased incidence of gram-positive sepsis, which theoretically could be related to changes in the immune system following splenectomy. Whether postsplenectomy infection is a significant problem in adults with Hodgkin's disease remains controversial (22). Wagener et al. tested the response of peripheral blood lymphocytes to PHA and PWM stimulation before and 10 days after splenectomy (88). PHA stimulation was unchanged in patients with Stage I or II but increased significantly in Stage III or IV. PWM stimulation was unchanged in all patients. No change in skin test reactivity, E rosettes, EAC rosettes, or proliferation following incubation with antigens or allogeneic cells was observed (89). However, patients whose spleens weighed more than 240 grams had decreased E rosettes and increased EAC rosettes in the peripheral blood following operation. The authors did not analyze cells in those large spleens to determine whether increased numbers of E rosetting lymphocytes were removed by splenectomy. They concluded that there was no major immunosuppression observed shortly after splenectomy. The effect of splenectomy on humoral immunity was described by Hancock et al. (41). Levels of IgG, IgA, and IgM were unchanged 2 to 4 weeks postsplenectomy from presplenectomy levels. The results of these studies do not provide an immunologic reason to suspect an increased incidence of gram-positive sepsis in patients with Hodgkin's disease following splenectomy. However, as noted below, the effects of treatment on antibody levels in splenectomized patients might explain the increased incidence of infection.

RADIOTHERAPY AND CHEMOTHERAPY. Detailed analysis of the effects of radiotherapy on the immune responses of patients with

Hodgkin's disease have been published recently. Hancock *et al.* reported that immediately after radiotherapy or chemotherapy IgA and IgM levels fell significantly only in splenectomized patients (41). Skin test immunocompetence decreased in all patients but the greatest decrease was seen after chemotherapy. Kun and Johnson analyzed 71 patients treated with radiotherapy who had remained disease free for 5 or more years (56). Quantitative immunoglobulins were within the normal range. The percent of anergic patients (10–13%) was unchanged since the pretreatment evaluation.

Fuks *et al.* analyzed multiple *in vitro* immune assays in 79 patients who were in long-term complete remission (one to ten years) following radiation therapy (32). A result which was more than two standard deviations below the mean for normal donors was defined as abnormal. Immediately following the completion of radiotherapy, all patients had severe lymphopenia while only 27% of patients studied 12–111 months following radiation had lymphopenia. Peripheral blood B lymphocytes were reduced in all patients immediately following radiation, but by 12–111 months, 61% actually had an absolute B lymphocytosis. Blood T lymphocytes were significantly reduced after radiotherapy and remained reduced in all long-term remissions. Null lymphocytes (small lymphs without B or T cell markers) increased significantly after treatment. Lymphocyte stimulation by PHA or ConA was significantly reduced in all long-term remitters. In contrast, the ability of a patient's lymphocyte to respond in a MLC was significantly reduced during the first 2 years after treatment but returned to normal after 5 or more years of continuous remission.

Therefore, radiation therapy, as used in treating Hodgkin's disease, significantly reduces B and T lymphocyte subpopulations immediately following therapy. All assays of lymphocyte function are likewise reduced. Thereafter a gradual increase in B lymphocytes occurs so that by one year after radiation therapy B cells are present in normal numbers. However, B cells continue to increase subsequently leading to a B lymphocytosis. In contrast, total T cells and T cells stimulated by PHA or Con A remain depressed for up to 10 years. However, the subset of T cells that responds in a MLC are restored to normal by 5 years. In summary, intensive radiation therapy for Hodgkin's disease (involved field, extended field, or total nodal) causes rapid, profound immunosuppression. The kinetics of restoration of immune function vary for each subpopulation of lymphocytes.

The effects of combination chemotherapy on the immune response have not been studied intensively. DeVita *et al.* reported the delayed hypersensitivity responses of 30 patients with advanced stages of Hodgkin's disease who were treated with MOPP chemotherapy (nitrogen mustard, vincristine, procarbazine, and prednisone) (23). Sixty percent of these patients were anergic to recall antigens and DNCB prior to treatment. Once again, the complete remission rate, duration of remission, and survival did not vary according to skin test responsiveness. However, 8 previously anergic patients entered a complete remission and had repeat skin testing after at least 10 months in complete remission. Five of the 8 patients had become reactive to at least one recall antigen.

Therefore, although the number of patients studied remains small, anergic patients achieving a complete remission may develop some evidence of restored immune competence. Detailed studies of multiple in vitro assays are needed to determine whether chemotherapy induces the same type of prolonged immune suppression that was reported in patients treated with radiotherapy.

IMMUNOTHERAPY. In 1969, Sokal and Aungst studied 32 patients with negative skin tests (79). Most of the patients were Stage IV and had either recently completed chemotherapy or radiotherapy or were receiving maintenance chemotherapy. These patients were immunized with living Bacillus Calmette-Guerin (BCG). Only 1 of 24 patients who converted to a positive I-PPD skin test died within one year, while 7 of 8 who remained anergic died. The authors suggested that the ability to convert to a positive I-PPD skin test might have prognostic significance. The authors acknowledged that this study preceded the development of effective regimens of radiotherapy or chemotherapy for the treatment of Hodgkin's disease. As noted above, studies of anergic patients treated with effective therapeutic regimens have not demonstrated that anergy had any prognostic significance. Sokal et al. later reported the results of a clinical trial which included 32 patients with Hodgkin's disease who were randomized after treatment to receive no maintenance treatment or BCG (80). The mean time to relapse was 13.1 months for the controls or 31.7 months for the vaccinated patients. Unfortunately no detailed analysis of the results in patients with Hodgkin's disease matched for stage and/or histology was provided. In addition the authors acknowledged that the treatment regimens utilized in 1965 were inadequate by present standards. Thus no conclusion concerning the value of BCG in these patients can be reached.

The Eastern Cooperative Oncology Group is attempting to determine the value of maintenance BCG in the treatment of Hodgkin's disease (8). Patients who achieved a complete remission are randomized to receive no further treatment, intradermal injections of BCG or maintenance chemotherapy. To date there are no differences between the maintenance regimens. Ramot et al. studied the in vitro and in vivo effects of levamisole, an antihelminthic agent which restores delayed hypersensitivity responses in anergic patients with cancer, on E rosette formation in patients with Hodgkin's disease (74). Twenty-eight patients, most of whom were undergoing therapy, had increased E rosettes after *in vitro* incubation with levamisole. Administration of 150 mg of levamisole to patients for 3 days also increased the percent of E rosettes to normal levels. This increase was maintained for 2 months. No clinical results of this effect were analyzed.

In summary, there is little information available concerning the effects of staging and treatment on the immune response in patients with Hodgkin's disease. Splenectomy does not appear to alter immunoglobulin levels, skin tests, or the proportion of T and B cells in the peripheral blood. More specific functional assays of immune response have not been studied. The exact immunologic effects of combination chemotherapy on the immune system are unknown. Radiotherapy causes profound and prolonged immunosuppression. Immunotherapy remains largely an unproven modality of therapy for Hodgkin's disease. Future studies need to determine whether immunotherapy can increase the initial complete remission rate or prevent relapse after attaining a complete remission.

Conclusion

The initial observations, that patients with Hodgkin's disease had an increased susceptibility to certain infections and often remained unresponsive to tuberculin testing during active infection with tuberculosis, suggested that an immunologic defect might be associated with Hodgkin's disease. Progress in defining the immunologic abnormalities was limited until the necessity of studying untreated, staged patients was realized. Results of recent *in vivo* and *in vitro* immunologic testing now enable us to define the immune abnormalities and often resolve inconsistencies that were evident from the older literature. Although patients with advanced disease have certain easily detectable abnormalities of immune function, the same alterations can generally be detected in patients with localized disease when more sensitive assays are used.

Patients with advanced stages of Hodgkin's disease have severely impaired delayed hypersensitivity skin tests while patients with localized disease also have abnormal skin tests when tested with lower doses of antigen. Numbers of circulating T cells are normal when detected by anti-T cell antibodies but reduced in the E rosette assay. The discrepancy between the two tests probably reflects the presence of an inhibitor of the sheep erythrocyte-T cell binding. Recent evidence suggests that the Reed-Sternberg cell is of monocytoid and not lymphoid origin.

Thus consistent abnormalities of T cell function can be detected in most patients with Hodgkin's disease. The fundamental question of what role these abnormalities have in the pathogenesis of Hodgkin's disease remains unresolved. Several authors have postulated that Hodgkin's disease results from an autoimmune reaction against a virus infected T cell. If future studies can define and characterize the tumor associated antigens, then investigators may be able to study immunologic reactions occurring early in the development of Hodgkin's disease. In addition, controlled trials can now be established to determine whether modulation of these defects by immunotherapy has any therapeutic efficacy.

REFERENCES

1. Aisenberg, A. C., and Leskowitz, S. 1963. Antibody formation in Hodgkin's disease. N. Engl. J. Med. 268: 1269–1272.

2. Aisenberg, A. C. 1964. Hodgkin's disease: prognosis, treatment, and etiologic and immunologic consideration. N. Engl. J. Med. 270: 617–622.

3. Aisenberg, A. C. 1965. Lymphocytopenia in Hodgkin's disease. Blood. 25: 1037–1042.

4. Aisenberg, A. C. 1966. Manifestations of immunologic unresponsiveness in Hodgkin's disease. Cancer Res. 26: 1152–1160.

5. Aisenberg, A. C., and Long, J. C. 1975. Lymphocyte surface characteristics in malignant lymphoma. Amer. J. Med. 58: 300–306.

6. Aiuti, F., and Wigzell, H. 1973. Function and distribution pattern of human T lymphocytes. II. Presence of T lymphocytes in normal humans and humans with various immunodeficiency. Clin. Exp. Immunol. 13: 183–189.

7. Andersen, E. 1974. Depletion of thymus dependent lymphocytes in Hodgkin's disease. Scand. J. Haematol. 12: 263–269.

8. Bakemeier, R. F., DeVita, V. T., and Horton, J. 1975. Chemotherapy and immunotherapy of Hodgkin's disease. Proc. Amer. Soc. Clin. Onc. 17: 293.

9. Barr, M., and Fairley, G. H. 1961. Circulating antibody in reticulons. Lancet i: 1305–1310.

10. Bieber, C. P., and Bieber, M. M. 1973. Detection of ferritin as a circulating tumor-associated antigen in Hodgkin's disease. Natl. Cancer Inst. Monogr. 36: 147–158.

11. Bjorkholm, G., Holm, G., Mellstedt, H., and Pettersson, D. 1976. Immunological capacity of lymphocytes from untreated patients with Hodgkin's disease evaluated in mixed lymphocyte culture. Clin. Exp. Immunol. 22: 373–377.

12. Bobrove, A. M., Fuks, Z., Strober, S., and Kaplan, H. S. 1975. Quantitation of T and B lymphocytes and cellular immune function in Hodgkin's disease. Cancer. 36: 169–179.

13. Braylan, R. C., Jaffe, E. S., and Berard, C. W. 1974. Surface characteristics of Hodgkin's lymphoma cells. Lancet ii: 1328–1329.

14. Brown, R. S., Haynes, H. A., Foley, H. T., Godwin, H. A., Berard, C. W., and Carbone, P. P. 1967. Hodgkin's disease: immunologic, clinical and histologic features of 50 untreated patients. Ann. Intern. Med. 67: 291–302.

15. Case, D. C., Hansen, J. A., Corrales, E., Young, C. W., Dupont, B., Pinsky, C. M., and Good, R. A. 1976. Comparison of multiple in vivo and in vitro parameters in untreated patients with Hodgkin's disease. *Cancer* 38: 1807–1815.

16. Casazza, A. R., Duvall, C. P., and Carbone, P. P. 1966. Infection in lymphoma. *JAMA* 197: 710–724.

17. Chang, T. C., Stutzman, L., and Sokal, J. E. 1975. Correlation of delayed hypersensitivity responses with chemotherapeutic results in advanced Hodgkin's disease. *Cancer.* 36: 950–955.

18. Chin, A. V., Saiki, J. H., Trujillo, J. M., and Williams, R. C. 1973. Peripheral blood T and B lymphocytes in patients with lymphoma and acute leukemia. *Clin. Immunol. Immunopathol.* 1: 499–510.

19. Cohnen, G., Augener, W., Brittinger, G., and Douglas, S. D. 1973. Rosette forming lymphocytes in Hodgkin's disease. *N. Engl. J. Med.* 289: 863.

20. Corder, M. P., Young, R. C., Brown, R. S., and DeVita, V. T. 1972. Phytohemagglutinin induced lymphocyte transformation: the relationship to prognosis of Hodgkin's disease. *Blood* 39: 595–601.

21. DeGast, G. C., Halie, M. R., and Niewig, H. O. 1975. Immunologic responsiveness against two primary antigens in untreated patients with Hodgkin's disease. *Eur. J. Cancer* 11: 217–224.

22. Desser, R. K., and Ultmann, J. E. 1972. Risk of severe infection in patients with Hodgkin's disease or lymphoma after diagnostic laparotomy and splenectomy. *Ann. Intern. Med.* 76: 143–146.

23. DeVita, V. T., Serpick, A. A., and Carbone, P. P. 1970. Combination chemotherapy in the treatment of advanced Hodgkin's disease. *Ann. Intern. Med.* 73: 881–895.

24. DeVita, V. T. 1973. Lymphocyte reactivity in Hodgkin's disease: a lymphocyte civil war. *N. Engl. J. Med.* 289: 801–802.

25. Dubin, J. N. 1947. Poverty of immunologic mechanism in patients with Hodgkin's disease. *Ann. Med.* 27: 898–913.

26. Eltringham, J. R., and Kaplan, H. S. 1973. Impaired delayed-hypersensitivity responses in 154 patients with untreated Hodgkin's disease. *Natl. Cancer Inst. Monogr.* 36: 107–116.

27. Engeset, A., Froland, S. S., Bremer, K., and Host, H. 1973. Blood lymphocytes in Hodgkin's disease. *Scand. J. Haematol.* 11: 195–200.

28. Eshhar, Z., Order, S. E., and Katz, D. H. 1974. Ferritin, a Hodgkin's disease associated antigen. *Proc. Nat. Acad. Sci. (U.S.)* 71: 3956–3960.

29. Faguet, G. B. 1975. Quantitation of immunocompetence in Hodgkin's disease. *J. Clin. Invest.* 56: 951–957.

30. Fairley, G. H., Crowther, D., Powles, R. L., Sewell, R. L., and Balchin, L. A. 1973. Circulating lymphoid cells in Hodgkin's disease. *Natl. Cancer Inst. Monogr.* 36: 95–98.

31. Fuks, Z., Strober, S., and Kaplan, H. S. 1976. Interaction between serum factors and T lymphocytes in Hodgkin's disease. *N. Engl. J. Med.* 295: 1273–1278.

32. Fuks, Z., Strober, S., Bobrove, A. M., Sasazuki, T., McMichael, A., and Kaplan, H. S. 1976. Long term effects of radiation on T and B lymphocytes in peripheral blood of patients with Hodgkin's disease. *J. Clin. Invest.* 58: 803–814.

33. Fuks, Z., Strober, S., King, D. P., and Kaplan, H. S. Reversal of surface

abnormalities of T lymphocytes in Hodgkin's disease after in vitro incubation in fetal sera. *J. Immunol.* (in press).

34. Gaines, J. D., Gilmer, M. A., and Remington, J. S. 1973. Deficiency of lymphocyte antigen recognition in Hodgkin's disease. *Natl. Cancer Inst. Monogr.* 36: 117–122.

35. Gajl-Peczalska, K. J., Bloomfield, C. D., Sosin, H., and Kersey, J. H. 1976. B and T lymphocytes in Hodgkin's disease: analysis at diagnosis and following therapy. *Clin. Exp. Immunol.* 23: 47–55.

36. Garvin, A. J., Spicer, S. S., Parmley, R. T., and Munster, A. M. 1974. Immunohistochemical demonstration of IgG in Reed-Sternberg cells and other cells in Hodgkin's disease. *J. Exp. Med.* 139: 1077–1083.

37. Goldman, J. M., and Hobbs, R. J. 1967. The immunoglobulins of Hodgkin's disease. *Immunology* 13: 421–431.

38. Goldman J. M., and Aisenberg, A. C. 1970. Incidence of antibody to EB virus, Herpes Simplex, and Cytomegalovirus in Hodgkin's disease. *Cancer* 26: 327–331.

39. Han, T., and Sokal, J. E. 1970. Lymphocyte response to phytohemagglutinin in Hodgkin's disease. *Amer. J. Med.* 48: 728–734.

40. Han, T. 1972. Effect of sera from patients with Hodgkin's disease on normal lymphocyte response to phytohemagglutinin. *Cancer* 29: 1626–1631.

41. Hancock, B. W., Bruce, L., Ward, A. M., and Richmond, J. 1976. Changes in immune status in patients undergoing splenectomy for the staging of Hodgkin's disease. *Brit. Med. J.* 1: 313–315.

42. Hancock, B. W., Bruce, L., and Richmond, J. 1976. Cellular immunity to Hodgkin's splenic tissue measured by leukocyte migration inhibition. *Brit. Med. J.* 1: 556–557.

43. Hancock, B. W., Bruce, L., and Richmond, J. 1976. Sensitization to Hodgkin's disease spleen tissue in patients with malignant lymphoma. *Brit. Med. J.* 2: 351–352.

44. Henry, L., Knowelden, J., and Swan, H. T. 1973. Relationship of the pretreatment peripheral lymphocyte count to histology in Hodgkin's disease. *Brit. J. Haematol.* 24: 773–776.

45. Hersh, E. M., and Oppenheim, J. J. 1965. Impaired *in vitro* lymphocyte transformation in Hodgkin's disease. *N. Engl. J. Med.* 273: 1006–1012.

46. Hoffman, G. T., and Rottino, A. 1950. Studies of immunologic reactions of patients with Hodgkin's disease: antibody reaction to typhoid immunization. *Arch. Int. Med.* 86: 872–876.

47. Holm, G., Mellstedt, H., Bjorkholm, M., Johansson, B., Killander, D., Sundblad, R., and Soderberg, G. 1976. Lymphocyte abnormalities in untreated patients with Hodgkin's disease. *Cancer* 37: 751–762.

48. Huber, C., Michlmayr, G., Falkensamer, M., Fink, U., Zur Nedden, G., Braunsteiner, H., and Huber, H. 1975. Increased proliferation of T lymphocytes in the blood of patients with Hodgkin's disease. *Clin. Exp. Immunol.* 21: 47–53.

49. Jackson, S. M., Garrett, J. V., and Craig, A. W. 1970. Lymphocyte transformation changes during clinical course of Hodgkin's disease. *Cancer* 25: 843–850.

50. Kadin, M. E., and Asbury, A. K. 1973. Long term cultures of Hodgkin's

tissue: a morphologic and radioautographic study. *Lab. Invest.* 28: 181–184.

51. Kadin, M. E., Newcom, S. R., Gold, S. B., and Stites, D. P. 1974. Origin of Hodgkin's disease cells. *Lancet ii*: 167–168.

52. Kaplan, H. S. 1976. Hodgkin's disease and other human malignant lymphomas: advances and prospects. *Cancer Res.* 36: 3863–3878.

53. Kasakura, S. 1975. MLC stimulatory capacity and production of a blastogenic factor in patients with chronic lymphatic leukemia and Hodgkin's disease. *Blood* 45: 823–832.

54. Kaur, J., Spiers, A. S., Catovsky, D., and Galton, D. A. 1974. Increase of T lymphocytes in the spleen of Hodgkin's disease. *Lancet ii*: 800–802.

55. Kelly, W. D., Lamb, D. L., Varco, R. L., and Good, R. A. 1960. An investigation of Hodgkin's disease with respect to the problem of homotransplantation. *Ann. N.Y. Acad. Sci.* 87: 187–202.

56. Kun, L. E., and Johnson, R. E. 1975. Hematologic and immunologic status in Hodgkin's disease 5 years after radical radiotherapy. *Cancer* 36: 1912–1916.

57. Lamb, D., Pilney, F., Kelly, W. D., and Good, R. A. 1962. A comparative study of the incidence of anergy in patients with carcinoma, leukemia, Hodgkin's disease and other lymphomas. *J. Immunol.* 89: 555–558.

58. Lang, J. M., Oberling, F., Tangio, M. M., Mayer, S., and Waitz, R. 1972. MLR as assay for immunologic competence of lymphocytes from patients with Hodgkin's disease. *Lancet i*: 1261–1263.

59. Langenhuysen, M. M., Cazemier, T., Houwen, B., Brouwers, T. M., Halie, M. R., The, T. H., and Nieweg, H. O. 1974. Antibodies of Epstein-Barr virus, cytomegalovirus, and Australia antigen in Hodgkin's disease. *Cancer* 34: 262–267.

60. Leech, J. 1974. Immunoglobulin positive Reed-Sternberg cells in Hodgkin's disease. *Lancet ii*: 265–266.

61. Levine, A. S., Schimpff, S. C., Graw, R. G., and Young, R. C. 1974. Hematologic malignancies: programs in management of complicating infections. *Sem. Hemat.* 11: 141–202.

62. Levine, P. H., Ablashi, D. V., Berard, C. W., Carbone, P. P., Waggoner, D.E., and Malan, L. 1971. Elevated antibody titers to Epstein-Barr virus in Hodgkin's disease. *Cancer* 27: 416–421.

63. Levy, R., and Kaplan, H. S. 1974. Impaired lymphocyte function in untreated Hodgkin's disease. *N. Engl. J. Med.* 290: 181–186.

64. Long, J. C., Aisenberg, A. C., and Zamecnik, P. C. 1974. An antigen in Hodgkin's disease tissue cultures: radioiodine-labelled antibody studies. *Proc. Nat. Acad. Sci. (U.S.A.)* 71: 2605–2609.

65. Longmire, R. L., McMillan, R., Yelenosky, R., Armstrong, S., Lang, J. E., and Craddock, C. G. 1973. *In vitro* splenic IgG synthesis in Hodgkin's disease. *N. Engl. J. Med.* 289: 763–767.

66. Lukes, R. J., and Collins, R. D. 1974. Immunologic characterization of human malignant lymphomas. *Cancer* 34: 1488–1503.

67. Matchett, K. M., Huang, A. T., and Kremer, W. B. 1973. Impaired lymphocyte transformation in Hodgkin's disease: evidence for depletion of circulating T-lymphocytes. *J. Clin. Invest.* 52: 1908–1917.

68. Order, S. E., Porter, M., and Hellman, S. 1971. Hodgkin's disease: evidence for a tumor associated antigen. *N. Engl. J. Med.* 285: 471–474.

69. Order, S. E., and Hellman, S. 1972. Pathogenesis of Hodgkin's disease. *Lancet* i: 571–573.

70. Order, S. E., Chism, S. E., and Hellman, S. 1972. Studies of antigens associated with Hodgkin's disease. *Blood* 40: 621–633.

71. Order, S. E., Colgan, J., and Hellman, S. 1974. Distribution of fast and slow migrating Hodgkin's tumor-associated antigens. *Cancer Res.* 34: 1182–1186.

72. Parker, F., Jackson, H., Fitzhugh, G., and Spies, T. D. 1932. Studies of diseases of the lymphoid and myeloid tissues. IV. Skin reactions to human and avian tuberculin. *J. Immunol.* 22: 277–282.

73. Peckham, M. J., and Cooper, E. H. 1969. Proliferation characteristics of the various classes of cells in Hodgkin's disease. *Cancer* 24: 135.

74. Ramot, B., Biniaminov, M., Shoham, C., and Rosenthal, E. 1976. Effect of Levamisole on E-rosette-forming cells *in vivo* and *in vitro* in Hodgkin's disease. *N. Engl. J. Med.* 294: 809–811.

75. Reed, D. M. 1902. On the pathological changes in Hodgkin's disease, with special reference to its relation to tuberculosis. *Johns Hopkins Hosp. Rep.* 10: 133–196.

76. Ruhl, H., Vogt, W., Bochert, G., Schmidt, S., Moelle, R., and Schaoua, H. 1975. Mixed lymphocyte culture stimulatory and responding capacity of lymphocytes from patients with lympho proliferative diseases. *Clin. Exp. Immunol.* 19: 55–65.

77. Saslow, S., Carlisle, N. H., Bouroncle, B. 1961. Antibody response in hematologic patients. *Proc. Soc. Exp. Biol. Med.* 106: 654–656.

78. Schiffer, C. A., Levi, J. A., and Wiernik, P. H. 1975. The significance of abnormal circulating cells in patients with Hodgkin's disease. *Brit. J. Haemat.* 31: 177–183.

79. Sokal, J. E., and Aungst, C. W. 1969. Response to BCG vaccination and survival in advanced Hodgkin's disease. *Cancer* 24: 128–134.

80. Sokal, J. E., Aungst, C. W., and Snyderman, M. 1974. Delay in progression of malignant lymphoma after BCG vaccination. *N. Engl. J. Med.* 291: 1226–1230.

81. Steiner, P. E., 1934. Etiology of Hodgkin's disease; skin reaction to avian and human tuberculin proteins. *Arch. Int. Med.* 54: 11–17.

82. Sternberg, C. 1898. Über eine eigenartige unter dem Bilde der Pseudoleukamie verlaufende Tuberculose des lymphatischen Apparats. *Z. Heilkunde* 19: 21–90.

83. Swain, A., and Trounce, J. R. 1974. Rosette formation in Hodgkin's disease. *Oncology* 30: 449–457.

84. Swan, H. T., and Knowelden, J. 1971. Prognosis in Hodgkin's disease related to lymphocyte count. *Brit. J. Haemat.* 21: 343–349.

85. Taylor, C. R. 1974. The nature of Reed-Sternberg cells and other malignant reticulum cells. *Lancet* ii: 807.

86. Trubowitz, S., Masek, B., and Del Rosario, A. 1966. Lymphocyte response to phytohemagglutinin in Hodgkin's disease. *Cancer* 19: 2019–2023.

87. Twomey, J. J., Laughter, A. H., Farrow, S., and Douglass, C. C. 1975. Hodgkin's disease: an immunodepleting and immunosuppressive disorder. *J. Clin. Invest.* 56: 467–475.

88. Wagener, D. J., Geestman, E., and Wessels, H. M. 1975. The influence of

splenectomy on the *in vitro* lymphocyte response to phytohemagglutinin and pokeweed mitogen in Hodgkin's disease. *Cancer* 36: 194–198.

89. Wagener, D. J., Geestman, E., Borgonjen, A., and Haanen, C. 1976. The influence of splenectomy on cellular immunologic parameters in Hodgkin's disease. *Cancer* 37: 2212–2219.

90. Winkelstein, A., Mikulla, J. M., Sartiano, G. P., and Ellis, L. D. 1974. Cellular immunity in Hodgkin's disease: comparison of cutaneous reactivity and lymphoproliferative responses to phytohemagglutinin. *Cancer* 34: 549–553.

91. Young, R. C., Corder, M. P., Haynes, H. A., and DeVita, V. T. 1972. Delayed hypersensitivity in Hodgkin's disease. *Amer. J. Med.* 52: 63–72.

92. Young, R. C., Corder, M. P., Berard, C. W., and DeVita, V. T. 1973. Immune alterations in Hodgkin's disease. *Arch. Intern. Med.* 131: 446–454.

CHAPTER 2

TUMOR IMMUNITY IN HUMAN AND MURINE LEUKEMIA

Kendall A. Smith

Department of Medicine
Dartmouth Medical School
Hanover, New Hampshire 03755

Although tumor-specific transplantation antigens (TSTA) have been demonstrated in experimental animals, the data supporting the existence of leukemia-specific antigens (LSA) in man are less convincing. There is little serological evidence for human recognition of LSA, and tests for cell-mediated immunity have been positive in only a fraction of cases. Animal studies support the concept that the tests for *in vitro* cell-mediated immunity correlate with the immune state and therefore may be defining (TSTA). Whether the leukemia antigens, which have been found to function as TSTA in experimental animals, are similar to leukemia antigens in man is ill-defined. Most evidence suggests that human LSA may be antigens unique to each leukemia and not cross-reactive with similar morphological types of leukemias.

INTRODUCTION

With the demonstration by Gross in 1943 that methycholanthrene-induced sarcomas carried unique tumor-specific antigens, there was a rebirth of the concept that tumor immunity might play a role in host responses against neoplastic cells (14). Others confirmed and extended Gross's findings and it became evident that chemically induced tumors were strongly antigenic (19, 28, 29). Through various techniques it was demonstrated that histocompatible inbred strains of mice could be immunized and protected against a lethal challenge of tumor cells. These studies precluded a universal tumor vaccine, however, since each tumor was uniquely antigenic. There was no cross-reactivity between independently induced tumors, even if produced by the same chemical carcinogen. The immunization techniques used by these investigators, however, were soon adopted by others studying tumors induced by oncogenic viruses. Klein and Klein demonstrated tumor-specific antigens on cells from leukemias and lymphomas induced by Moloney leukemia virus, an RNA, type-C virus (18). In contrast to the immunity to chemical-carcinogen-induced tumors, all leukemia cells induced by the Moloney agent were shown to be cross-reactive. Later the cross-reactivity was shown to include leukemias induced by Rauscher and Friend leukemia viruses as well (5). Initial experiments employed Gross's tumor-transplantation-resistance technique to demonstrate immunity, and thus the antigens involved in these reactions were termed tumor-specific transplantation antigens (TSTA). Because these antigens were shown to be common to all leukemias induced by these viruses, it was postulated that similar agents might be responsible for leukemias of man. Accordingly, the search for putative human oncogenic viruses and leukemia associated antigens has been strongly influenced by these animal models. Acting on the hypothesis that human leukemias might share antigenic specificities, Mathe et al. reported a therapeutic benefit of active immunotherapy in acute lymphocytic leukemia (ALL) (22). It was reported that the disease free interval could be significantly prolonged after a remission induced chemotherapeutically by the injection of allogeneic irradiated leukemia cells, together with the administration of Bacillus Calmette Guerin (BCG), a strain of *Mycobacterium bovis*. This report stimulated a veritable explosion of interest in tumor immunology and today there are currently hundreds of clinical trials in progress designed to test the efficacy of immunotherapy in leukemia as well as other human cancers[1].

The success of this approach rests upon an hypothesis which, however, remains unproven; that is, the existence of human tumor-specific antigens. Since the techniques of transplantation resistance used by early investigators dealing with animal models are not applicable to human experimentation, the evidence for the existence of human leukemia antigens rests on the utilization of indirect methods. Furthermore, to demonstrate the presence of antigens, it is necessary to detect an immune response to the leukemia cells. Transplantation resistance is one way to demonstrate an immune response; however, in animal models it has also been possible to detect tumor-specific antibodies as well as in vitro evidence of cell-mediated immunity. At this point, it is critical to examine the data accumulated by studies of human leukemia which suggest the existence of leukemia antigens. In addition, it is imperative to re-examine the nature of the antigens in animal models, which have been termed TSTA.

HUMORAL IMMUNITY IN HUMAN ACUTE LEUKEMIA

Surprisingly few well-documented instances of specific antibodies against autologous human acute leukemia cells have been reported. A variety of techniques has been utilized in the search for human antibodies, all of which have been successful in demonstrating antibodies in animal models. In 1954 Seligman et al. found that sera from 8 of 54 patients with acute leukemia had immunoprecipitation reactions with leukocyte lysates (32). In these 8 cases, the specificity of the reactions was not explored nor was there any attempt to demonstrate cross reactivity with leukemias of similar morphologic types. Greenspan et al. used passive cutaneous anaphylaxis, immunodiffusion, microprecipitation, and immunofluorescence techniques and failed to demonstrate positive reactions from sera of 6 patients with acute myelogenous leukemia (AML) and 4 patients with ALL (13). Dore et al. reported studies of 22 patients with acute leukemia (8). Utilizing complement fixation, one positive test was found; and using complement mediated cytotoxicity, sera from 2 patients were found positive. By immunofluorescence one serum sample from a patient with acute monocytic leukemia was positive. In all of these tests, however, the sera tested were either undiluted or diluted 1:2. Absorptions using normal cells or leukemia cells were not performed, nor were the substances yielding the positive test results shown to be immunoglobulins. Yoshida and Imai tested the sera of 30 patients for antibodies to autologous leukemia cells by the immune adherence technique (39). They found many positive reactions with higher titers for patients when in remission. Once again, however, the positive reactions were not shown to be due to immunoglobulins and the phenomenon of immune adherence could be demonstrated with only a minor proportion of the leukemia cells.

Herberman found no evidence for positive reactions when sera from patients with ALL were tested by the sensitive isotopic antiglobulin technique (17). It should be noted that experiments were successful using this technique to detect tumor-specific antibodies in experimental animals (34). Similar negative results have been found using the assay of antibody-dependent, cell-mediated cytolysis, testing sera from patients with both AML and ALL (I. Maclennan, personal communication). This test has been shown to be positive in experimental animal systems in serum dilutions of 10^{-10}, where conventional complement-mediated cytotoxicity using the same serum ceases to function at dilutions of 10^{-3} (41). Therefore, despite the use of extremely sensitive assays, there has been a failure to detect the existence of leukemia-specific antibodies in the sera of patients with acute leukemia. The failure to find antibodies, however, does not necessarily mean that leukemia antigens do not exist. It is possible that there exists a state of antigen excess in the leukemia patient such that all antibody is complexed to either cell surface or circulating soluble antigen. If this were the case, one might expect to find evidence of antigen–antibody complex deposition in the kidneys of leukemia patients. Indeed, Sutherland and Mardiney did find immunoglobulin and complement deposition in 6 of 37 cases of AML (37). Also, Gutterman et al. reported that the blast cells of 8 patients with AML were coated with immunoglobulins, primarily IgG (15). However, there was no evidence presented that the immunoglobulins represented specific antibodies.

In addition to the possibility that there exists a state of antigen excess, it is also possible that there is a specific immune deficiency on the part of the host to mount an effective humoral immune response. It is this possibility which led to the rationale for the use of nonspecific immunologic adjuvants such as BCG in human cancer therapy. Unfortunately, where successful clinical trials have been reported with the use of this agent in ALL, there have been no reports of attempts to demonstrate leukemia-specific antibodies in the sera of patients. Recently, Klouda et al. have used BCG and allogeneic leukemia cell injections during the remission therapy of AML (20). Although these investigators were able to detect the induction of humoral immune responses to the allogeneic, immunizing leukemia cells, no cross-reactivity was found when the patient's autologous leukemia cells were tested. These findings are particularly distressing, since they suggest that, contrary to some experimental animal leukemias, there may not be cross reactive antigens in human leukemia.

Failure to demonstrate specific antibodies in human sera has led some investigators to search for leukemia-associated antigens by inoculating heterologous species with human leukemia cells (16, 26). Using this technique, some cell surface changes have been detected on leukemia cells which are not found on normal cells. The immunologic significance of these cell surface changes, however, remains unclear. Structures which are recognized as foreign by a heterologous species may not be so recognized by the human host. The heterologous immune response may be directed against fetal, differentiation, or species antigens which are preferentially expressed on the leukemia cells. If man is tolerant to these antigens or if these cell surface changes are present normally on early hemopoietic precursor cells, there would be no human recognition of antigenicity. It is critical in the conduct of these experiments to test the heterologous sera on normal hemopoietic precursor cells and this has not been reported (16, 26). The sera have only been tested on mature peripheral blood leukocytes. Therefore, it remains to be defined what antigens are involved in these reactions, and what relationships exist between normal hemopoietic precursor cells and leukemia cells.

CELL-MEDIATED IMMUNITY IN HUMAN LEUKEMIA

In contrast to the failure to detect leukemia-specific humoral immunity, cell-mediated immunity to human leukemia cells has been demonstrated (3, 11, 21, 24). Utilizing the mixed tumor-lymphocyte culture (MTLC), lymphocytes obtained after a patient has attained a chemotherapeutically induced remission, have been shown to proliferate when cocultured with autologous, irradiated leukemia cells. However, the degree of proliferation has been small as measured by tritiated thymidine incorporation into DNA. This fact, together with the absence of any correlation of a positive MTLC with a good prognosis, leads one to be cautious in the interpretation of this data.

Since the MTLC measures only the afferent or recognition arm of the immune response, others have searched for evidence of immune reactivity utilizing lymphocyte-mediated cytolysis (LMC). This test, shown to be mediated by activated thymid-dependent lymphocytes (T cells) has been found to correlate with in vivo graft rejection in transplantation experiments (6). As such, it reflects the efferent or effector arm of the immune response. When this assay has been used in human acute leukemia, however, there has not been convincing evidence that circulating cytotoxic cells exist. Cytotoxicity has only been demonstrated in a fraction of the patients studied, and furthermore when found, the degree of cytotoxicity has been very low (1–10%) (21). Again, no correlation has been found between a positive test and a favorable prognosis.

Recently Taylor *et al.* have combined the MTLC and LMC in the hope of detecting reactivity to human-leukemia-associated antigens (38). MTLC consisting of remission lymphocytes and autologous AML blasts were performed prior to the testing of the lymphocytes for cytotoxicity. Unfortunately, no positive reactions could be demonstrated. Since these same patients were undergoing immunotherapy with BCG and allogeneic leukemia cells, these investigators also attempted to demonstrate cross reactive leukemia-associated antigens. Lymphocytes were first stimulated in MTLC using the same allogeneic blasts used for the *in vivo* immunizations. Lymphocytes from these cultures were then tested for cytotoxic activity on allogeneic and autologous blast cells. Although allogeneic cytotoxicity was easily demonstrated, no cytotoxic activity was found in using the autologous leukemia cells as targets. Similar experiments and results have been related by Powles (personal communication). These experiments are important because, like the findings with sera, they do not support the concept that cross-reactive antigens exist in human leukemia. More extensive studies are needed, since it is always possible that only a fraction of morphologically similar leukemias share antigens. Additionally, it would be critical to demonstrate cross-reactive antigens prior to the use of allogeneic cells for immunotherapy.

Zarling *et al.* have recently utilized a similar experimental approach and reported evidence that at least some human leukemia cells may have unique antigens similar to the antigens of chemically induced sarcomas in mice (40). Taking advantage of the observation that a mixed lymphocyte culture can enhance the generation of cytotoxic lymphocytes to other, third-party antigens, "three cell" MTLC were performed (2). Remission lymphocytes were co-cultivated with autologous leukemia blasts from a patient with acute myelomonocytic leukemia. To this culture, mitomycin-treated allogeneic lymphocytes were added. Surviving lymphocytes were found to be cytotoxic for the autologous leukemia cells. Cytotoxic cells were not generated when the allogeneic lymphocytes were omitted or when allogeneic leukemia cells were utilized in a two-cell MTLC. Thus, this report provides the most convincing evidence to date that human leukemia-associated antigens exist and that they can be detected by *in vitro* cell-mediated immunologic assays. Confirmation of these findings must be demonstrated and more extensive similar studies, hopefully, will answer the questions of whether all human-leukemia-associated antigens are unique.

TUMOR IMMUNITY IN MURINE LEUKEMIA

Although considerable work has been reported concerning the various aspects of immune reactions in murine leukemia models, this review will be concerned with only two critical questions. (1) In murine models, where leukemia cells have been shown to be clearly antigenic by transplantation experiments, do the *in vitro* tests of MTLC and LMC correlate with the immune state? (2) What is the evidence that tumor-specific neo-antigens exist distinct from virus or virus structural proteins? These questions are important since, of all the *in vitro* immunologic tests available, only the MTLC-LMC has been found to be positive when tested in human leukemia. It is important, therefore, to be sure that these tests are detecting host immunologic recognition and reactivity to tumor-specific antigens. In addition, although much circumstantial evidence has accumulated in the past five years suggesting that RNA tumor viruses may be associated with human leukemia, mature type-C viral paricles have not been identified from fresh leukemia cells (23). It is important, therefore, when examining animal models to critically evaluate the evidence that the immune responses detected, are directed toward nonviral antigens.

The MTLC, with the measurement of tritiated thymidine incorporation into newly synthesized DNA after lymphocyte blastic transformation, is patterned after similar systems where antigen-induced lymphocyte transformation has been shown to be immunologically specific. That is, the *in vitro* test has been found to be positive only if the host has had prior *in vivo* exposure (33). Theoretically, then, if the tumor cell is antigenic, the MTLC will be positive only if the host has been exposed to the tumor cells prior to the culture. In human leukemia, since the leukemic cells arise in the host, there has certainly been prior exposure. However, in this situation, other factors may come into play which block the ability of the host to generate enough antigen-reactive cells to allow a detectable *in vitro* response. Since, in general, only peripheral blood lymphocytes are tested, a negative test might be due to a paucity of antigen-reactive cells in the peripheral blood because of compartmentalization of the cells to other lymphoid organs, such as the bone marrow. Using animal models, these factors may be overcome. It is possible to expose the host to subtumorigenic doses of cells or to large doses of X-irradiated cells. In this setting, then, one can perform the MTLC with lymphoid cells derived from the various lymphoid organs. When experiments of this nature have been done, a positive MTLC reaction has been found to occur (12). Furthermore, the antigen reactive cells have been found to persist for long periods after the primary *in vivo* exposure. In addition, the degree of reactivity has been shown to vary according to the route of exposure. For example, if animals are injected intraperitoneally, the peritoneal exudate cells are more reactive than spleen or regional lymph node cells (27). Similarly, if a subcutaneous route is used, the regional lymph node contains the highest numbers of antigen reactive cells. Animals that have not received prior *in vivo* exposure do not yield lymphocytes that give a positive reaction in the MTLC as measured by tritiated thymidine incorporation. Therefore, from these experiments, there certainly is correlation of this test with the immune state. Other experiments have solidified this interpretation. Adoptive transfer of immune lymphocytes after activation in an MTLC has been shown to protect unimmunized animals against a lethal tumor cell challenge (30). Since there is greater protection with the immunized lymphocytes if an MTLC is performed than if lymphocytes are transferred without MTLC, the culture step presumably selects for a greater proportion of tumor-specific antigen reactive cells.

Since the MTLC tests only the afferent or recognition arm of the immune response, a positive interpretation of the test depends upon the demonstration of tumor antigen specificity. That is, a mouse immunized with tumor A should only react with tumor A and not others, unless they too share antigens with tumor A. Unfortunately, since most MTLC performed in human leukemia have yielded borderline positive results, one cannot be sure these tests have actually measured immunologic recognition of tumor-specific antigens. Since the lymphocyte-mediated cytolysis test measures the effector capacity of lymphocytes, this test offers an additional means to search for antigen-specific reactions. When this test has been performed using lymphocytes from immunized animals, a sharp peak of reactivity has been detected several days after immunization (7). The reactivity then becomes undetectable and remains so. These findings could account for the low levels of reactivity which have been found when human peripheral blood lymphocytes have been tested after the tumor mass has been reduced by chemotherapy.

Because of these findings, investigators have combined MTLC and the LMC assays as previously related in human leukemia. Our laboratory has found that prior MTLC enhances the degree of cytolysis measured by LMC. Furthermore, if the lymphocytes are harvested after one MTLC and reactivated in a second reaction, the cytolytic capacity can be increased still further. These secondary and tertiary *in vitro* immunizations presumably enrich the population for specific-antigen-reactive cells. Similar studies are underway using human cells to see if the sensitivity for detection of tumor-specific antigens can be increased.

From these studies, therefore, MTLC and LMC tests do appear to correlate with the immune state and have been shown to detect tumor-specific antigens. Whether the antigens involved in these animal models are similar to human leukemia antigens remains unknown. Unfortunately, most, if not all, of the studies that have dealt with murine RNA virus-induced leukemias, have utilized virus-producing tumor cells. In most instances, virus type–specific immunity has been demonstrated to these tumors, but it has not been clearly defined whether the immune response has been directed toward the tumor cell, or toward antigens associated with the budding viral particle. As already pointed out, this is an important question, since human leukemia cells have not been shown to bud mature viral particles.

It has been established that mammalian sarcoma viruses are replication-defective and require genetic information from helper leukemia viruses to complete the replicative cycle to bud mature viral particles (31). Replication-defective cell lines have been cloned which contain the MSV genome, but lack the genetic information for full virus production. These "nonproducer" cells have been studied by several investigators to ascertain if neo-antigens exist and further to discern if tumor transplantation resistance can be demonstrated. All of the cells that have been studied to date have been transformed fibroblast cells. Malignant, nonproducing hemopoietic cells have not been available until recently.

The data accumulated on the transformed fibroblastoid cells are controversial. Aoki et al., using immunoelectron microscopy, found tumor-associated cell surface antigens on nonproducing cells of Kirsten-MSV–transformed BALB/c 3T3 cells, Kirsten–transformed normal rat kidney cells, and Simian sarcoma virus–transformed normal rat kidney cells (1). These investigators used heterologous antisera raised in rabbits against the respective cells, followed by absorption with nonvirus-transformed cell lines. In this experimental approach, again one tests the immunologic recognition of the heterologous host, which may not be the same as the homologous host. No studies were reported relating these antigens to tumor transplantation resistance.

McCoy et al. (25) were able to demonstrate transplantation resistance to nonproducing Harvey sarcoma virus–induced hamster fibrosarcomas utilizing immunization experiments in histocompatible hosts. Protection against a lethal challenge was afforded by immunization with lethally irradiated (15,000 r) tumor cells. Furthermore, the tumors grew more readily in X-ray immunodepressed animals. No studies were reported, however, using in vitro tests for either humoral or cellular reactivity of the immunized hosts against cell surface antigens of the nonproducing cells.

Contrasting evidence was found in the experiments reported by Strouk et al. (36), studying the Sarcoma virus–positive, leukemia virus–negative (S+, L–) cell lines, isolated by Bassin (4). These cells are Moloney-MSV–transformed BALB/3T3 cells which have been cloned and selected to produce no infectious MSV or murine leukemia virus. They do, however, produce a small amount of noninfectious C-type particles, which may be detected by electron microscopy and ^{3}H-uridine labeling. Two different experimental approaches were utilized to try to demonstrate immunoreactive surface antigens on these cells. Syngeneic BALB/c mice were innoculated with MSV, to induce sarcomas. Serum and lymphocytes were then taken from regressor animals and tested for reactivity against the nonproducing cells, using the mixed hemabsorption test and the microcytotoxicity assay. In addition, allo-antisera were obtained by immunizing C57B1/6 mice with S+, L− cells, followed by adsorption with nontransformed BALB/3T3 cells. No evidence was obtained by either of these approaches for a new MSV-induced surface antigen on the nonproducing tumor cells.

Similar but more extensive studies were reported by Stephenson and Aaronson (35). Kirsten-MSV−transformed nonproducing cells were clonally derived from BALB/3T3 cells (K-BALB). A parallel, virus-producing cell line was obtained by infection of the MSV-transformed nonproducer cells with Rauscher leukemia virus (RLV). Preimmunization of syngeneic mice with low, nontumorigenic doses of the virus-producing line or with UV-inactivated RLV, resulted in transplantation resistance to subsequent challenge with the virus-producing line but not with the nonproducing line. In contrast, mice preimmunized with nonproducer cells were not made resistant to subsequent challenge with homologous cells. Antisera prepared from mice immunized with the virus-producing line were cytotoxic for that line but not the nonproducing line. These investigators concluded that MSV nonproducer cells lack detectable tumor-transplantation antigens and suggested that the transplantation resistance to the producing cells was attributable to maturing virus at the cell surface.

Recently Freedman and Lilly (10) have reported on the loss of virus-producing capacity of Friend virus erythroleukemia cells after prolonged passage in vitro. Interestingly, when the cell line became nonproducing it became much more tumorigenic and more difficult to induce transplantation resistance by immunization. Equally as interesting was the fact that nonproducing cells still expressed gp-71 and p-15 virus structural protein antigens on the cell surface. With continued passage even these antigens were lost and with them transplantation resistance was lost as well. Thus, the immunogenicity of leukemia cells induced by RNA tumor viruses may depend, in large part, on the antigenic density of virus structural proteins on the nonproducing cells.

Because of these considerations, we have recently employed the MTLC-LMC tests in experimental situations to ascertain if tumor-specific antigens could be detected on nonproducer cells. BALB/c mice were immunized with an RLV-induced acute myelogenous leukemia designated TNF (9). We have characterized this cell line to be producing mature virus particles as measured by X-C assay, and assay for reverse transcriptase activity. In addition, using antisera directed toward the RLV proteins gp-71 and p-12, we have found positive cytotoxic reactions, suggesting that this cell line expresses these virus structural proteins on the cell surface. Mice immunized with large doses of X-irradiated cells reject a lethal challenge of cells, thus demonstrating transplantation resistance and, by definition, TSTA. Splenic lymphocytes from these immunized animals activated in an MTLC specifically kill TNF cells in the LMC assay. To ascertain if these splenic cells also recognize antigens on non-producing cells we have characterized the antigenic expression of the K-BALB cells. These cells are negative for virus production as tested by reverse transcriptase activity of culture fluids, the X-C assay of culture fluids, and the co-cultivation of K-BALB cells with SC-1 mouse embryo fibroblasts used in the X-C assay. In addition, K-BALB cells are negative for cell surface expression of gp-71, p-30 and p-12 when tested by a complement-mediated cytotoxicity assay. Having characterized the K-BALB as a nonproducer, we next co-cultivated the K-BALB cells with mitomycin-treated TNF cells. This resulted in a virus-producing subline of K-BALB designated K-BALB (T). This cell line is positive by X-C assay and reverse transcriptase assay and like TNF, there is a cell surface expression of gp-71 and p-12.

When these cells are used as targets in an LMC assay after an MTLC using spleen cells from immunized animals and TNF cells, there is definite cytotoxicity of both the K-BALB and the K-BALB (T). Interestingly, there is considerably more cytolysis of the K-BALB (T) than of K-BALB. This evidence suggests that nonproducing cells may demonstrate cell surface TSTA which are definitely not related to budding virus or cell surface viral proteins. In addition, the fact that there is less reactivity of lymphocytes when tested against the nonproducer cells, as compared to the producer cells, suggests that these antigens may be considerably weaker than the viral antigens.

Further studies are needed to isolate and characterize antigens from nonproducer cells in murine leukemia models, and similar studies employing the MTLC-LMC in human leukemia are needed to search for leukemia-specific antigens. In addition, more work is needed to define methods to isolate tumor antigen specific lymphocytes. It may be possible to cultivate such cells in vitro for immunotherapeutic use. Certainly the studies in animals regarding the adoptive transfer of in vitro activated lymphocytes are promising. If a similar approach could be shown to be practical for human leukemia, it would offer a new means of tumor-specific immunotherapy.

NOTE

1. Compendium of Tumor Immunotherapy Protocols, International Registry of Tumor Immunotherapy. Number 4, August, 1976.

BIBLIOGRAPHY

1. Aoki, T., Stephenson, J. R., Aaronson, S. A., and Hsu, K. C., 1974. Surface antigens of mammalian sarcoma virus-transformed nonproducer cells. *Proc. Natl. Acad. Sci.* 71: 3445–3449.

2. Bach, F. H., Bach, M. L., and Sondel, P. M., 1976. Differential function of major histocompatibility complex antigens in T-lymphocyte activation. *Nature* 259: 273–281.

3. Bach, M. L., Bach, F. H., and Joo, P., 1969. Leukemia-associated antigens in the mixed leukocyte culture test. *Science* 166: 1520.

4. Bassin, R. H., Phillips, L. A., Kramer, M. J., Haapala, D. K., Peebles, P. T., Nomura, S., and Fischinger, P. J., 1971. Transformation of mouse 3T3 cells by murine sarcoma virus: release of virus-like particles in the absence of replicating murine leukemia helper virus. *Proc. Natl. Acad. Sci.* 68: 1520–1524.

5. Bianco, A. R., Glynn, J. P., and Goldin, A., 1966. Induction of resistance against the transplantation of leukemias induced by Rauscher virus. *Cancer Res.* 26: 1722–1728.

6. Brunner, K. T., Mauel, J., Cerottini, J. C., and Chapuis, B., 1968. Quantitative assay of the lytic action of immune lymphoid cells on ^{51}Cr-labelled allogeneic target cells *in vitro*; inhibition by isoantibody and by drugs. *Immunology* 14: 181–196.

7. de Landazuri, M. O., and Herberman, R. B., 1972. Immune response to gross virus-induced lymphoma. III. Characteristics of the cellular immune response. *J. Natl. Cancer Inst.* 49: 147–154.

8. Dore, J. F., Marholev, L., Motta, R., Hrsak, I., de Vassal, F., Seman, G., Mathe, G., and Colas de la Noue, H., 1967. New antigens in human leukaemic cells, and antibody in the serum of leukaemic patients. *Lancet* 2: 1396.

9. Fredrickson, T. N., LoBue, J., Alexander, Jr., A., Schultz, E. F., and Gordon, A. S., 1972. A transplantable leukemia from mice inoculated with Rauscher leukemia virus. *J. Natl. Cancer Inst.* 48: 1597–1605.

10. Freedman, H. A., and Lilly, F., 1975. Properties of cell lines derived from tumors induced by Friend virus in BALB/c and BALB/c-H-2^b mice. *J. Exp. Med.*, 142: 212–223.

11. Fridman, W. H., and Kourilsky, F. M., 1969. Stimulation of lymphocytes by autologous leukaemic cells in acute leukaemia. *Nature* 224: 277–228.

12. Glaser, M., Herberman, R. B., Kirchner, H., and Djeu, J. Y., 1974. Study of the cellular immune response to Gross virus-induced lymphoma by the mixed lymphocyte-tumor interaction. *Cancer Res.* 34: 2165–2171.

13. Greenspan, I., Brown, E. R., and Schwartz, S. O., 1963. Immunologically specific antigens in leukemic tissues. *Blood* 21: 717–728.

14. Gross, L., 1943. Intradermal immunization of C3H mice against a sarcoma that originated in an animal of the same line. *Cancer Res.* 3: 326–333.

15. Gutterman, J. U., Rossen, R. D., Butler, W. T., McCredie, K. B., Bodey, G. P., Freireich, E. J., and Hersh, E. M., 1973. Immunoglobulin on tumor cells and tumor-induced lymphocyte blastogenesis in human acute leukemia. *N. Engl. J. Med.* 288: 169–173.

16. Halterman, R. H., Leventhal, B. G., and Mann, D. L., 1972. An acute-leukemia antigen: correlation with clinical status. N. Engl. J. Med. 287: 1272–1274.

17. Herberman, R. B., 1974. Immune responses to virus induced experimental leukemia and to human leukemia. Johns Hopkins Med. J. Suppl., 3: 3–14.

18. Klein, E., and Klein, G., 1964. Antigenic properties of lymphomas induced by the Moloney agent. J. Natl. Cancer Inst. 32: 547–568.

19. Klein, G., Sjogren, H. O., Klein, E., Hellstrom, K. E., 1960. Demonstration of resistance against methylcholanthrene-induced sarcomas in the primary autochthonous host. Cancer Res. 20: 1561–1572.

20. Klouda, P. T., Lawler, S. D., Powles, R. L., Oliver, R. T. D., and Grant, C. K., 1975. HL-A antibody response in patients with acute myelogenous leukaemia treated by immunotherapy. Transplantation 19: 245–249.

21. Leventhal, B. G., Halterman, R. H., Rosenberg, E. B., and Herberman, R. B., 1972. Immune reactivity of leukemia patients to autologous blast cells. Cancer Res. 32: 1820–1825.

22. Mathé, G., Amiel, J. L., Schwarzenberg, L., Schneider, M., Cattan, A., Schlumberger, J. R., Hayat, M., and de Vassal, F., 1969. Active Immunotherapy for acute lymphoblastic leukaemia. Lancet 1: 697–699.

23. Maugh, T. H., 1975. Leukemia: a second human tumor virus. Science 187: 335–336.

24. Mavligit, G. M., Hersh, E. M., and McBride, C. M., 1973. Lymphocyte blastogenic responses to autochthonous viable and nonviable human tumor cells. J. Natl. Cancer Inst. 51: 337–343.

25. McCoy, J. L., Ting, R. C., Morton, D. L., and Law, L. W., 1972. Immunologic and virologic studies of a nonproducer tumor induced by murine sarcoma virus. J. Natl. Cancer Inst. 48: 383–391.

26. Metzgar, R. S., Mohanakumar, T., and Bolognesi, D. P., 1976. Relationships between membrane antigens of human leukemia cells and oncogenic RNA virus structural components. J. Exp. Med., 143: 47–63.

27. Plata, F., MacDonald, H. R., and Sordat, B., 1976. Studies on the distribution and origin of cytolytic T-lymphocytes present in mice bearing Moloney murine sarcoma virus (MSV)-induced tumors. Comparative Leukemia Research, 1975, Bibl. Haemat., No. 43, J. Clemmensen and D. S. Yohn (eds.), pp. 274–277 (Karger, Basel, 1976).

28. Prehn, R. T., and Main, J. M., 1957. Immunity to methycholanthrene-induced sarcomas. J. Natl. Cancer Inst. 18: 769–778.

29. Revesz, L., 1960. Detection of antigenic differences in isologous host-tumor systems by pretreatment with heavily irradiated tumor cells. Cancer Res. 20: 443–451.

30. Rollinghoff, M., and Wagner, H., 1973. In vitro protection against murine plasma cell tumor growth by in vitro activated syngeneic lymphocytes. J. Natl. Cancer Inst. 51: 1317–1318.

31. Rowe, W. P., 1971. The kinetics of rescue of the murine sarcoma virus genome from a nonproducer line of transformed mouse cells. Virology 46: 369–374.

32. Seligman, M., Grabar, P., and Bernard, J., 1954. Mise en évidence dans le

serum de sujets atteints de leucose aigue d'anticorps précipitants anti-leucocytaires (leucoprécipitaines). *Comptes Rendus Acad. Sciences* 239: 1559–1561.

33. Smith, K. A., Chess, L., and Mardiney, M. R., 1972. The characteristics of lymphocyte tritiated thymidine incorporation in response to mumps virus. *Cell. Immunol.* 5: 597–603.

34. Sparks, F. C., Ting, C. C., Hammond, W. G., and Herberman, R. B., 1969. An isotopic antiglobulin technique for measuring antibodies to cell-surface antigens. *J. Immunol.* 102: 842–847.

35. Stephenson, J. R., and Aaronson, S. A., 1972. Antigenic properties of murine sarcoma virus-transformed BALB/3T3 nonproducer cells. *J. Exp. Med.* 135: 503–515.

36. Strouk, V., Grundner, G., Fenyo, E. M., Lamon, E., Skurzak, H., and Klein, G., 1972. Lack of distinctive surface antigen on cells transformed by murine sarcoma virus. *J. Exp. Med.* 136: 344–352.

37. Sutherland, J. C., and Mardiney, M. R., 1973. Immune complex disease in the kidneys of lymphoma-leukemia patients: the presence of an oncornavirus-related antigen. *J. Natl. Cancer Inst.* 50: 633–641.

38. Taylor, G. M., Harris, R., and Freeman, C. B., 1976. Cell-mediated cytotoxicity as a result of immunotherapy in patients with acute myeloid leukaemia. *Brit. J. Cancer* 33: 137–143.

39. Yoshida, T. O., and Imai, K., 1970. Auto-antibody to human leukemia cell membrane as detected by immune adherence. *Rev. Eur. Etud. Clin. Biol.,* 15: 61–65.

40. Zarling, J. M., Raich, P. C., McKeough, M., and Bach, F. H., 1976. Generation of cytotoxic lymphocytes *in vitro* against autologous human leukaemia cells. *Nature* 262: 691–693.

41. Zighelboim, J., Bonavida, B., and Fahey, J., 1973. Evidence for several cell populations active in antibody dependent cellular cytotoxicity. *J. Immunol.* 3: 1737–1742.

CHAPTER 3

HUMAN LEUKEMIA ANTIGENS

Bernice Schacter,
Paul N. Anderson and
Bert C. DelVillano

Case Western Reserve University
Cleveland, Ohio/44106
Penrose Cancer Hospital
Colorado Springs, Colorado/80907
and The Cleveland Clinic Foundation
Cleveland, Ohio/44106

The exploration of human leukemia antigens has proven of relevance to the question of the etiology of leukemia and has provided support for the role of oncogenic viral information in the etiology of leukemia.

I. INTRODUCTION

The search for human leukemia-specific antigens is a venerable one, dating from the 1916 study of Tyzzer, in which he immunized a patient with acute myelocytic leukemia with autologous tumor cells (104, 199, 251). The subject of human leukemia-associated antigens (LAA) has particular importance in three major areas of study: (1) in the understanding of the biology of normal blood elements and their abnormal counterparts; (2) in evaluation of evidence relating to the etiology and pathogenesis of leukemia; and (3) in the pragmatic clinical areas of diagnosis, clinical correlation, prognosis, and therapy of human leukemia.

The demonstration and characterization of leukemia-specific or -associated antigens could provide clinical tools for the monitoring tumor load. If patients can be shown to mount protective immune responses to leukemia-specific antigens, specific stimulation of such responses by immunotherapy will become a therapeutic maneuver in the maintenance of remission and possibly in the induction of remission in concert with chemotherapy. Sufficient experience in immunotherapy in human leukemia has accumulated to allow some reasonable promise. The application of specific immunotherapy in human leukemia requires not only the expression of accessible antigens by the tumor, but also the ability of the host to mount an effective immune response to the tumor. Assessment of other host factors, such as immunocompetence, type and timing of chemotherapy, clinical status, and tumor type may prove critical to the application of leukemia immunotherapy.

The search for human leukemia-specific or -associated antigens also has much interest from a basic research point of view. A most intriguing question centers on the relationship between the human leukemia-associated antigens and putative etiologic agents. Related to this question are the clues that can be drawn from cell surface biology about the cell line of origin of the tumor. Recent data has suggested that the "lesion" in leukemia is not one of loss of control of proliferation, but one of loss of control of differentiation (41, 45, 86, 134, 158). The leukemia cell may be blocked in its normal differentiation path, either because it is receiving no signal or an inappropriate one, or because it has been rendered unable to respond to the normal signal. Viewed in this way, changes in the cell surface markers in leukemia, immunogenic in the host or not, may provide clues to those interactions between hematopoietic cells and their environment, cellular or humoral, which regulate the normal differentiation pathways. Definition of the normal topological language of the cell may provide tools for understanding the point in differentiation where loss of control occurs in the various leukemias, and the point where a suspected etiologic agent might effect that diversion, as well as possibly suggesting points where the cell might be switched back onto its normal pathway. Thus, beyond the promise of immunotherapy in human leukemia, a study of the cell surface changes in leukemia may provide conceptual tools for physiological intervention in leukemia.

Most of this review will consist of the formulation of questions about human leukemia antigens rather than the presentation of answers. Clearly, several general questions can be formulated at the outset:

1. Are there specific, immunologically detectable changes in human leukemia?
2. Are these changes detectable and/or detected by the host?
3. Are the antigens leukemia-specific antigens (LSA), defined here as present only on leukemic cells and absent at all times from all non-malignant host tissues, or leukemia-associated antigens (LAA), defined here as present on leukemic cells, absent from a reasonable normal counterpart, but present on some normal cells or tissues at some point in embryogenesis or differentiation?
4. Do the antigens offer clues to the etiology and/or cell line of origin of leukemias?
5. Does specific or general immunotherapy hold any promise in leukemia?

We will discuss evidence of human leukemia antigens from animal studies, evidence of human humoral and cellular immune response to leukemia antigens, other tumor and animal models of relevance, and the results of the limited immunotherapy trials in leukemia. In addition, we will discuss the immunological data relevant to a putative viral etiology of human leukemia.

II. SEROLOGICAL DETECTION OF HUMAN LEUKEMIA ANTIGENS

A. Sera from Animals Immunized with Human Leukemic Material (Heterologous Sera)

There are two interrelated requirements posed for the human host to perceive leukemia neo-antigens: (1) new surface markers must appear on leukemia cells: (2) these new surface markers must be immunogenic in the host. Many laboratory and *in vivo* studies interweave questions related to these requirements. Evidence for human leukemia-associated or -specific antigens uncomplicated by questions of their immunogenicity in man has been obtained by immunizing an experimental animal with human leukemic material and studying the animal sera for specific reactivity with leukemic cells (104, 199). The variables in these systems are the selection and processing of immunogen, the species of the immunized animal, the application of absorption and other techniques to render the sera operationally specific, and the test used to assay the immune response. Most of the early workers immunized rabbits and assayed their serum using gel diffusion or immunoelectrophoresis. These studies produced evidence of detectable antigenic differences between normal and leukemic-derived soluble material (52, 53, 127, 148, 174, 254, 255) by the appearance of new bands by immunodiffusion or immunoelectrophoresis.

The question of specificity of these heteroantisera to leukemias of different cell lines remains unanswered by the early studies since the sera were not rigorously tested for cross-reactivity on different leukemia cells.

Garb et al. induced tolerance to normal tissue antigens prior to immunization of the rabbits with leukemic cell materials, but concluded that this had little effect on the development of a specific leukemic reaction (83). Mice, treated with cyclophosphamide and remission leukocytes to induce partial tolerance prior to immunization with myelogenous leukemic blasts, produced antisera with complement dependent cytotoxicity to the blasts after absorption with normal WBC or marrow (13). The blasts of a patient with ALL* were also sensitive to these sera which had been raised against the AML blasts. Greaves, Brown, and coworkers have reported rabbit antisera raised to ALL blasts which carried neither of the standard T or B lymphoid cell surface markers (E rosettes and surface Ig) (38, 39, 87). These sera detected, by immunofluorescence, antigens which were restricted to similar "null" ALL blasts.

Further possibilities that the "null" ALL antigen is either (a) fetal or oncofetal, (b) cell cycle restricted, (c) a normal cryptic antigen, (d) or a normal antigen present on a rare cell have been tested by absorption (39). The absorption studies appeared to exclude the first three alternatives but the last could not be rigorously eliminated—and awaits antigen isolation and tests with purified cell populations from normal marrow. Rabbits immunized with a soluble cell surface fraction from a lymphoblastoid cell line, RAJI (derived from a patient with Burkitts' lymphoma) produced an antiserum which reacted with tumor cells of patients with acute myelocytic and acute lymphocytic leukemia (101, 163). Cells of patients in remission were unreactive with the anti-Raji serum and tumor cells of patients

*Abbreviations are explained at the end of the chapter.

with chronic lymphocytic and chronic myelocytic leukemia were also unreactive. Billing and Terasaki have also immunized rabbits with papain-solubilized membrane components from Raji or from fresh human lymphoma tissue producing antisera which react at high titer with cells of leukemias and lymphoblastoid cell lines though they are unreactive with normal peripheral blood lymphocytes, phytohemagglutinin-induced lymphoblasts, or normal marrow cells (32). Although normal lymphocytes could absorb the antileukemia reactivity, this effect appeared nonspecific. The purified antigen is a glycoprotein with an apparent molecular weight on SDS gel of 27,000 (33). Since these authors have recently shown that all leukemia cells carry B cell antigens, the possibility that the rabbit sera with antileukemia activity are detecting a public determinent of B cell alloantigens must be considered (31) (see Section V).

In these studies with antisera raised in species distant from humans (rabbits, mice), there is no consistent pattern of cross reactivity between myelogenous and lymphocytic antigens, although in general some crossreactivity was found. This may, in part, reflect only the polyspecificity of the sera, since Greaves was able to remove the little anti-AML activity in his anti-ALL sera by absorbing with normal marrow, although the ALL reactivity was retained, as was reactivity with some chronic granulocytic leukemia cells and some acute undifferentiated leukemia cells (39). These authors have argued that the cross-reactivity between some CML tumors and some ALL tumors suggest a common cell of origin for these tumors (129). This interesting model has not been tested rigorously but does demonstrate the potential power of serological probes. These authors suggest as an alternative explanation of the cross-reactivity of these two tumors that ALL and some CMLs may share a common etiologic agent. A third possibility is that these tumor cells share a common defect in the control of differentiation in that a cell surface molecule which plays a role in modulating differentiation is similarly expressed on these two tumors.

Metzgar et al. have immunized nonhuman primates with human leukemic cells or soluble antigens from leukemic cells producing a set of sera which should prove extraordinarily useful and informative for diagnosis and classification of leukemias as well as providing elegant structural probes (178, 183). As with many recent studies, Metzgar has used the complement-dependent microcytotoxicity assay to test these sera, which requires small numbers of cells for each test and allows many tests to be conducted even with small or leukopenic blood samples. Metzgar's nonhuman primate antisera after absorption have operational specificity for leukemic vs. normal cells and are able to discriminate a lymphoid leukemia from a myeloid leukemia. Cross-absorptions suggested that acute and chronic lymphocytic leukemias shared antigens detected by these sera. Some cross-reactivity between acute myeloid leukemia and chronic myeloid leukemia is also apparent from cross absorption experiments (183). In fact, the serology, particularly for the myeloid leukemias, is complex, as might be expected with sera raised in the closely related primates. Unlike species distant from humans, primates may fail to respond to primate antigens shared with humans and thus respond to the weaker leukemic and alloantigenic determinants. The advantage of the primate sera is that distant cross-species immunization will be minimized but the cross-reactivity of human and nonhuman primate alloantigenic systems may result in complex sera detecting both leukemia and alloantigens.

A number of workers have tested for cross-reactivity between human leukemia antigens detected by heterologous sera and murine and other animal leukemia viral antigens (72, 73, 128). In an early study Fink raised rabbit antisera against viruslike particles present in the plasma of leukemia patients, which after absorption showed reactivity by immunofluorescence restricted to leukemia cells (72, 73). These sera were also tested in parallel with an antiserum raised against MuLV-Rauscher. Cross-reactivity between the human and MuLV-Rauscher antigens was suggested by the reactivity of some leukemic bone marrows with both antisera (72). There was, however, no definitive correlation of reactivity of these sera. A later study by Yohn showed that normal human marrow, although unreactive by direct testing with a similarly prepared antiserum to human leukemic particles, could absorb the antileukemic reactivity (264). This points to a major problem of such studies using crude antigen preparations: sera with complex cross-reactivity to normal and leukemic antigens are likely to result.

Mann et al. have shown that the rabbit antiserum raised against a membrane fraction of a cultured lymphoblastoid line, Raji, with specific reactivity with acute leukemia cells, reacted with a human embryonic kidney cell line infected with MuLV-Rauscher, but did not react with uninfected human embryonic kidney cell line (162). The MuLV-Rauscher infected human cells absorbed the antileukemia activity of this serum but other cell lines could not, including mouse fibroblasts infected with MuLV-Rauscher. Brown et al. have reported that their rabbit serum with specificity for "null" ALL shows no cross-reactivity with MuLV-Gross or MuLV-Moloney, feline leukemia virus, New Castle disease virus, influenza virus, and HL23V-1, a C-type particle derived from a cultured human myeloid leukemia (39). Three antisera to viral antigens, one with specificity for interspecies determinants of p30, the major internal structural protein of oncornaviruses, one with specificity for simian sarcoma virus p30, and a third antiserum to whole simian sarcoma virus also did not react with ALL cells in this study (39). Also negative in Brown's studies were antisera to the DNA viruses: EBV, CMV, herpes saimiri, and rubella virus.

Metzgar, Mohanakumar, and Bolognesi have reported extensive positive evidence for cross-reactivity between some human leukemia membrane antigens and components of mammalian RNA tumor viruses (175, 176). The data on cross absorptions with antisera directed against viral antigens (Table 1) suggest that there is cross-reactivity between a myeloid leukemia-associated differentiation antigen and gp70, the major envelope glycoprotein of MuLV, and between a possibly leukemia-specific antigen of AML and p30, a major internal protein of MuLV. Reciprocal experiments with the primate antileukemia sera are less clear but are consistent with these interpretations. Further studies by this group with the primate RNA virus-simian sarcoma virus (SSV-1), and Gibbon ape leukemia virus (GALV) have suggested shared antigenic determinants between these viruses and ALL and CLL cells and the absence of these determinants from normal cells (175).

These more recent studies of cross-reactivity between human leukemia cells and viral antigens have benefited by advances in animal tumor virology providing relatively pure antigen preparations for study. The problem remains of the significance of the observed cross-reactivity between human leukemia antigens and animal tumor viral or virus-associated antigens, with particular reference to a viral etiology of human leukemia. (See Section VI.) The animal sera raised against human

Table 1. Serological cross-reactivity of Leukemic cells and RNA Tumor virus antigens

Tested on Cells from	Antiserum to				
	FLVgp71	FLVgp71 Absorbed With Platelets or Neutrophils	FLV	FLV Absorbed With Platelets or Neutrophils	FLV Absorbed With FeLVp30 or FLVp30
	Cells Reactive				
AML	None	None	All	All	None
CGL	All	None	All	None	All
AMML	Some	N.T.	All	All	None
ALL	None	None	Some	N.T.	N.T.
CLL	None	None	None	N.T.	N.T.

FLV = Friend leukemia virus; FeLV = Feline leukemia virus; gp71 = 71,000 dalton molecular weight glycoprotein; p30 = 30,000 dalton molecular weight protein.
  N.T. = not tested.
  Source: Data from Ref. 172, 173.

leukemia material have provided overall, the strongest evidence of the expression of new antigenic determinants on leukemia cells. The available data, however, are insufficient to establish absolute leukemia specificity.

Several of the animal antisera raised against human leukemia antigens have been exploited for the partial purification of the antigens they detect. No antigen of known leukemia specificity has been completely purified and, in fact, no such preparation has been shown to be devoid of HLA-A, -, B, or other alloantigenic specificity (33, 177, 255). These data are presently too immature to allow any substantive conclusions to be drawn about the biochemical nature of any human leukemia-associated antigen.

B. Human Sera Reactive with Leukemia Cells

1. AUTOLOGOUS REACTIVITY.   In comparison with the progress made in developing and exploiting heterologous antihuman leukemia sera, there is relatively less solid information about a human humoral immune response to leukemia. Dore et al. have reported that of 51 patients with leukemia or lymphoma, 12 had serum antibodies to their own tumor cells (63). These antibodies could be demonstrated by cytotoxicity, immunofluorescence, complement fixation, or immune adherence. There was little correlation among the results with each of the different methods and no correlation of any test with the detection of electron microscopy of C-type virus particles in the leukemic blasts. Yoshida et al. similarly reported autoantibody to leukemic cells in 22 of 30 leukemic patients using an immune adherence test (265). Specific cytophilic antibodies which stimulate the adherence of naive macrophages to autochthonous or allogeneic tumor cells were found by Mitchell in the serum of patients with acute leukemia (182). Dreesman et al. reported that some children with ALL develop cytotoxic antibodies to autologous peripheral blood leukocyte cells in relapse (64). In addition, some reactivity was found to autologous remission cells.

Gutterman et al. reported in a study of the cellular immune response to autologous leukemia cells that 8 of 24 patients with AML had IgG bound to their tumor cells (96). Positive IgG by immunofluorescence correlated well with a positive blastogenic response to autologous tumor and with an inhibition of that response by autologous serum. Interestingly enough, these three factors (mixed lymphocyte response to autologous blasts, surface IgG, and serum blocking of the mixed culture response) correlated positively with a good prognosis (90, 94, 96).

These data suggest that the patient's ability to mount a cellular and humoral immune response to a tumor-associated antigen is of prognostic significance. The factors which control the immune response to leukemia may include the nature of the leukemia antigen, the ability of the host to respond specifically to that antigen, or his overall immune status. The critical factor is difficult to isolate. It is unclear why a surface antitumor antibody, if it is such, is of positive prognostic significance unless it indicates that the tumor is capable in that host of stimulating an effective cellular immune response. These studies do suggest, however, that the humoral immune response of the patient is significant in a positive way, and is not necessarily involved only in the production of antibodies which block cellular immune response as has been described by the Hellstroms et al. for several animal and human systems (105). Recently Cotropia and co-workers have studied the immunoglobulins eluted from acute myeloblasts and have found that immunoglobulin fragments are found on the cell surface probably due to the activity of proteases at the tumor cell surface (47). The proteolysis could render the antibodies incapable of activating complement and may be a mechanism by which the tumor is protected from complement dependent immunolysis.

While there is evidence of an autologous humoral immune response to leukemia there are a number of technical problems in assessing the specificity and significance of this data. The technique used to detect humoral reactivity to leukemic cells is a critical factor since the cells are fragile and often very sensitive to manipulation and reagents. A critical factor in the cytotoxic tests can be the serum used as a complement source. In addition, in tests that employ macrophage adherence or hemagglutinating immune adherence or its inhibition, the presence of new or modified cell surface receptors (i.e., F_c or C3 receptors) on leukemic cells could give rise to a nonspecific sensitivity of leukemic cells. It may also be argued that leukemia patients because of concurrent infections, tumor or chemotherapy altered immune responsiveness, or antigenic stimulation through transfusion have non-specific serum alterations which give rise to the observed reactivity to autologous tumor. Thus, operational leukemia specificity may be demonstrated for autologous sera, yet it may be most difficult to rule out nonspecific effects with the use of sera from patients. Often only vigorous cross absorption studies, if feasible, can achieve this end. These problems discourage further study in this area, though certainly the interesting data of Hersh, Gutterman et al. suggest that the patient's humoral response to his leukemia is of key importance to the clinical course (90, 96).

2. SERUM FROM INDIVIDUALS WITHOUT LEUKEMIA. Evidence that people without leukemia express a humoral immune response to a leukemia specific or leukemia associated antigen could support a role

for the transmission of a putative leukemic infectious agent in the etiology of leukemia. Such data has been difficult to obtain for technical and conceptual reasons. A recent report has suggested that human sera often contain detectable antibody to primate C-type RNA viruses and virus-infected cells; however, the specificity of these sera has not been clearly delineated, and the relevance to malignant transformation as opposed to virus infection remains unresolved (7, 46). Stephenson and Aaronson were unable to find evidence in human sera to antigens of the type-C viruses of the woolly monkey and Gibbon ape (235). Greenspan, in experiments not likely to be repeated, showed that normal humans immunized with cell-free extracts from leukemic brain and Hodgkin's lymphoma developed tumor-specific antibodies to leukemia tissue extracts when tested by (1) passive cutaneous anaphylaxis in the guinea pig, (2) immunodiffusion, (3) immunoprecipitation, and (4) immunofluorescence (89).

We have described several human sera from healthy individuals which demonstrate complement-dependent cytotoxicity to the cells of patients with acute leukemia, particularly acute lymphocytic leukemia. We have designated these sera HUNAT (see Table 2) (28, 29, 221, 222). These reactions are operationally leukemia-specific in that all of the fol-

Table 2.   Reactivity of HUNAT sera[a] with cells of patients with leukoproliferative disorders

Peripheral Cells from Patients (Diagnosis)	Number of Reactive Cell Samples/Total Tested				
	(1)	(2)	(3)	(4)	(5)
Normal lymphocytes	0/76	0/76	0/76	0/36	0/23
ALL	9/64	16/64	8/64	8/60	6/28
AML	2/51	4/51	2/51	5/48	2/20
AMOL	1/8	0/8	0/8	0/6	0/3
AMMOL	0/7	0/7	0/7	0/5	0/3
Infectious mononucleosis	0/7	0/7	0/7	0/7	0/7
CLL	0/6	0/6	0/6	1/6	0/6
CML	0/5	0/5	0/5	0/5	0/2

a. HUNAT sera were obtained from healthy individuals with no history of alloimmunization: HUman NATural.

Source: Data from Ref. 218.

lowing cells will not react with the HUNAT sera: lymphocytes from normal individuals, remission lymphocytes, enriched normal T and B cell fractions, and PHA transformed normal lymphocytes. Some established lymphoblastoid cell lines are reactive, with no correlation with T/B surface properties (222). There is no correlation between reactivity with the HUNAT sera and age, sex, race, or peripheral blood count of the patient. There is strong correlation between HUNAT reactivity and peripheral lymphoblast count. Some lymphoblastoid cell lines (e.g., Raji, CCRF-CEM) will absorb the antileukemia reactivity of the HUNAT sera though normal or remission lymphocytes will not. Whole buffy coat from a single normal individual would remove the antileukemic reactivity from one HUNAT serum. These data suggest that the HUNAT sera are detecting a blast-associated antigen of acute lymphoblastoid leukemia, which may be present on a nonlymphoid leukocyte. The nature of the exposure responsible for the development of this reactivity is unknown. All donors of HUNAT sera have no history of alloimmunization through transfusion, pregnancy or transplantation. A systematic study of sera from healthy individuals for such antibody has not been performed to determine the frequency of such reactivity in the normal population. Dreesman et al. have reported cytotoxic antibody to peripheral blasts of ALL in the serum of 8 of 22 family contacts of ALL patients (64). Yoshida has reported a low-level reactivity of normal sera to leukemic cells in the hemagglutination immune adherence test (265). Bertoglio has reported a family in which the sibling of the proband with immunoblastic lymphosarcoma demonstrated antibody to the proband's tumor cells (27). This family is an especially interesting one since two siblings died of "unconfirmed hemopathies." This includes a fraternal twin of the sibling with the antitumor cytotoxic antibody. Whether this family expresses a genetic disorder, either in susceptibility or immune reactivity, an infectious disease with low-grade infectivity passed by horizontal transmission, or a vertically transmitted infectious disease is a matter for speculation.

These few studies provide the scant documentation of the development of a humoral immune response in healthy individuals to leukemia-associated antigens. Further systematic population studies are required in concert with progress in the identification and characterization of leukemia-associated antigens detected by heterologous antisera. The alloantisera often have weak reactivity by the usual immunological tests which discourages further work in antigen isolation. Such studies, however, may provide important evidence that human leukemia-associated antigens have at least limited immunogenicity in humans and that there is exposure to leukemia-associated antigens (or material which cross-reacts with leukemia-associated antigens) of individuals who do not have lymphoproliferative disorders.

III. CELLULAR IMMUNITY TO LEUKEMIA-ASSOCIATED ANTIGENS

Many studies of human acute leukemia have suggested that leukemia blasts have tumor-specific antigens, and that human immune reactions to these antigens can be demonstrated by assays of cellular immunity (104, 199). Nonspecific cellular immune competence has been correlated in some studies with a good prognosis in leukemia. Hersh has reported that patients in chemotherapy-induced remission of their leukemia who have strong established delayed hypersensitivity skin test reactions to bacterial and fungal antigens have prolonged remissions, and that a decline in such nonspecific immunocompetence may precede hematological relapse (116, 117). Additionally, adequate responses by remission patients, when evaluated using in vitro assays for cellular immune responsiveness to phytohemagglutinin or to a primary antigen (keyhole limpet hemocyanin), were associated with good prognosis. Baker also demonstrated that cutaneous reactivity to established delayed hypersensitivity antigens was somewhat correlated with good clinical prognosis (14). Char and Greene, however, could not correlate nonspecific immune competence, as demonstrated by skin testing, to duration of remission in leukemia (42, 88).

It is even more difficult to document that specific antileukemia cellular immunity is associated with prolonged survival. Positive skin tests to extracts of autologous leukemic blasts have been associated with good prognosis in the studies of Herberman (111, 112, 113). Baker reported that positive skin test reactions to whole irradiated autologous leukemia blasts did not correlate with prognosis (14), a finding confirmed in other reports (111, 112).

In vitro cellular immune reactivity to leukemic blasts has been studied using several techniques including the mixed lymphocyte culture blastogenesis (MLC) assay which tests the ability of the responding lymphocytes to recognize foreign antigens, as well as the migration inhibition factor (MIF) assay and the ^{51}chromium release cytotoxicity (CRC) assays, which presumably measure prior sensitization when conducted as short-term assays. In these assays responder and/or effector cells have been from leukemia patients, their family members, and unrelated normal controls.

In vitro cellular reactivity of leukemia patients in remission to leukemic blasts has been reported in the mixed lymphocyte culture (MLC) assay in a number of studies (40, 75, 96, 154, 200, 254). Gutterman showed that a proliferative response to autologous leukemic blasts in mixed leukocyte culture, accompanied by presence of associated inhibitory serum factors, was correlated with prolonged remission (90, 93, 94). Gutterman also demonstrated lymphocyte blastogenesis in response to a hypertonic potassium chloride extract of the autogenous leukemic blasts (93). Using the CRC assay, Herberman and Leventhal have demonstrated killing of autologous labeled leukemic blasts by lymphocytes of patients in remission (111, 112, 154). Hillberg (119), and Neidhart and LoBuglio (186), have reported evidence of response to leukemia antigens (extracted from autologous tumors) by the use of the MIF assay. Gutterman reported that 25% of leukemic patients in remission responded to their own tumor by MIF production (96). Studies of adult acute leukemics in remission have shown that 43% of patients respond in the MLC assay, 57% in the MIF test, and 74% in the CRC test to autologous leukemic blasts (stored in liquid nitrogen, prior to therapy) (3, 4, 5, 138, 217). We also tested about thirty sera collected from patients at various times in their courses for possible "blocking" effects on MLC and CRC reactions but no consistent effects were found, in contrast to the results of Gutterman (217). We could not demonstrate correlation of the responses to autologous blasts with remission duration although a correlation between strong reactions and longer remission was noted by Gutterman (90, 104, 105).

Further evidence suggesting the existence of leukemia-associated antigens in human leukemia comes from studies in which lymphocytes from family members of patients with leukemia, from patient contacts, and from unrelated normal controls are tested using the in vitro assays, for antileukemia immune reactivity. Han reported that a normal twin responded in MLC to his identical twin's leukemic lymphoblasts but not to his remission lymphocytes, indicating new antigens on the leukemic blasts (102). Another study of normal twins for antileukemia reactivity against identical twin leukemic blasts did not show the same result (211). Antileukemia reactivity demonstrable in HLA identical non-twin siblings using the MLC was first described by Bach (12), although this finding was not confirmed by Halterman and Leventhal (100) or by Schweitzer (228). We have found that over 80% of siblings HLA identical to the patient react in MLC to leukemic blasts from their sibling (3, 217). Evidence was found indicating that the normal HLA identical siblings could distinguish between the patient's leukemic blasts and his remission cells. We could not find evidence that normal bone marrow cells, or normal peripheral lymphocytes stimulated by phytohemagglutinin to express presumptive normal blast antigens (T cell?) were stimulatory to autologous normal peripheral lymphocytes. Because of the low frequency of recombination between the serologically detectable HLA antigen loci and the loci controlling the MLC, HLA identical siblings are generally reciprocally nonstimulatory to each other in MLC testing. The positive response to "HLA identical" blasts supports, but does not prove, the concept of specific tumor antigens on leukemic blasts which are recognized by, and stimulatory to, HLA identical normal lymphocytes.

Studies of antileukemia reactions of family members and normal controls using the CRC and MIF assays have suggested presentization to leukemia antigens in some nonleukemic individuals. Rosenberg (211), Levine (156), and McCoy (170) have reported that significant numbers of family members and of unrelated normal controls did demonstrate significant lymphocyte mediated cytotoxicity to ^{51}chromium-labeled leukemic blasts. Rarely do such family members or controls react to normal allogeneic cells, but occasionally they have been demonstrated to react to the remission cells of leukemic patients. Family member responses to leukemic cell antigen extract using the MIF assay were reported by Hillberg (119). In our laboratory, 51% of family members react to the leukemic blasts of their family member in the CRC assay (138) and 47% using the MIF assay (5). Those same family members also responded with CRC to unrelated leukemic blasts in 73% of the cases tested, and in 58% of the cases tested with the MIF assay.

The MIF and CRC reactions have been used to study the reactions of nonfamily normal controls to leukemic blasts (5, 138, 170). Essentially all normal controls react in MLC to leukemic blasts. This is the expected result based on HLA differences and does not imply or require prior antigenic sensitization. The MIF and CRC presumably measure prior antigenic sensitization when conducted as short-term assays: the MIF using 24–48 hours for reaction, and the CRC performed with a 4 hour incubation. These tests were used in our laboratory in an effort to describe the extent and prevalence of antileukemia immune reactivity in a normal population (5, 138). Using the CRC technique, 37 of 46 (80%) normal unrelated controls reacted to leukemic blasts. Our first hypothesis, because most of our initial controls were physicians, nurses, technicians, etc., was that exposure to leukemic patients conferred in vitro anti-leukemia reactivity. Very early studies in a few controls had suggested to us that persons who did not know of any exposure to leukemic patients, cells, or other suggested cancer associated exposure, might have less reactivity than those with known exposure to such patients or materials. Further so-called "unexposed controls" were found, who gave a negative history of known exposure to leukemic or other cancer-associated material and were compared in these assays with "exposed controls" with known clinical or family contact. Using the CRC assay, 23 of 28 (82%) of "exposed" controls, and 14 of 18 (78%) of "unexposed" controls responded with cytotoxicity to at least one sample of leukemic blasts. Similarly, the MIF assay demonstrated that 18 of 23 (78%) of "exposed" and 11 of 14 (78%) of "unexposed" controls gave evidence of prior sensitization to leukemic cell antigens. It should be noted that "exposed" versus "unexposed" was determined by subject recollections. That persons claiming nonexposure actually have accurate medical information about distant family or other casual contacts seems unlikely. Recollection of exposure is a notoriously poor way to determine actual exposure. However, using this crude distinction, no difference could be seen in the two groups as evidenced by the similar percentage of responders in the two groups. Thus, another hypothesis could be entertained: that "exposure" is ubiquitous in the environment, and that the agent inciting the immune reactivity is related to oncogenesis only infrequently.

The extent of an individual's response to leukemic blasts was tested using responders as sources of effector cells in the MIF and CRC assays against a variety of leukemic blasts from different patients and of different histological leukemic subtypes. Any consideration of tumor antigen reactivity or of tumor immunotherapy requires evaluation of the important question of cross-reactivity. In the studies reported by McCoy many patient relatives and normal unrelated controls responded in the CRC assay to leukemic blasts of different types (170). Herberman also reported significant skin reactivity and CRC reactivity of remission patients to allogeneic leukemic cells (111, 112). In our laboratory, most remission patients respond in MIF and MLC to allogeneic as well as autologous leukemic blasts. They often respond, however, also to allogeneic normal cells, and all of these responses by remission patients may reflect alloantigen sensitization by the multiple erythrocyte, platelet, and leukocyte transfusions given during induction chemotherapy (225, 226, 244). Family members and unrelated normal controls have been studied for cross reactivity to leukemic blasts of different cell types (4, 138). In essentially every case where the responder was tested against several samples of leukemic blasts, he reacted to more than one cell type, and to more than one sample of a given cell type. Not all reactors react to all cell samples, but in general, these reactions appear to demonstrate a broad cross reactivity to leukemic blasts of different origin and morphological cell type. This broad reactivity in cellular immunity to leukemic blasts suggests that various histological types share cross-reacting antigens, or that the cell population of the responder has subpopulations of cells each capable of responding individually to broad classes of antigens on leukemic cells even if those antigens are not identical. Theoretically, normal humans (unless sensitized by pregnancy, blood transfusions or specific immunization) essentially should never respond in these tests to normal allogeneic cells. The responses to leukemic cells in assays that require presensitization may imply prior exposure to some relatively common immunogen related to leukemia.

In summary, the above studies of antileukemia cell mediated immune responses have been interpreted as supporting the evidence for leukemia associated antigens, and demonstrating a lack of tolerance of remission patients, or the population at large, to these antigens. Reactions in family members and unrelated controls in the MIF and CRC assays are consistent with responses caused by prior sensitization of these persons who have not been purposely immunized. As such, evidence for prior sensitization can be used to support the concept of widespread exposure and response to an immunizing agent, such as a virus. Such an agent would presumably be widely spread in terms of exposure, but only rarely be associated with the occurrence of the clinical state recognized as leukemia.

The problems of specificity and significance of a positive response in these assays has been raised in other human and animal systems (20). At present, without further studies, these questions in relation to leukemia cannot be firmly resolved, although leukemia-specific reactivity can be operationally demonstrated. For the mixed lymphocyte studies, the responses of remission patients and/or their HLA identical siblings to leukemic blasts may be leukemia specific as suggested or may be in response to rare, tissue specific or embryonic antigens derepressed on leukemia. An animal model of autochthonous tissue-specific responses in the MLC has been reported (74) and Kuntz has reported blastogenic response of human peripheral T lymphocytes to autologous B lymphocytes (149). Thus the responses of normal lymphocytes in the MLC to leukemic blasts may reflect the quantitatively or qualitatively modified expression on the blast of a normal "differentiation" antigen.

IV. LEUKEMIA ANTIGENS AND STUDIES OF STRUCTURAL CHANGES IN TRANSFORMED CELL MEMBRANES

The study of cell surfaces and their changes in malignancies including in leukemia has been approached from a biochemical and structural as well as immunological point of view (54, 203). VanBeek et al. have recently reported that the surface glycoprotein composition is altered in human leukemia cells as detected by a shift in the chromatographic elution profile of surface glycopeptides (252). Except for cells from the CML patients, the profile from leukemic samples of all histologic types was rendered similar to the normal profile by treatment of the preparations with neuraminidase to decrease the sialic acid content. This change is unlikely to be due simply to a general change in blasts since PHA-stimulated normal blasts did not show a similar shift. This increase in surface sialyzation of leukemic blasts may be relevant to the observation that the detectable level of blood group substance A is decreased on the leukocytes of leukemia patients while blood group substance M and N appear on leukemic cells though they are absent from normal leukocytes (135). While several explanatory mechanisms for the blood group changes can be entertained, including somatic mutation, Kassulke et al. have found that the changes in expression on leukemic blast cells of blood group substances A, M, and N are sensitive to neuraminidase (135). These authors suggest that increased sialic acid units on the leukemic cells may interfere with the detection of antigens or alter their antigenicity.

Sahasrabudhe et al. have produced a horse antiserum which showed operational leukemia specificity using agglutination and immunoprecipitation by immunizing the animal with white blood cells from a normal blood group O donor, which had been tagged with fluorodinitrobenzene (FDNB). Tagging with FDNB was used to reduce the net surface charge of the cells and thus presumably nonspecifically increase the immunogenicity of the cells (215). This maneuver was also employed by these workers to immunize an ALL patient on maintenance chemotherapy with tagged allogeneic white cells (214). This patient produced an isoantibody which showed leukemia specificity by agglutination and immunodiffusion. This intriguing study suggests that a modification of net surface change may be a significant property of leukemic blasts.

Mintz, Sachs, and co-workers studied cell surface properties of normal peripheral lymphocytes and chronic lymphocytic leukemia cells and found that the leukemic cells had decreased cap formation and increased agglutinability with Con A, and increased ability to attach to a Petri dish (19, 168). Cap formation requires extensive lateral movement of ligand receptors in the membrane while agglutinability reflects only short range mobility and thus these differential changes in the membrane response to Con A by CLL cells suggests a specific structural modification. Vlodarsky and Sachs have shown a change in the phospholipid/cholesterol ratio in CLL cells which is consistent with an increase in membrane fluidity (256). The decrease in phosphopid/cholesterol ratio probably results from a marked increase in cholestrol rather than a decrease in phospholipid content. Evidence has been obtained of increased sterol synthesis in human non-myeloid leukemia cells and animal models have suggested that the increased sterol synthesis is leukemia specific and not blast associated since chemotherapy induced marrow proliferation in normal mice does not result in increased sterol synthesis (106).

Metzgar's primate anti-CLL, AML, and CGL sera are not reactive to tumor cells pretreated with neuroamindase or trypsin (177, 178, 183). These treatments do not render normal lymphocytes reactive to the antileukemia sera. Treatment of leukemic cells with trypsin resulted in release from the cell surface of antigens detected by primate antileukemia sera and allowed their detection in the supernate by inhibition of cytotoxicity. Treatment of target cells with neuraminidase, however, resulted in complete absence of antigen on cells and in the supernate. Treatment of subcellular membrane antigens (or soluble antigens prepared by proteolysis) with neuraminidase did not destroy antigenic activity. These results suggest that the antigens detected by the primate antisera consist of both carbohydrate and protein. The anomolous disappearance of antigenicity by treatment of whole cells with neuraminidase in contrast to the retention of antigenicity after treatment of partially purified antigen with neuraminidase may be a technical artifact or may result from proteolytic activity by a component of intact cell membranes which is lost upon membrane fragmentation or antigen solubilization, allowing survival of the antigen after neuraminidase solubilization. The "null" ALL antigen of Brown, Hogg, and Greaves is not neuraminidase sensitive (39). These authors have, however, shown that the antigen detected by this serum cocaps with the lentil lectin receptor but not the PHA receptor, which may suggest a relationship between the antigen and a specific glycoprotein receptor.

These data support a concept of changes in the cell surface of leukemic cells which are related to changes in glycoprotein and phospholipid composition and overall membrane structure. These changes may comprise the antigenic modification on leukemic cells which are detected by the various immunological probes. Alternatively, the changes in composition may reflect, along with those antigenic changes, the pleiomorphic effects of altered gene expression which occurs in leukemia. There are several studies of comparisons of glycolipid and glycoprotein composition of normal and tumor cell membranes. Much of this data has been recently reviewed (54, 203). Few consistent patterns have emerged. It has been suggested that the integration of oncogenic DNA virus may result in the change in expression of the gene controlling the enzyme N-acetylgalactosaminyl-glycolipid N-acetylgalactosaminyl transferase, but the situation with oncornavirus induced or spontaneous transformation is less clear in terms of alternation of the glycolipid of transformed cells (54).

Much of the most intriguing information about cell surface changes in malignancy relate specifically to changes in adherence and density-dependent growth control (203). These properties may be of little direct relevance to hemopoietic malignancies. Cell surface changes detected by agglutinens, and immunological probes in model systems of "normal" cultured cells and their in vitro transformed counterparts and the relationship of these changes to transformation, malignancy, cell cycle, or metabolic state is an active area of study. These studies have spoken more to the general questions about the nature and function of exposed cell surface components than to changes uniquely associated with in vivo malignancy. Progress is being made in understanding the functional topography of cells in culture and the functional language of that topography. What remains to be elucidated are the specific functions of cell surface components in the interaction of the cell with its *in vivo* humoral and cellular environment. Models of cell surface function relevant to *in vivo* cell surface changes in malignancy or differentiation can then be formulated and tested. Leukemia neo-antigens may themselves play a role in the pathological misdirection of the control of differentiation and thereby offer powerful tools for understanding the structure and function of the cell surface in the control of differentiation.

V. LEUKEMIA ANTIGENS, ALLOANTIGENS, AND CELL SURFACE MARKERS

There have been a number of studies of the frequency of specific HLA antigens in patients with leukemia (W. E. Braun, *HLA and Disease: A Critical Review*. Critical Reviews in Clinical Laboratory Sciences, in preparation). HLA is the name given to the human, major histocompatibility complex: that region of the genome which appears to code for or control expression of the major transplantation antigens. The HLA complex is large, has four known, and probably many unknown, polymorphic loci, and appears to play a role not only in the allograft response, but also in control of immune responsiveness and susceptibility to certain diseases. The genetics and biology of HLA have been recently well reviewed (9–11). There is a growing appreciation of the complexities of the host response to the gene products of the known loci of HLA, and two general classes of HLA loci whose products are detectable on nucleated cells have been formulated: SD and LD. The serologically detectable (SD) antigens controlled by loci HLA-A, -B, -C are defined using selected alloantisera, and the lymphocyte-defined (LD) or MLC-detected antigens controlled by the HLA-D, and possibly other loci, are typed using a variation of the mixed lymphocyte culture technique. Recently a third type of alloantigen locus (loci) has been identified whose products like HLA-A, -B, and -C are detected using alloantisera but which show limited tissue distribution of expression (10). These antigens which may be analogous to the Ia antigens of I region of the H-2 complex of the mouse, are expressed on B lymphocytes and monocytes, but are not directly detectable on T lymphocytes (?32). These so-called B cell alloantigens are presently under extensive study and the number of loci, within or without the HLA genetic region and their relationship to other antigenic systems is not fully understood (10, 160, 161, 258).

Overall, a weak but significant association between HLA-A2 and ALL has been seen in several studies with an increased frequency of A2 of less than 10% in comparison with controls (85, 209, 210, 216, 254). This has not been consistently reproduced (15, 23, 61, 130, 131, 147). It has been suggested that by necessity these studies have involved newly diagnosed cases and "survivors" of ALL and may reflect an association between HLA-A2 and survival (145). In studies with freshly diagnosed ALL cases this association with A2 is not seen (209). Our own data with 43 caucasian ALL patients corroborates the observation of no shift in HLA-A or -B antigen frequency in freshly diagnosed ALL, with a frequency of A2 of 26% which approximates the control caucasian frequency (Schacter, Kaiser, and Bias, unpublished observations). The difference in prospective and retrospective data has suggested that this is an association between HLA-A2 (and the related antigens A28, A9) and factors such as response to leukemia and/or disease severity which effect survival but not with susceptibility (145, 209). Several reports have suggested that the strength of the HLA associations varied not only with time elapsed since diagnosis but also with peripheral WBC at diagnosis, which may reflect that there are several biological forms of ALL of different severity, and susceptibility to one form or the other is associated with an A2 or non-A2 antigenic determinant (145, 209).

In analyzing the reactivity of the allogeneic antileukemia sera described above (HUNAT) with cells of 30 ALL patients, we have found a significant negative correlation ($P < 0.005$) between reactivity with one serum we call HUNAT 2 and HLA-A2 (222). This may reflect a relationship between the antigen detected by HUNAT and a supertypic determinant of the non-A2 A locus antigens directly, or indirectly through an association between HLA-A locus antigenic determinants and a particular form or line of ALL. Larger numbers are needed to confirm this observation, but the correlation in reference to the HLA data is intriguing. In a recent study including C locus typing, Johnson et al. have reported a weak association in a prospective study between ALL and the C locus antigen Cw3 (132).

For other leukemias there is little reproducible evidence for even a weak association with any HLA-A, -B, or -C antigen (55, 130, 192).

"Extra" reactions of leukemic cells are often found during routine HLA typing (28, 29, 51, 259). This finding is similar to the "extra reactions" found in HLA typing of cultured lymphoblastoid cell lines (26, 62, 65). "Extra reactions" in this context means that an HLA typing serum whose operational specificity has been well defined on normal peripheral lymphocytes may react with leukemic cells although family studies and phenotyping of remission cells suggests that the patient did not inherit the antigen detected by the serum in question. Only one of several standard typing sera detecting a single specificity may give extra reactivity with a particular cell suggesting that the extra reactivity is not directly related to an HLA specificity. "Extra reactivity" often also occurs with sera detecting HLA antigens known to cross-react with HLA antigens carried by the leukemia patient (e.g., an A2 serum may react with an A28, non-A2 blast). Such known HLA cross-reactivity however does not account for all extra reactions. The extra reactions may have several explanations: 1) the overall increased sensitivity of blasts to the microcytotoxicity assay giving rise to random false positives; 2) the presence in HLA typing sera of HLA-directed antibodies not strong enough to react with normal lymphocytes, but reactive with leukemic cells because of an increased density or qualitative change in expression of HLA antigens; 3) the presence of alloantigens or differentiation antigens of restricted distribution on leukemic cells; 4) the presence of truly leukemia-specific neoantigens of either viral or cellular origin on the leukemic cells.

Explanations 1 and 2 are easily tested by analysis of the reproducibility of the extra reactions with a given cell, absorption studies, and analysis of the HLA phenotype of cells giving extra reactions. Leukemic blasts are in general more sensitive to the manipulations required for microcytotoxicity testing, and careful control of time, temperature and reagents during the test may be critical. The source of complement can be a problem since some rabbit sera used for complement have a "natural" cytotoxicity for blasts. Several studies of "extra reactions" of leukemia blasts and lymphoblastoid cell lines have analyzed for these technical variables and concluded that there is extra reactivity to human blasts in some alloantisera which cannot be accounted for by these technical explanations (49, 62, 65, 68, 259).

Recent progress in exploring the Ia-like antigens in humans has directed interest in leukemia or blast-associated extra reactivity to these alloantigens of restricted distribution. It has become apparent that the extra reactivity of CLL cells with HLA typing sera is in large part due to the presence in many HLA-A, -B, or -C antisera of antibodies to alloantigens absent from T lymphocytes and present on B lymphocytes (49, 258, 259). There has been much interest in characterizing leukemia cells for the presence of the lymphoid cell surface markers of the two arms of the immune system to aid in understanding the biology of leukemia. An examination of the expression of characteristic markers of normal T and B lymphocytes (Table 3) on leukemia cells has led to some interesting suggestions (25, 76, 133, 231).

For the lymphoid leukemias it has become apparent that most CLL tumors carry B cell markers, and that most ALL tumors are non-B cells, the majority also non-T cell type, using the surface Ig to define B cells and E rosettes to define T cells (1, 2, 25). Using the "extra reactions" of CLL cells, Walford has identified a new alloantigenic system which is expressed on CLL cells and by absorption is found on some normal lymphocytes (258, 259). Further studies have suggested that these sera are detecting an HLA-linked alloantigenic system restricted in its distribution in

Table 3. Surface markers of normal human peripheral lymphocytes

Lymphocyte Type	Surface Ig[a]	E− Rosette[b]	C_3 Receptor	F_c Receptor	Ia-Like Antigen	Human T Cell Antigen[c]
T	−	+	−	−	−	+
B	+	−	+/−	+/−	+	−
"Null"	−	+/−	−	+	+	−

a. Definitive marker for peripheral B lymphocyte.
b. Definitive marker for peripheral T lymphocyte.
c. Sera with T cell specificity have been raised using as immunogen human thymus, peripheral E-rosetting lymphocytes, and human brain (25, 37, 44, 131, 176, 256).

Source: Data for this table compiled from Ref. 25, 75, 131, 222, 226, 256.

normal individuals to B lymphocytes, monocytes and possibly other non-lymphoid cells, but absent from T lymphocytes (10). The expression of these antigens on CLL cells is consistent with the expression of other B cell markers on CLL cells. The genetics and serology of this system are under intensive study but present data suggests at least two loci within the HLA region which code for normal B cell alloantigens possibly analogous to the mouse Ia antigens coded for in the I or immune response regions of H-2 complex (9, 10, 11, 160, 161). Such antibodies are often found in sera devoid of HLA antibodies (49, 77).

B cell determinants on acute leukemic cells have also been studied using heterologous and allogeneic sera. Billings has reported that a rabbit serum raised against malignant and cultured lymphoid cells reacts with normal B cells and most ALL cells (31). Schlossman et al. raised a rabbit antiserum to p23,30, a glycoprotein isolated from a human lymphoblastoid B cell line, and found that the serum reacted with normal B and null cells, 21 of 24 ALL cells, 10 of 10 AML cells, 7 of 7 CLL cells and 0 of 2 CML cells suggesting the presence of normal B cell determinants on these leukemic cells (227). In contrast they raised a serum against whole lymphoblasts from a patient with ALL, which after absorption reacted only with thymocytes (not peripheral T cells) and the 3 of 24 ALL cells which failed to react with the anti p23,30. Chechik and Gelfand found that a human thymus antigen absent from peripheral lymphocytes was present on E rosette positive leukemic lymphoblasts and in the serum of patients with E rosette positive ALL (44). Interestingly, the antigen was found in the serum of one patient with AML.

This data suggest that leukemia cells express public determinants of lymphoid differentiation antigens, that is, determinants recognized by cross-species antisera. Leukemia cells have also been studied for alloantigenic determinants of lymphoid differentiation antigens using sera from humans, immunized by transplantation or pregnancy. Fu et al. have reported the presence of B cell alloantigens on non-T ALL cells (77). Billings has reported the presence of B lymphocyte alloantigens on most leukemia cells, acute and chronic, lymphocytic and myeloid. One B cell antigen called Group 2, however, was absent from leukemic cells though found on the B cells of 22% of normal controls (34). Further studies are necessary on remission cells and families of leukemic patients, but the absence of a specificity from leukemic cells suggests the possibility of an unknown B group antigen associated with leukemia. Alternatively, genetic studies and tests with remission cells may show repression of selected B cell alloantigens in leukemia. In either case these observations do suggest that what appears to be a leukemia specific or associated antigen, may be the product of a "normal," nonleukemic gene which has undergone depression or modification on the leukemic cell or alternatively which confers susceptibility to leukemia.

Further data point out that discordant expression of "normal" cell surface markers of restricted tissue distribution may occur on leukemia blasts including not only the expression of lymphoid markers on non-lymphoid tumors, but also in that ALL tumor cells, devoid of surface Ig and/or the ability to form E rosettes may express other B or T associated markers (37, 78, 229, 262). Indeed Brouet et al. have examined ALL tumor cells for several T and B markers and have found that some but not all E rosette forming ALL tumors will react with a rabbit antiserum specific for human peripheral thymocytes (37). A rabbit serum raised with fetal thymocytes reacted with all E rosetting ALL cells, but also reacted with 1) the non-T, non-B ALL cells; 2) the ALL tumors bearing surface Ig; and 3) AML cells. Absorption with AML cells removed reactivity with the non-T, non-B ALL cells. An antiserum raised against CLL cells reacted with 30 of 33 non-T, non-B ALL cells, 2 of 2 B type ALL cells, but only 1 of 19 T type ALL cells. At least two antigens are involved since absorption with normal thymus removed the reactivity with the non-T, non-B ALL cells, though leaving reactivity with CLL and normal peripheral B lymphocytes. In contrast Greaves' rabbit antisera, discussed above, raised against non-T, non-B ALL, did not react with either CLL cells or normal peripheral B cells, though it did react with blasts from patients with CML (39, 87, 129).

There is a mouse alloantigen system which may prove of some relevance to human leukemia antigens—the TL system (35, 36, 190, 191, 233). The TL system consists of four antigens—TL.1, TL.2, TL.3, TL.4. In normal mice, the TL antigens are exclusively expressed on thymocytes and three phenotypes have been identified—TL−, TL.2, and TL.1, 2, 3. TL.4 is never expressed on normal cells. Some, but not all, leukemias of all mouse strains, are TL⁺ regardless of whether normal cells are TL⁺ or TL−. Table 4

Table 4. TL antigen phenotypes of mice

Phenotype of Normal Thymocytes (Strain)	Phenotype of Leukemias in Such Mice
TL⁻ (e.g. AKB)	TL⁻ or TL.1, 2, 4
TL.2 (e.g. BALB/C)	TL⁻, or TL.2, or TL.1, 2, or TL.1, 2, 4
TL.1, 2, 3 (e.g. A)	TL⁻, or TL.1, 2, 3

Source: Compiled from Ref. 36.

describes the possible TL antigens of leukemias of mice of different thymocyte TL phenotypes.

Since some leukemias of all strains may express TL antigens, the TLa locus, mapped to linkage group IX, probably governs the expression of structural genes present in all mice at an unknown location. Bone marrow transplantation experiments between TL⁻ and TL⁺ have shown that the recipient thymus was repopulated by donor cells of donor TL phenotype (35). Mouse leukemia passaged into TL-mismatched unimmunized recipients retains its TL phenotype. If, however, a TL⁺ leukemia is passaged into an immunized TL⁻ host, the TL antigens are antibody modulated or repressed, though on removal to an unimmunized host or to *in vitro* culture minus anti-TL antibody, the TL⁺ phenotype is re-expressed (191).

There is no absolute correlation of expression of the TL antigens with the means of induction of leukemia. For example, in C57B/6 (a TL⁻ strain) ¾ spontaneous leukemias are TL⁻, and ⅝ of Gross virus induced leukemias are TL⁺. Generally, however, spontaneous leukemias of high incidence strains are usually TL⁻ and spontaneous leukemias of low incidence strains (which may be the most relevant to humans) are rarely TL⁻ (35). In contrast, most human lymphoid leukemias, chronic and acute, do not express T cell markers, and do express some B cell markers (1, 2, 25).

From the studies of the human lymphoid leukemia antigens detected by animal and human sera, one could suggest that what is being detected is properly called a leukemia-associated antigen, with public antigenic determinants, and private or alloantigenic determinants, with limited distribution on normal cells as a marker of a particular differentiation step, and with anomolous or discordant expression on leukemia cells. The locus of genes controlling the B cell alloantigens of humans and the gene controlling TL expression lie in or near the major histocompatibility complex of their respective species (10, 36, 77, 160, 161, 232).

Thus the TL system possesses many properties which may be relevant to human leukemia associated antigens: a polymorphic alloantigen of restricted distribution which is anomously expressed on leukemic cells.

Like the B cell alloantigen system in humans, the TL system is not leukemia specific though one antigen TL 4 is expressed only on leukemia cells (cf absence of B cell group 2 from leukemia cells) (34, 36). The expression of TL antigens is not related to the means of leukemogenesis and certainly not restricted to specific viral induction of leukemia. Thus if the TL model speaks to human leukemia it would suggest that discordant expression of polymorphic markers of differentiation may constitute many of the detectable leukemia associated antigens. This may be of little direct relevance to the etiology of leukemia but may offer clues to the cell line of origin or the natural biology of the leukemic line.

Thus studies of leukemia specific or associated antigens must be explored in the context of normal or non-malignant markers of a particular differentiated state. It is clear that the lack of correlation between a putative leukemia antigen and a particular marker (e.g., with E rosetting ability in ALL) does not necessarily demonstrate the leukemia specificity of the antigen but may only reflect the discordant expression of cell surface markers of leukemia cells. We do not know the significance of the expression of these markers. Sen and Borella have suggested that the patients with E rosette forming ALL have a different age distribution, more severe disease, and poorer prognosis than the non-T, non-B ALL patients (229), but this was not corroborated by Brouet et al. (37). Clearly, further coordinated studies of immunological markers, including leukemia associated antigens, alloantigens, and clinical course in leukemia are necessary.

VI. ANIMAL LEUKEMIA VIRUSES AND THEIR ANTIGENS IN RELATION TO HUMAN LEUKEMIA

A. Herpes Virus and Human Tumor Antigens: A Model System?

One model for exploring the relationship in humans between oncogenic viruses and tumor antigens could be that of herpes virus. There are at least two herpes viruses with suspected oncogenicity in humans, Epstein-Barr virus (EBV) and HSV-2, and several more in animals. Data on the oncogenic potential of these viruses have recently been reviewed and will not be detailed here (67, 140, 204, 245). EBV and herpes virus have been shown to be associated in vivo with neoplastic transformation and to demonstrate the ability to transform cells in vitro (140, 245). We will deal here only with the relevance to human leukemia antigens that these models present in terms of the antigens associated with virally infected and/ or transformed cells.

Infection in vitro and in vivo with EBV has been associated with development of one or more classes of antigens: VCA (viral capsid antigen), EA (early antigen), S (soluble antigen), EBNA (Epstein-Barr nuclear antigen), MA (membrane antigen) (Table 5) (140, 141, 142, 194, 206, 261). Clearly infection with EBV does not, in all cases, give rise to tumors or to virus production. The data in Table 5 on the expression of the various EBV associated antigens on cells on different paths of infection, taken together with data on the humoral immune response of patients to EBV antigens (Table 6) suggest that no antigen associated with EBV infection is uniquely associated with *in vivo* transformation. Indirectly there is evidence that antibody to the methanol resistant early antigen of restricted distribution [EA(R)] may be uniquely correlated *in vivo* with Burkitts' lymphoma (109, 140, 141, 142). Most detectable antigens with the exception of the EB nuclear antigen (EBNA) require virus production for their expression if only abortively so (67). Virus production appears to occur at most in a small fraction of infected cells and since it leads in

Table 5.   Epstein-Barr virus antigen expression in human cells

| Cell | Antigens | | | | | | | |
| | VCA | MA | EA | | | EBNA | EBV DNA | EBV particles |
			R	D	S			
Burkitt's lymphoma	rare	+	−	−	+	+	+	−
Nasopharyngeal carcinoma	−	+	−	−	?	+	+	−

Infectious mononucleosis
  Unfractionated peripheral
  blood lymphocytes
  (predominately T cells)
	−	−	−	−	−	−	−	−

Peripheral B lymphocytes	?	?	?		?	+	?	−
Lymphoblastoid cell lines T lines	−	−	−	−	−	−	−	−
B lines EBV producer	+	+	+		+	+	+	+
nonproducer	−	−	−		+	+	+	−

VCA—viral capsid antigen; MA—membrane antigen; EA—early antigen; R—restricted staining; D—diffuse staining; S—soluble antigen; EBNA—Epstein-Barr virus nuclear antigen.
   + = present;   − = absent;   ? = not tested.
   Source: Data for this table compiled from Ref. 137, 138, 139, 190, 202.

Table 6. Antibodies to Epstein-Barr virus antigens in serum from patients

| Antibody in Patients with: | Antigens Detected by Patient Serum | | | | | |
| | VCA | MA | EA | | S | EBNA |
			R	D		
Burkitts' lymphoma	++	++	+	+/−	+	+
Nasopharyngeal carcinoma	++	++	+/−	+	+	+
Infectious mononucleosis	+ (IgM)	−	−	+	+	+
Controls	+	−	−	−	+	+
Acute/chronic leukemia	+	−	−	−	+	?

VCA—viral capsid antigen; MA—membrane antigen; EA—early antigen; R—restricted staining; D—diffuse staining; S—soluble antigen; EBNA—Epstein-Barr virus nuclear antigen.

++ = present at high titer;   + = present;   +/− = present in some patients;   − = absent from all patients tested; ? = not tested.

Source: Data for this table compiled from Ref. 107, 108, 138, 139, 202.

general to cell death is not compatible with transformation. For EBV, and in general from a theoretical view, it is the latent form of virus infection which may be the most relevant to viral tumorigenesis, and no unique antigen has been found in nonproductively infected transformed cells (Table 5). No antigen carried by the virus is found in transformed cells not producing virus (67, 143, 144). All cells in which EBV DNA is found by hybridization, including B cells in infectious mononucleosis, do express EBNA (140, 143). Whether the infected B lymphocytes in infectious mononucleosis are transformed is open to question and may be semantic. Epstein and Achong have suggested that the two kinds of herpes virus infections in man, BL (Burkitts' lymphoma) and IM (infectious mono-nucleosis), exemplify the transformed and non-transformed state of viral infection (62).

Immunologically there is no absolute ability to distinguish these states, though cytogenetics may provide a tool with the observation that a chromosome 14 abnormality is uniquely associated with Burkitts' lymphoma and possibly with EBV transformation (266). Why infection in some individuals results in a benign condition (IM) but in others is associated with a malignant uncontrolled growth of infected cells is unknown. If EBV infection is necessary but not sufficient for transformation, the *sine qua non* for transformation is unknown and may lie in a genetic factor in the host or in the ability of the host to immunologically control infected cells. As suggested by Klein, the finding of a unique cytogenetic marker in biopsies of malignant infected cells may lend support to the role of genetic factors (139). The suggestion may be made from the EBV-tumor system that among the many virus-associated antigens found, the immune response of the affected patient may offer the only clue for those antigens associated uniquely with transformation.

A similar lesson may be learned from the studies of herpes virus and squamous cell carcinomas. Serum IgM antibody to Ag-4, a non-capsid virion antigen expressed early in cells infected by HSV-2, has been associated in patients with cervical carcinoma. Ag-4 is present in cervical tumor tissue but not in normal tissue (8). Hollinshead et al. have reported a high frequency of antibody to herpes virus non-virion membrane antigens (HSV-TAN) in the serum of patients with squamous cell carcinomas at different locations (124). HSV-TAN can be demonstrated in squamous cell tumors. Melnik and co-workers have also found that cervical cancer patients have an increased titer of serum antibody to an HSV early nonstructural protein (173). Thus, for this suspected oncogenic herpes virus evidence suggests that the tumor bearing host mounts a specific immune response to an early cellular antigen of viral infection which may also be present in the virion as a low level, nonstructural antigen. In the search for immunological evidence to support or deny a viral etiology for human leukemia, it may, therefore, be necessary to search not for viral antigens or an immune response to viral antigens, but to look for viral-associated cellular antigens restricted to transformed cells.

B. Viruses, Leukemia, and Human Leukemia Antigens

One of the major objectives in studies of human leukemia cell surface antigens is to identify viral agents which may be involved in the etiology of this disease.

Viral etiology of leukemias and lymphomas has been shown in several species, such as chickens, mice, cats, cattle, and nonhuman primates, but despite a concerted effort by numerous laboratories, the role oncornaviruses play in human leukemia is not clear. There is a long history of reports of virus isolations from a variety of human tissues. A detailed review of these reports is well beyond the scope of this chapter, and will be covered in other chapters in this series.

Three approaches have been used in the identification of putative human leukemia viruses, each of which is subject to criticism and has severe limitations. First, direct isolation of viruses has been accomplished by many investigators. In many of these studies, the virus was subsequently shown to be a laboratory contaminant; in many others, the virus was probably present in the leukemic tissue as a passenger, and not involved in the etiology of the disease. The second major approach is to identify virus specific proteins in leukemic tissues, either immunologically or biochemically. In both cases, it is essential to show that the antibody that is used, or that the enzyme activity that is observed is truly virus specific. The studies with gp70 and p30 presented below suggest the complexities that may be revealed by such an effort. Finally, nucleic acid hybridization has been used to show the presence of viral genetic material in leukemic tissues. The exquisite sensitivity of this method requires equally exquisite specificity controls—controls which are often not presented.

A virus was isolated by Gallo and co-workers that satisfies all the requirements to confirm its association with a human leukemia (79, 80, 81, 82, 207). This virus, HL 23V, was first isolated from cultured blood cells of a patient with acute myelogenous leukemia, and was infectious for other cell strains. HL 23V is a C-type oncornavirus which has a reverse transcriptase that is immunologically related to the reverse transcriptase of a primate C-type virus Simian Sarcoma Virus (SiSV). By nucleic acid hybridization, HL 23V is closely related to SiSV. In addition, viruses isolated from secondary passage of HL 23V also contained nucleic acid sequences related to the endogenous C-type virus of baboons (BaEV). Recently, Reitz et al. showed that viral nucleic acids were present in the spleen of the patient when the HL 23V virus was isolated (207). SiSV RNA was present in cytoplasmic fractions and BaEV DNA was present as a provirus in the DNA from these cells.

The study of HL 23V points out one of the unresolvable dilemas facing those who are attempting to define the role of oncornaviruses in human leukemias. In this case, there is overwhelming evidence that a primate oncogenic virus (or viruses) are present in a leukemic individual, but the question of the significance of that virus in the etiology of the disease in general, remains unknown. Extension of these studies, in parallel with immunological studies of leukemic material, are necessary to determine if a viral or viral-related oncogene product can be found in human leukemic material. The demonstration of an infectious agent and the rigorous fulfillment of Koch's postulates may not be possible in human leukemia, not only because of the ethical considerations but also because intact, nondefective virus production may be a rare event in human leukemia. Lapin et al. have reported that innoculation of human leukemic material (whole blood or filtered plasma) produced malignant lymphoma in two nonhuman primate species (Macaca arctoides and Papio hamadryas) (150). The disease could be passaged with the tumor and C-type virus particles were found in plasma, leukocytes and other tissue of affected monkeys. Natural transmission of the disease occurred to healthy baboons housed with the innoculated animals. And these workers reported that membrane antigen of human leukemia detected by rabbit and hamster antisera was expressed on cells of affected animals.

These remarkable experiments are consistent with a viral etiology of human leukemia but do not prove such a relationship. The C-type virus could have been derived and "rescued" from the nonhuman primates after derepression by an earlier oncogenic event. Critical here may be hybridization experiments to show that new viral genetic information was introduced with the human material. Further efforts in this area are needed to define the mode or modes of transmission of human leukemia.

In 1969, Huebner and Todaro proposed the "oncogene theory" to explain the role of oncornaviruses in human cancers (126). It was hypothesized that oncornaviruses had two sets of genes: 1) virogenes, which coded for viral structural molecules, and 2) oncogenes, which were responsible for oncogenic transformation. Further, they proposed that virogenes and oncogenes need not be coordinately expressed. That is, in some cases, infectious virus (or viral proteins) could be expressed in cells which are not cancerous; and conversely, the oncogenes could cause transformation of some cells in the absence of expression of other viral genetic information. Although these ideas are attractive on a theoretical basis, they have not yet been proven by experimentation, and indeed, it may not be possible to subject the oncogene theory to critical experimental test.

In recent years, there have been two major conceptual advances which support the oncogene theory. The first is the finding that viral structural molecules can be normal cellular differentiation antigens, such as the thymocyte differentiation antigen G_{ix} (239). This is analogous to one of the predictions of the oncogene theory—that viral genes can be expressed in the absence of viral particles. The second supporting advance is the identification of endogenous, integrated oncornaviruses in several species (43). These viruses have been useful in studies of the evolutionary relationships among oncornaviruses (247).

In the relationship between mice and their endogenous oncornaviruses, the distinction between cellular and viral molecules is often quite arbitrary because the viral genome(s) may be physically integrated into the host genome, and because during the replication of oncornaviruses, viral molecules must be a part of the host cell surface at some point in the formation of an infectious particle. Nevertheless, it is useful to make the distinction between "viral" and "cellular" molecules. For the following discussion it is useful to define viral molecules as those which are expressed coordinately with the production of virus particles, and cellular molecules as those which are expressed in the absence of virus particles. Of course, there are many examples of oncogenic and nononcogenic viruses in which there is overlap between these classes. For example, polyoma virus particles contain cellular histones (70) and viral proteins are found on the surface of cell cultures which are infected with influenza virus (208).

The importance of the distinction between viral and cellular molecules is illustrated in the case of the major envelope glycoprotein of murine leukemia virus, gp70 (MuLV) (glycoprotein of molecular weight 70,000 daltons). Gp70 is located on the viral envelope as the spike protein and is the molecule by which oncornaviruses absorb to cells (224, 241). In addition, gp70 is also present on the surface of infected cells and some normal cells (57, 136). These latter findings are not surprising since, as pointed out above, oncornavirus molecules are associated with the surface of the cell during the formation of the infectious particle.

Immunologic studies of MuLV gp70 have shown that gp70s have three sets of antigenic determinants, which can be identified by their cross reactions in radioimmune assays: The first set is "interspecies," which includes those determinants shared by gp70s of viruses from different species; the second is "group specific," shared only by gp70s of viruses from the same species; the third is "type specific," unique to an individual virus (240). The interspecies determinants have been particularly useful in studies of MuLV gp70 expression because these determinants are present on essentially all strains of leukemia virus (152, 240, 243). Thus, with the interspecies radioimmune assay, it is possible to quantitate the expression of RNA leukemia virus gp70s regardless of the source. Conversely, using the interspecies assay, it is not possible to identify the source of gp70 (see Fig. 1).

The concept that gp70 could also be a "cellular" molecule was developed in three sets of experiments. First, gp70 was shown to be present on the surface of MuLV infected cells, normal lymphoid cells, and sperm by lactoperoxidase cell surface labeling, immune precipitation and SDS-gel electrophoresis (57, 58, 152, 249). Further, combining these methods with immunoelectronmicroscopy, Kennel and Feldman showed that gp70 was present in areas of the cell surface in which no morphological evidence of virus particles or buds were recognizable (137).

Second, several laboratories have studied the expression of endogenous gp70s using radioimmune assays (56, 152, 240, 242, 243). By the interspecies assay, very high concentrations of gp70 were found in sera and tissue of all mouse strains tested, ranging from 1 to 200 μg/ml for serum. The concentration of gp70 was much higher than that of the major internal protein of MuLV, p30, which is usually less than 0.1 μg/ml. From the ratio of gp70 to p30, it was concluded that the gp70 was not present in these sera and cells as a part of virus particles, and that the expression of these two viral molecules was not coordinate. In addition, these studies also showed that the serum concentration of gp70 was considerably higher in mice which were positive for the thymocyte differentiation alloantigen, G_{IX}, than in mice which did not express this antigen. Using a type-specific radioimmune assay, Hino et al. found that the serum gp70s of several mouse strains reflected the viral flora of these strains (121). However, the concentration of these gp70s is lower than those found by other investigators, raising the possibility that these type specific assays measure only one of a set of gp70s present in these sera. In toto, the radioimmune assay data suggest that in the mouse there are several genes which code for different gp70s. Some of these may be components of infectious viruses as shown by Hino et al. and others may be expressed apparently in the absence of viral particles (137). Our present understanding of the antigenic relationships of the various gp70s is summarized in Fig. 1.

The third, and probably most important set of experiments showing that gp70 may be a cellular molecule, is by Boyse and colleagues. In 1971, Stockert et al. (239) described an antigen, G_{IX}, which can be detected on thymocytes of some mouse strains, but not others. This antigen is detected using an antiserum prepared by immunization of rats with syngeneic, MuLV-induced tumor cells, and was considered to be a virus-related antigen, but not a component of virus particles. G_{IX} was regarded as a differentiation antigen because by cytotoxicity tests it could only be found on thymocytes but not on other lymphoid cells from bone marrow, spleen or lymph nodes. Subsequent studies, using cell surface labeling methods and absorption techniques, have shown that the G_{IX} antigen represented exposed type-specific antigen determinants which were present on certain classes of gp70s (187, 188, 249). More recently, Tung et al. (248, 250) have extended these studies by identifying two other classes of cell surface gp70s, 0-gp70 and X-gp70, which are serologically and genetically distinct from the G_{IX}-gp70. 0-gp70 may be found on the surface of thymocytes from some strains of mice such as C57B6 which are negative for G_{IX} antigen; but no cell surface gp70 has been found on thymocytes from other G_{IX}^- strains, such as BALB/C or congenic 129 G_{IX}^-. Thus, 0-gp70 is a component of the surface of C57B6 thymocytes as shown by the lactoperoxidase cell surface labeling methods, but this molecule differs from the G_{IX}-gp70 in the so called type specific antigenic determinants. The third class of gp70, X-gp70, is associated with the expression of MuLV (220). Two kinds of antisera are used to detect X-gp70. The first was originally used for the identification of TLA, i.e., thymus leukemia antigen (190) which was prepared by immunization of mice with a spontaneous strain A leukemia. Secondly, X-gp70 may be identified using X1 typing sera (220). In this case sera are also raised in certain strains of mice by immunization with leukemia cells. These X1 antisera probably recog-

EXPRESSION OF ANTIGENIC DETERMINANTS OF gp70

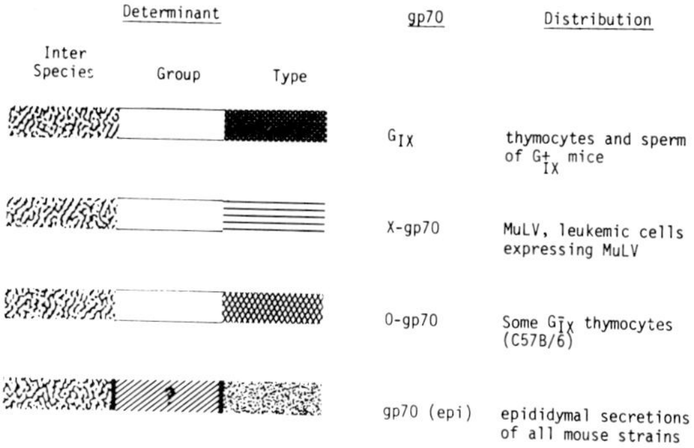

Reagents	Inter Species	Group	Type
Goat anti FeLV			
Reacts with	+	-	-
Discriminates	-	-	-
Goat anti gp70			
Reacts with	+	+	+/-
Discriminates	-	+	+
Rat anti MuLV			
Reacts with	+/-	+	+
Discriminates	+/-	+	+
Mouse anti MuLV			
Reacts with	-	-	+
Discriminates	-	-	+

Fig. 1. A schematic representation of antigenic composition of MuLV related gp70s, indicating that all four classes share inter-species antigens, three share group-specific antigens, and each has unique type-specific antigens. Typing sera used to distinguish among these sets of antigenic determinants are presented in the lower part. Taken in part from Refs. 56–58, 121, 232, 237–239, 248–250.

nize highly type specific determinants found exclusively on some classes of viral gp70s.

A fourth class of gp70, which is serologically distinct from all the others in that it does not react with rat typing sera and thus does not have the major group-specific determinants of murine leukemia virus gp70s, was originally described in the epididymal secretions from several strains of mice (56). As in the case of the other MuLV gp70s, it does have the interspecies determinants of gp70s as shown by competition radioimmune assay goat antifeline leukemia virus and ^{125}I MuLV gp70.

Gp70, as a class of molecules, links normal differentiation and leukemogenesis and lends support and interest to the oncogene theory. The role of the gp70s in leukemogenesis and lymphoid differentiation are unknown. The number of different genes responsible for the structural variants of gp70 is unknown, though Tung *et al.* (248) have suggested on the basis of finding O-gp70 that there are at least two genes. This question may be of fundamental interest to our understanding of leukemogenesis and differentiation. The possibility of post transcriptional modification giving rise to the gp70 variants has not been eliminated though the data presently available is more consistent with a multiple gene model. Relevant here may be the TL antigen system described in Section V. The implications of this question to the evolutionary and symbiotic relationship between virus and host are intriguing.

Our present knowledge of the expression of oncornavirus related antigens in mammalian tissue suggests that at least two antigens are of relevance in leukemia and differentiation; gp70 and p30. For mice, the expression of gp70 antigenic determinants has been detected in normal and leukemia material and thus this class of molecules is not unique to transformed cells. An examination of the pattern of expression of the various known antigenic determinants of gp70 (Fig. 1, Table 7) also suggests that no antigenically distinct gp70 molecule as presently known is uniquely expressed on transformed cells and absent both from virus and all normal cells. Thus gp70 is probably not the product of a oncogene in mice (30). The major MuLV internal protein p30 is also expressed on leukemias and some normal cells during embryogenesis and thus does not appear leukemia specific (125). In man limited data is available to suggest that these molecules are expressed in a limited (controlled) way on specific leukemias, on normal cells as differentiation markers and on the cells of patients with certain disorders (Table 7) (172, 175, 176, 242).

Thus at our present understanding in man and mice these viral molecules are not leukemia specific, but may be differentiation markers. The fact that they are also found in a similar form on or in leukemia viruses may reflect the 1) adaptation of the virus to the host by means of mimicry of a host antigen to minimize the host immune response to the virus or 2) the incorporation of host genes into the virus and their transduction into new hosts. This relationship between the oncornaviruses and host thus may be vestigal or functional. Through evolution, oncornaviruses and their hosts may have established a symbiotic relationship which could have benefits to both the virus and the host. Obviously, the virus is dependent upon the host for replication and horizontal spread. Whether benefit derives to the host is a matter of speculation. A clear evolutionary benefit of oncornaviruses to the host is not immediately apparent, but one attractive hypothesis is that oncornaviruses could "transduce" genes from one species to another—that is, an integrated viral genome could acquire a set of genes (either DNA or RNA) as the viral genome is excised from the cellular DNA, and then carry these cellular genes to another host. This could result in the addition of new, functional host genes to species, thereby accelerating the rate of evolution. In this

Table 7. Expression of murine oncornavirus-related antigens on murine and human tissues

	Mouse		Human	
Antigen	Normal Tissue	Leukemia	Normal Tissue	Leukemia
p30	During embryogenesis	+	? Lupus kidney	AML?
gp70	Differentiation antigen of G_{IX}^+ thymocytes and gp70$^+$ epithelium	Usually	? platelets/neutrophils	CGL

Source: This table compiled from Ref. 55, 56, 57, 157, 173, 244.

case, oncogenesis would be an unfortunate consequence of an otherwise beneficial symbiosis between oncornaviruses and their hosts.

The mechanism for the action of such a selective pressure to retain oncornaviruses is not immediately clear, since the trait retained would be viral infection which would, itself, confer no advantage on the individual. An alternative model to explain the evolutionary retention of the oncogenic viruses might invoke the elimination of elderly or unfit competitors for food, but it is also unclear how such selective pressure would be exercised except if two populations, one with the virus, one without, were competing for the same food source.

It is not possible to more closely define a putative agent for leukemia by immune reactions at this time. The source of the antigens involved is speculative. Certainly a primary oncogenic virus is a possibility. Murine studies, for example, show widespread cellular and humoral immunity against murine leukemia viruses in strains with a low incidence of leukemia, as well as in those strains with high leukemia susceptibility (103, 114, 115, 123, 189). The widespread cellular immune response pattern to leukemic cells by humans might represent a similar type of widespread exposure and reactivity as that demonstrated in the murine system where the antigen/oncogene is better defined.

Another possibility is that nononcogenic viruses, with widespread infectivity in humans, contain or induce identical or cross-reacting antigens to those on leukemia cells to which reactions can be demonstrated. Studies in other laboratories showing that bacterial antigens (i.e., streptococcal) may induce cross reactions to histocompatibility or tumor antigens, suggest a third source of nonspecific immunization or infection which might be detected as antileukemia reactivity in our assays (122, 205, 236). Viruses have been demonstrated by electron microscope in relation to leukemic cells, (72, 73, 159, 185) and presumed viral products have been found in leukemia cells and even in remission cells (82, 105, 159, 230, 253). Evidence for the presence of C-type viral information in human leukemic material has been discussed by Gallo and others (17, 18, 19, 79, 80, 81, 82). Our laboratory has collaborated with such studies, and many of the samples of leukemic blasts to which we have demonstrated human in vitro immune reactions have also been shown to have evidence of viral nucleic acids and reverse transcriptase. Many healthy gibbon apes have natural antibody to gibbon ape leukemia virus which can at least be partially absorbed by blast cells from a patient with chronic myelogenous leukemia in blast crisis, suggesting cross antigenicity between a known oncogenic primate virus and human leukemia antigens (6). A similar argument is raised by the cross-reactivity between human leukemia membrane antigens and the membrane antigens of C-type virus producing malignant lymphomas arising in nonhuman primates after innoculation with human leukemia material (150). The isolation of an RNA virus, with characteristics of nonhuman primate leukemia sarcoma viruses provides further support for the concept for a viral etiology for human leukemia (79, 207). The key point of determining whether such viruses, or viral products, represent the etiologic agent in leukemia remains to be unequivocally determined.

VII. IMMUNOTHERAPY OF LEUKEMIA

Although the specific physical or chemical structure of the leukemia-associated antigens has not been defined, the multiple examples of human reactivity to human leukemia has prompted the use of immunotherapy in the clinical treatment of leukemia patients. For theoretical reasons, and from experimental data in animals, it has been appreciated that immunotherapy is most effective when tumor burden has been reduced to a very low level. Acute leukemia in remission provides a clinical correlate in which residual tumor is minimal. The multiple studies mentioned previously established that patients in remission generally are immunocompetent, and can have demonstrable anti-tumor reactivity to their own leukemia by several assay techniques. Two kinds of immunotherapy have been used to treat leukemics in remission: nonspecific immunotherapy, in which the patient's immune system is stimulated by adjuvants, usually Bacillus Calmette-Guerin (BCG) or its derivatives; or specific immunotherapy in which patients are immunized with whole killed autologous and/or allogeneic leukemic blasts in an attempt to increase anti-leukemia protective immunity. Often both BCG and leukemic blasts are used, usually in a schedule combined with intermittent maintenance chemotherapy, using prolongation of duration of complete remission and length of survival as the criteria of effectiveness.

Initial experiments in mice with L1210 lymphatic leukemia, in which vaccination with BCG and irradiated leukemic blasts was done after initial reduction of tumor load with induction chemotherapy, showed that such immunotherapy could prolong survival of the leukemic mice (168). A similar study was undertaken in children with acute lymphoblastic leukemia (ALL), after initial induction of complete remission with chemotherapy (166). In the first human study, patients were treated with either no maintenance therapy, BCG alone, BCG plus irradiated allogeneic ALL blasts, or irradiated ALL blasts alone. All ten controls relapsed by 130 days, but of those thirty treated with any of the three immunotherapy protocols, only nine relapsed in the same period, and there were seven long term (over seven years) survivors (169). Mathé's group has used BCG and irradiated allogeneic ALL blasts in many subsequent immunotherapy trials, as well as testing some other nonspecific immunostimulants (165, 167). Each of these subsequent trails have also included maintenance chemotherapy, and have not had randomization of immunotherapy versus no immunotherapy, so that whether the improved remission durations and survivals reported in these studies are due to immunotherapy or due to improved maintenance chemotherapy is not completely clear (164).

A similar study of immunotherapy of childhood ALL in remission was done in England (171). After induction chemotherapy, patients were randomized to BCG, to methotrexate maintenance chemotherapy, or to no maintenance therapy. Results showed that BCG alone was not better than no maintenance therapy, but that methotrexate was better than either BCG alone or no therapy. Another study, by the Children's Cancer Research Study Group A in the United States, randomized childhood ALL patients, in remission after induction chemotherapy, to either BCG alone, chemotherapy (methotrexate, vincristine, and prednisone), or no maintenance therapy (118). Again chemotherapy was better than either of the other treatments, and BCG alone was no better than no treatment. These results were the same whether the patients were randomized soon after achieving complete remission, or were started on immunotherapy after eight months of chemotherapy-maintained remission. These studies using BCG alone comparing it to chemotherapy in the maintenance of remission in childhood ALL have not shown similar results to the initial study of Mathé. Whether this results from different BCG strains, preparations, or dosages, or to other factors is not clear. Only in the initial Mathé study has BCG alone been superior to maintenance chemotherapy in acute lymphocytic leukemia.

Nonspecific immunostimulation with BCG and specific immunization with allogeneic leukemic cells plus BCG have received further study. Elkert and Gutterman have independently reported no difference in remission duration in two groups of ALL patients maintained either with chemotherapy alone or maintenance chemotherapy plus BCG (66, 95). Leventhal has reported that the duration of remission between groups of ALL patients maintained either with allogeneic leukemic blasts plus BCG or allogeneic leukemic blasts plus methotrexate did not differ (155). A study of ALL patients by Guyer using a Bordetella pertussis vaccine as the immunostimulant in addition to maintenance chemotherapy demonstrated no improvement in remission duration when the immunostimulant was added to standard chemotherapy (97). These four studies indicate that remission duration is not statistically improved by either BCG (or, in the one case, B. pertussis) immunotherapy alone, or, BCG plus leukemic blast vaccination. That immunotherapy plus maintenance chemotherapy is better than maintenance chemotherapy alone was indicated by Mathé's work, but awaits further confirmation.

Generally, passive immunotherapy using immune serum has been ineffective in treating human tumors, including leukemia. In one single case, several of our HUNAT sera, with strong complement-dependent cytotoxic activity against the patient's ALL blasts, were used in a patient with early relapse. Three pints of such cytotoxic sera, obtained from the normal donors, were given during two days to the patient, with no apparent helpful effect against the progression of his leukemic relapse (Bias, Anderson, Mullins, Santos, unpublished observations).

Three patients with ALL were reported to have been treated with transfer factor extracted from lymphocytes of normal donors with demonstrable MIF reactivity to an antigen extract of ALL blasts, but no apparent benefit could be shown (157).

In acute myelogenous leukemia (AML), immunotherapeutic maneuvers in the attempt to prolong remission have shown somewhat more promise. In an initial study, reported by Crowther, patients induced into complete remission by chemotherapy were randomized to immunotherapy (allogeneic irradiated leukemic blasts alone, or blasts plus BCG, or BCG alone) or chemotherapy (6-mercaptopurine and methotrexate) (48). Patients receiving each of the maintenance protocols had approximately equivalent durations of remission. Further studies in Britain have indicated that immunotherapy with BCG and irradiated allogeneic leukemic blasts, when added to maintenance chemotherapy, did statistically increase remission duration and survival when compared to maintenance chemotherapy alone (196, 198, 201, 213). Vogler reported that short-term BCG immunotherapy at the beginning of maintenance chemotherapy improved remission duration when compared to chemotherapy alone (257). Vigorous prolonged repeated immunization with

BCG, combined with maintenance chemotherapy was also shown by Gutterman to prolong remission duration, compared to chemotherapy without immunotherapy (91, 95).

Current studies using MER (methanol extractable residue of BCG) as the immunostimulant also indicate that immunotherapy is efficacious in prolonging remission duration in AML (50, 262). Studies using nouraminidase treated allogeneic AML blasts as immunotherapy, showed that immunotherapy plus chemotherapy resulted in longer remission duration than maintenance chemotherapy alone (21). It has not yet been demonstrated that nonspecific immunotherapy with BCG alone provides better immunotherapy in AML than specific immunotherapy employing either allogeneic leukemic blasts alone, or blasts plus BCG, or, that specific is superior to non-specific immunotherapy. It does seem, however, that non-specific BCG immunotherapy, with or without specific tumor immunization, is of value in AML in prolonging duration of chemotherapy maintained remission and of survival, although questions about the statistical analysis of these studies persist (196).

In one study of chronic myelogenous leukemia the addition of BCG and allogeneic chronic myelocytic leukemia cells in an immunotherapy regimen did improve the five year survival rate from less than 40% in the control group to about 60% in the immunotherapy treated group (223).

Throughout a review of immunotherapy of leukemia, the relevance of the leukemia associated antigens and protective immune responses to them remains difficult to interpret. Demonstrable patient responses to autologous leukemic cells are seen, and in vitro immune responses to these cells may sometimes be increased after immunotherapy (90, 200). There is, however, no conclusive evidence to date that non-specific enhancement of general immunocompetence is not solely responsible for any benefit rendered the patient by immunotherapy. It is still equivocal whether or not any of the assays for antileukemia reactivity reflect protective immunity. Also not firmly established is whether the initial stimulus which resulted in a positive response in these assays was in fact a leukemia antigen in origin. Although in Hersh's studies, anti-leukemia reactivity in vitro seemed to correlate with duration of remission, it was not always directly related, and could not be used as a basis upon which to make clinical decisions (94, 116). Certainly patients who have demonstrable antileukemia response may relapse at the same time they have strong in vitro reactions (MLC, MIF, CRC) to their own leukemic blasts (Anderson and Schacter, unpublished results).

Gutterman has reported that remission patients who had mixed leucocyte culture reactivity against their own simultaneously aspirated presumably remission marrow had poor prognosis related to remission duration, in that a positive response predicted early relapse (92). This is interpreted as a demonstration that leukemia-antigen-bearing cells persisted in the marrow, even though it appeared on histologic examination to be a remission marrow. Persistence of enough leukemic blasts in the marrow to cause a proliferative immune response by peripheral lymphocytes was the earliest sign of relapse, which took place in face of the immune response to the leukemic cells. Obviously, our techniques for assay of antileukemia reactivity in humans is not adequate to tell us why or when remission patients will relapse.

One possibility, that suppressor T cells might inhibit effective antileukemia reactivity and thus cause relapse, is suggested by the viral murine sarcoma system, where progression of tumor is associated with T-suppressor cell inhibition of cellular immunity (115). It must be noted, however, that with the exception of Gutterman's studies of serum factor effect on MLC reaction to leukemic blasts, assays of cellular immunity tell very little about the clinical interaction of cellular and humoral antileukemic reactions (47, 90, 96). The role in vivo of blocking serum factors as described by the Hellstroms, or of T cell suppression as described by Gershon and Mitchell in affecting patient course is unknown (84, 181).

Very little is known about the relationship of immune factors to other serum factors affecting leukemia cell proliferation (41, 134). Preliminary data has been obtained to show that serum factors affecting the proliferation of normal granulocyte precursors are not cytotoxic antibodies (223). And to date, although some statistically (and biologically) significant prolongation in duration of remission and survival have been achieved by active immunotherapy, the goal (hypothetically achievable using immune killing of the "last leukemic blast") of increasing the number of long-term survivors has not yet been achieved.

It might be anticipated that the use of specific leukemia antigens as immunostimulants may improve immunotherapy and enhance survival. It may be, however, that shortage of antigen is not the major problem, as most patients seem to have adequate antigenic exposure, and responses to such antigens to suggest that they recognize and respond to leukemia antigens. In that case, immunotherapy which increases ability to handle or process antigen, increases the numbers of cytotoxic antileukemic cells or antibodies or decreases the number of inhibitory serum factors or suppressor lymphoid cells may be the important factor. These may be the bases for the efficacy of immunotherapy with BCG. Overcoming chemotherapy induced immunosuppression may also be an important effect of immunotherapy (153). To the end that antigenicity may help define etiology, leukemia-associated antigens may provide specific targets for therapy directed against specific etiologic agents (120).

Another concept for exploiting leukemia cell antigenicity in leukemia immunotherapy comes from the experience in adoptive immunotherapy using the technique of bone marrow transplantation for the treatment of acute leukemia (67, 218, 219). In identical bone marrow grafts, leukemia is killed by chemotherapy and radiotherapy, and the patient's marrow replaced by normal HLA identical twin marrow. Similarly, marrow from an HLA identical (non-twin) sibling in some cases can cause apparent cure when used to repopulate the leukemic marrow previously destroyed by high dose chemotherapy and 1000-rad total body radiotherapy.

Hypothetically, this should be the ideal immunotherapy model: minimal residual tumor in the recipient, usual evidence for immunologic reactions to specific leukemia associated antigens (in vitro) in the HLA identical normal donor, presumed low dose leukemic antigen stimulus to the newly acquired normal marrow-derived cells by the minimal residual leukemia, and demonstrable in vitro antileukemia reactions in the recipients after recovery, which resemble those pretransplant reactions of the donor.

The problems with this therapeutic maneuver include 1) limitation in our ability to reduce the tumor load sufficiently, resulting in recurrence of the original recipient leukemia, 2) difficulty in the clinical management of the high-dose cytoreductive therapy and its resulting aplasia, 3) prior sensitization and graft rejection by the patient, 4) graft-versus-host disease, and 5) depression of posttransplant immunocompetence. These problems also confuse the question of passive transfer of immune reactivity to leukemia associated antigens. Technical and clinical improvements are expected to improve the "cure rate" using this formidable mode of therapy, and may well provide the best example of the clinical manipulation of leukemia associated antigens. The recurrence in two cases of leukemia in donor cells suggest involvement of an infectious agent present in the recipient (hypothetically a virus) which resulted in infection and malignant transformation of two different marrows (donor and recipient, different sex markers) into leukemia (71, 246).

VIII. CONCLUSION

The problem of experimental controls has seriously hampered the interpretation of research data related to leukemia cell antigenicity. It will be difficult to demonstrate the absence of any antigen from all normal cells at all points in development and differentiation. The most rigorous testing is possible with the serological probes and no compelling evidence of absolute leukemia specificity has been generated with the available serological probes. Yet the overwhelming body of evidence indicates that there are immunologically detectable alterations of the surface of leukemic cells when compared to normal, peripheral blood elements, and that at least some patients have evidence of having mounted an immune response to such changes. That leukemia-associated antigens may be differentiation antigens anomalously expressed on leukemia cells may prove of greater therapeutic and conceptual significance than the demonstration of absolute specificity. Several of the antileukemia sera, however, have been shown to be operationally specific and thus may prove of great clinical use in the identification and monitoring of tumor load.

In vitro studies of the human response to leukemia antigens and pilot studies of the application of immunotherapy have suggested that leukemia-associated antigens are detectable not only in the lab but by the patient. What we are now presented with is the unglamorous task of the isolation, purification, and characterization of those detectable antigenic changes so that we may better perceive their significance in the etiology and biology of leukemia. Further, we can pursue the early promise of immunotherapy not only to provide an extra margin of safety for the patient, but also to better understand the interaction between the host and his neoplastic autograft.

ACKNOWLEDGMENT

The authors wish to acknowledge the support of their respective institutions during the preparation of this manuscript. Partial support for work performed by two of us (Bernice Schacter and Paul Anderson) was derived from funds awarded to Johns Hopkins University: NOICP-33337 of the Special Virus Cancer Program, NCI grant CA06973, and the American Cancer Society, Maryland Chapter #73-12, 74-38. The work of B.C.D. was supported in part by a grant from the Coyahoga County Unit of the American Cancer Society and from the Cancer Center, Inc., Cleveland, Ohio. The excellent secretarial work of Ms. Maxine Shankman must be acknowledged. We also wish to thank Drs. George Santos and Wilma Bias of the Johns Hopkins University, who provided encouragement to formulate the basic questions relative to human leukemia antigens.

ABBREVIATIONS

ALL   Acute lymphocytic leukemia
AML   Acute myelogenous leukemia
BCG   Bacillus calmette-guerin
BL   Burkitts' lymphoma
CLL   Chronic lymphocytic leukemia
CML (CGL)   Chronic myelogeneous (granulocytic) leukemia
CRC   51-Chromium release cytotoxicity

EBV   Epstein-Barr virus
GALV   Gibbon ape leukemia virus
HLA   Human leukocyte antigen, marker for the major human histocompatibility complex
HSV   Herpes simplex virus
IM   Infectious mononucleosis
LAA   Leukemia-associated antigens
LSA   Leukemia-specific antigens
MIF   Migration inhibition factor

MLC   Mixed lymphocyte culture   SSV-1   Simian sarcoma virus
MuLV   Murine leukemia virus   TL   Thymus leukemia

REFERENCES

1. Aisenberg, A. C., and Bloch, K. J. 1972. Immunoglobulins on the surface of neoplastic lymphocytes. N. Engl. J. Med. 287: 272–276.

2. Aisenberg, A. C., Bloch, K. J., Long, J. C., and Colvin, R. B. 1973. Reaction of normal human lymphocytes and chronic lymphocytic leukemia cells with an antithymocyte antiserum. Blood 41: 417–423.

3. Anderson, P. N., Bias, W. B., and Santos, G. W. 1973. Mixed leucocyte culture responses of HL-A identical siblings to leukemia blasts. Proc. Amer. Assoc. Cancer Res. 14: 40.

4. Anderson, P. N., Klein, D. L., Bias, W. B., Mullins, S. M., Burke, P. J., and Santos, G. W. 1974. Cell-mediated immunological reactivity of patients and siblings to blasts from acute adult leukemia. Israel J. Med. Sci. 10: 1033–1051.

5. Anderson, P. N., and Santos, G. W. 1975. Macrophage migration inhibition factor (MIF) production in response to human leukemia associated antigens (LAA). Proc. Amer. Assoc. Cancer Res. 16: 149.

6. Aoki, T., Liu, M., Walling, M. J., Buchar, G. S., and Brandchaft, P. B. 1976. Specificity of a naturally occurring antibody in normal gibbon serum. Science 191: 1180–1183.

7. Aoki, T., Walling, M. J., Buchar, G. S., Liu, M., and Hsu, K. C. 1976. Natural antibodies in sera from healthy humans to antigens on surfaces of type C RNA viruses and cells from primates. Proc. Natl. Acad. Sci. 73: 2491–2495.

8. Aurelian, L., and Strand, B. C. 1976. Herpes virus type 2-related antigens and their relevance to humoral and cell mediated immunity in patients with cervical cancer. Cancer Res. 36: 810–820.

9. Bach, F. H., and vanRood, J. J. 1976. The major histocompatibility complex genetics and biology, first part. N. Engl. J. Med. 295: 806–813.

10. ibid., second part. N. Engl. J. Med. 295: 872–878.

11. ibid, third part. N. Engl. J. Med. 295: 927–936.

12. Bach, M. L., Bach, F. H., and Joo, P. 1969. Leukemia associated antigens in the mixed leukocyte culture test. Science 166: 1520–1522.

13. Baker, M. A., and Taub, R. N. 1973. Production of antiserum in mice to human leukemia associated antigens. Nature New Biology 241: 93–94.

14. Baker, M. A., Taub, R. N., Brown, S. M., and Ramachandar, K. 1974. Delayed cutaneous hypersensitivity in leukaemic patients to autologous blast cells. Brit. J. Haematol. 27: 627–634.

15. Batchelor, J. R., Edwards, J. H., and Stuart, J. 1971. Histocompatibility and acute lymphoblastic leukaemia. Lancet: 1: 699.

16. Bates, H. A., Bankole, R. O., and Swaim, W. 1969. Immunofluorescent studies in human leukemia. Blood 34: 430–440.

17. Baxt, W., Hehlmann, R., and Spiegelman, S. 1972. Human leukaemic cells contain reverse transcriptase associated with a high molecular weight virus-related RNA. Nature New Biology 240: 72–75.

18. Baxt, W. G., and Spiegelman, S. 1972. Nuclear DNA sequences present in human leukemic cells and absent in normal leukocytes. *Proc. Natl. Acad. Sci.* 69: 3737–3741.

19. Baxt, W., Yates, J. W., Wallace, H. J., Jr., Holland, J. F., and Spiegelman, S. 1972. Leukemia-specific DNA sequences in leukocytes of the leukemic member of identical twins. *Proc. Natl. Acad. Sci.* 70: 2629–2632.

20. Bean, M. A., Bloom, B. R., Herberman, R. B., Old, L. J., Oettgen, H. F., Klein, G., and Terry, W. D. 1975. Cell mediated cytotoxicity for bladder carcinoma: evaluation of a workshop. *Cancer Res.* 35: 2902–2913.

21. Bekesi, J. G., Roboz, J. P., and Holland, J. F. 1976. Therapeutic effectiveness of neuraminidase-treated tumor cells as immunogen in man and experimental animals with leukemia. *Ann. N.Y. Acad. Sci.* 277: 313–331.

22. Ben-Bassat, H., Goldblum, N., Manny, N., and Sachs, L. 1974. Mobility of conconavalin A receptors on the surface membrane of lymphocytes from normal persons and patients with chronic lymphocytic leukemia. *Int. J. Cancer* 14: 367–371.

23. Benbunan, M., Saglier, M., Owens, A., Husson, N., Bussel, A., Reboul, M., Dastot, H., and Czazar, E. 1976. Acute myelocytic leukemia (AML), chronic myeloid leukemia and HLA antigens. *Proceedings of First Int. Symp. on HLA and Disease,* INSERM, Paris, 217.

24. Bentwich, Z., Weiss, D. W., Sulitzeanu, D., Kodar, E., Izak, G., Cohen, I., and Eyal, O. 1972. Antigenic changes on the surface of lymphocytes from patients with chronic lymphocytic leukemia. *Cancer Res.* 32: 1375–1383.

25. Bentwich, Z., and Kunkel, H. G. 1973. Specific properties of human B and T lymphocytes and alterations in disease. *Transplant. Rev.* 16: 29–50.

26. Bernoco, D., Glade, P. R., Broder, S., Miggiano, I., Hirschhorn, K., and Ceppellini, R. 1969. Stability of HL-A and appearance of other antigens (Iiva) at the surface of lymphoblasts grown *in vitro. Hematologica* 54: 795–812.

27. Bertoglio, J., Dore, J., and Souillet, G. 1976. Leukaemia-associated antigens and related antibodies in the family of a lymphoma patient. *Lancet* 2: 204–205.

28. Bias, W. B., Santos, G. W., Burke, P. J., Mullins, G. M., and Humphrey, R. L. 1973. Normal human sera with cytotoxic reactivity to acute lymphocytic leukemia cells. *Transplant. Proc.* 5: 949–952.

29. Bias, W. B., Santos, G. W., Burke, P. J., Mullins, G. M., and Humphrey, R. L. 1972. Cytotoxic antibody in normal human serums reactive with tumor cells from acute lymphocytic leukemia. *Science* 178: 304–306.

30. Bilello, J. A., Strand, M., and August, J. T. 1974. Murine sarcoma virus gene expression: transformants which express viral envelope glycoprotein in the absence of the major internal protein and infectious particles. *Proc. Natl. Acad. Sci.* 71: 3234–3238.

31. Billing, R., Rafizadeh, B., Drew, I., Hartman, G., Gale, R., and Terasaki, P. 1976. Human B-lymphocyte antigens expressed by lymphocytic and myelocytic leukemia cells. I. Detection by rabbit antisera. *J. Exp. Med.* 144: 167–178.

32. Billing, R., and Terasaki, P. 1974. Human leukemia antigen production and characterization of antisera. *J. Natl. Cancer Inst.* 53: 1635–1638.

33. Billing, R., and Terasaki, P. 1974. Human leukemia antigen II. Purification. *J. Natl. Cancer Inst.* 53: 1639–1643.

34. Billing, R., Ting, A., and Terasaki, P. 1976. Expression of human B lymphocyte antigens by most lymphocytic and myelocytic leukemia cells. In: M. Stevenson and A. Brzytwa (eds.), *Abstracts of Sixth International Congress of the Transplantation Society*, p. 63. Grune and Stratton, N.Y.

35. Boyse, E. A, Old, L. J., and Stockert, E. 1965. The TL (Thymus Leukemia) antigen: a review. In: P. Grabeek and P. A. Miescher (eds.), *Immunopathology IV International Symposium*, p. 23–40. Schwabe and Co., Basel.

36. Boyse, E. A., Old, L. J., and Stockert, E. 1972. The relation of linkage group IX to leukemogenesis in the mouse, In P. Emmelot and P. Bentvelzens (eds.), *RNA Viruses and Host Genome in Oncogenesis.* pp. 171–185. North Holland Publishing Co., Amsterdam and London.

37. Brouet, J. C., Valensi, F., Daniel, M. T., Flandrin, G., Preud'homme, J. L., and Seligman, M. 1976. Immunological classification of acute lymphoblastic leukaemias: evaluation of its clinical significance in a hundred patients. *Brit. J. Haematol.* 33: 319–328.

38. Brown, G., Capellaro, D., and Greaves, M. 1975. Leukemia-associated antigens in man. *J. Natl. Cancer Inst.* 55: 1281–1289.

39. Brown, G., Hogg, N., and Greaves, M. 1975. Candidate leukemia-specific antigen in man. *Nature* 258: 454–456.

40. Bryan, J. H., Johnson, G. E., and Leventhal, B. G. 1974. The effect of autologous serum on lymphocyte response to human leukemia cells. *Blood* 43: 781–787.

41. Burke, P. J., Diggs, C. D., and Owens, Jr., A. H. 1973. Factors in human serum affecting the proliferation of normal and leukemic cells. *Cancer Res.* 33: 800–806.

42. Char, D. H., Lepouheit, A., Leventhal, B. G., and Herberman, R. B. 1973. Cutaneous delayed hypersensitivity response to tumor-associated and other antigens in acute leukemia. *Int. J. Cancer* 12: 409–419.

43. Chattapadhyay, S. K., Rowe, W. P., Teich, N. M., and Lowry, D. R. 1975. Definitive evidence that the murine C-type virus including locus AKV-1 is viral genetic material. *Proc. Natl. Acad. Sci.* 72: 906–910.

44. Chechik, B. E., and Gelfand, E. W. 1976. Leukaemia-associated antigen in serum of patients with acute lymphoblastic leukaemia. *Lancet* 1: 166–168.

45. Coggin, Jr., J. H., and Anderson, N. G. 1974. Cancer differentiation and embryonic antigens: some central problems. *Adv. Cancer Res.* 19: 106–165.

46. Cooper, N. R., Jensen, F. C., Welsh, R. M., and Oldstone, M. B. A. 1976. Lysis of RNA tumor viruses by human serum: direct antibody-independent triggering of the classical complement pathway. *J. Exp. Med.* 144: 970.

47. Cotropia, J. P., Gutterman, J. Y., Hersh, E. M., Granatek, C. H., and Mavligit, G. 1976. Antigen expression and cell surface properties of human leukemic blasts. *Ann. N.Y. Acad. Sci.* 276: 146–164.

48. Crowther, D., Powles, R. L., Bateman, C. J. T., Beard, M. E. J., Cauci, C. J., Wrigley, P. F. M., Malpas, J. S., Hamilton-Fairley, G., and Scott, R. B. 1973. Management of adult acute myelogenous leukaemia. *Brit. Med. J.* 1: 131–137.

49. Cullen, P. R., and Mason, D. Y. 1974. Leukaemia-associated antigens in man. Clin. Exp. Immunol. 17: 571–586.

50. Cuttner, J., Holland, J. F., Bekesi, J. G., Ramachandar, K., and Donovan, P. 1975. Chemoimmunotherapy of acute myelocytic leukemia. Proc. Amer. Assn. Cancer Res. 16: 264.

51. Davey, F. R., Henry, J. B., and Gottlieb, A. J. 1973. HL-A antigens in lymphatic leukaemia. Lancet 2: 802.

52. DeCarvalho, S. 1960. Segregation of antigens from human leukemic and tumoral cells by fluorocarbon extraction. J. Lab. Clin. Investigation 56: 333–341.

53. DeCarvalho, S. 1964. Identity of reaction of an autologous antibody in leukemic children in remission with a heterologous antibody produced with leukemic antigens. Proc. Amer. Assoc. Cancer Res. p. 114.

54. Defendi, V. H. Relationship between biochemical and immunological changes, in Peter T. Mora (ed.), Cell Surfaces and Malignancy, Fogarty International Center Proceedings, No. 24, DHEW Pub. No. NIH 75-796, pp. 229–240.

55. Degos, L., Drolet, Y., and Dausset, J. 1971. HL-A antigens in chronic myeloid leukemia (CML) and chronic lymphoid leukemia (CLL). Transplant. Proc. 3: 1309–1310.

56. DelVillano, B. C., and Lerner, R. A. 1976. Relationship between the oncornavirus gene product gp70 and a major protein secretion of the mouse genital tract. Nature (London) 259: 497–499.

57. DelVillano, B. C., Nave, B., Croker, B. P., Lerner, R. A., and Dixon, F. J. 1975. The oncornavirus glycoprotein gp 69/71: a constituent of the surface of normal and malignant thymocytes. J. Exp. Med. 141: 172–187.

58. DelVillano, B. C., Nave, B., and Lerner, R. A. 1975. Oncornavirus genes and host proteins. Bibl. Haematol. 43: 109–114.

59. deSchryver, A., Klein, G., Henle, W., and Henle, G. 1974. EB virus-associated antibodies in caucasian patients with carcinoma of the nasopharynx and in long term survivors after treatment. Int. J. Cancer 13: 319–325.

60. deSchryver, A., Rosen, A., Gonven, P., and Klein, G. 1976. Comparison between two antibody populations in the EBV system: anti-MA versus neutralizing antibody activity. Int. J. Cancer 17: 8–13.

61. Dick, F. R., Fortuny, I., Theologides, A., Greally, J., Wood, N., and Yunis, E. J. HL-A and lymphoid tumors. Cancer Res. 32: 2608–2611.

62. Dick, H. M., Steel, C. M., and Crichton, W. B. 1972. HL-A typing of cultured peripheral lymphoblastoid cells. Tissue Antigens 2: 85–93.

63. Doré, J. F., Motta, R., Marholev, L., Hrsak, I., Colas De la Noue, H., Seman, G., deVassal, F., and Mathé, G. New antigens in human leukaemic cells and antibody in the serum of leukaemic patients. Lancet 2: 1396–1398.

64. Dreesman, G. R., Brill, D. L., Fernbach, D. J., and Benyesh-Melnick, M. 1973. Cytotoxic antibody to autologous lymphocytes in childhood leukemia. Proc. Amer. Assoc. Cancer Res. 14: 85.

65. Dumble, L., Jack, I., and Morris, P. J. 1974. Serological studies of HL-A on continuous lymphoblastoid cell lines (CLC) and the definition of an antigen of CLC determined by a heat-liable antibody. Clin. Exp. Immunol. 16: 441–454.

66. Ekert, H., Jose, D. G., Wilson, F. C., Mathews, R. N., and Lay, H. 1975. Intermittent chemotherapy and immunotherapy with BCG in remission mainte-

nance of children with acute lymphocytic leukemia: effects on immunological function. *Int. J. Cancer* 16: 103–112.

67. Epstein, M. A., and Achong, B. G. 1973. Various forms of Epstein-Barr virus infection in man: established facts and a general concept. *Lancet* 2: 836–839.

68. Evans, C. A., and Pegrum, G. D. 1973. The reactivity of leukaemic cells to HL-A typing sera. *Tissue Antigens* 3: 454–464.

69. Fefer, A., Thomas, E. D., Buckner, C. D., Cheeves, M. A., Clift, R. A., Einstein, Jr., A. B., Neiman, P. E., Storb, R., and Weiden, P. L. 1976. Marrow transplantation for acute leukemia in man. *Ann. N.Y. Acad. Sci.* 277: 52–59.

70. Fez, G., and Hirt, B. 1974. Fingerprints of polyoma virus proteins and mouse histone. *Cold Spring Harbor Symposium on Quantitative Biology* 39: 235–241.

71. Fialkow, P. J., Thomas, E. D., Bryant, J. I., and Neiman, P. E. 1971. Leukaemic transformation of engrafted human bone marrow cells *in vivo*. *Lancet* 1: 251–252.

72. Fink, M. A., Karon, M., Rauscher, F. J., Malgrem, R. A., and Orr, H. C. 1965. Further observations on the immunofluorescence of cells in human leukemia. *Cancer Res.* 18: 1317–1321.

73. Fink, M. A., Malgren, R. A., Rauscher, F. J., Orr, H. C., and Karon, M. 1964. Applications of immunofluorescence to the study of human leukemia. *J. Natl. Cancer Inst.* 33: 581–588.

74. Finke, J. A., Ponzio, N. M., and Battisto, J. R. 1976. Isogeneic and allogeneic lymphocyte interactions may be controlled by cell surface immunoglobulin tropism. *Cell. Immunol.* 26: 284–294.

75. Fridman, W. H., and Kourilsky, F. M. 1969. Stimulation of lymphocytes by autologous leukaemic cells in acute leukaemia. *Nature (London)* 224: 277–279.

76. Froland, S. S., and Nativg, J. B. 1973. Identification of three different human lymphocyte populations by surface markers. *Transplant. Rev.* 16: 114–162.

77. Fu, S. M., Winchester, R. J., and Kinkel, H. G. 1975. The occurrence of the HL-B alloantigens on the cells of unclassified acute lymphoblastic leukemias. *J. Exp. Med.* 142: 1334–1337.

78. Gaji-Peczalski, K. J., Bloomfield, C. D., Nesbit, M. E., and Kersey, J. H. 1974. B-cell markers on lymphoblasts in acute lymphoblastic leukaemia. *Clin. Exp. Immunol.* 17: 561–569.

79. Gallagher, R. E., and Gallo, R. C. 1975. Type C RNA tumor virus isolated from cultured human acute myelogenous leukemia cells. *Science* 187: 350–353.

80. Gallagher, R. E., Mondal, H., Miller, D. P., Todaro, D. H., Gillispie, D. H., and Gallo, R. C. 1974. Relatedness of RNA and reverse transcriptase from human acute myelogenous leukemia cells and from RNA tumor viruses, in R. Neth, R. C. Gallo, S. Spiegelmann, and F. Stohlman, Jr. (eds.), *Modern Trends in Human Leukemia*, pp. 185–196. Grune and Stratton, New York.

81. Gallagher, R. E., Todaro, G. J., Smith, R. G., Livingston, D. M., and Gallo, R. C. 1974. Relationship between RNA directed DNA polymerase (reverse transcriptase) from human acute leukemic blood cells and primate Type-C viruses. *Proc. Natl. Acad. Sci.* 71: 1309–1313.

82. Gallo, R. C., Miller, N. R., Saxinger, W. C., and Gillispie, D. 1973. Primate

RNA tumor virus-like DNA synthesized endogenously by RNA-dependent DNA polymerase in virus-like particles from fresh human acute leukemic blood cells. *Proc. Natl. Acad. Sci.* 70: 3219–3224.

83. Garb, S., Stein, A. A., and Sims, G. 1962. The production of anti-human leukemic serum in rabbits. *J. Immunol.* 88: 142–152.

84. Gershon, P. K., Mokyr, M. B., and Mitchell, M. S. 1974. Activation of suppressor T cells by tumor cells and specific antibody. *Nature* 250: 594–596.

85. Gluckman, E., Lemarchand, F., Nunez-Roldan, A., Hors, J., and Dausset, J. 1976. Possible excess of HLA-A homozygous among aplastic anemia and acute lymphoblastic leukemia (ALL), *Proceedings of International Congress on HLA and Disease*, INSERM, Paris, 226.

86. Golde, D. W., and Cline, M. J. 1973. Human pre-leukemia: identification of a maturation defect *in vitro. N. Engl. J. Med.* 288: 1083–1086.

87. Greaves, M. F., Brown, G., Rapson, N. T., and Lister, T. A. 1975. Antisera to acute lymphoblastic leukemia cells. *Clin. Immunol. Immunopath.* 4: 67–84.

88. Greene, W. H., Schimpff, S. C., and Wiernick, P. H. 1974. Cell-mediated immunity in acute non-lymphocytic leukemia: relationship to host factors, therapy and prognosis. *Blood* 43: 1–14.

89. Greenspan, I., Brown, E. R., and Schwartz, S. O. 1963. Immunologically specific antigens in leukemic tissues. *Blood* 21: 717–728.

90. Gutterman, J. U., Hersh, E. M., Mavligit, G. M., Freireich, E. J., Rossen, R. D., Butler, W. T., McCredie, K. B., Bodey, G. P., Sr., and Rodriguez, V. 1973. Cell-mediated and humoral immune response to acute leukemia cells and soluble leukemia antigen—relationship to immunocompetence and prognosis. *Natl. Cancer Inst. Monogr.* 37: 153–165.

91. Gutterman, J. U., Mavligit, G. M., Burgess, M. A., Cardenas, J. O., Blumenschein, G. R., Gottleib, J. A., McBride, C. M., McCredie, K. B., Bodey, G. P., Rodriguez, V., Freireich, E. J., and Hersh, E. M. 1976. Immunotherapy of breast cancer, malignant melanoma, and acute leukemia with BCG: prolongation of disease free interval and survival. *Cancer Immunol. Immunother.* 1: 99–107.

92. Gutterman, J. U., Mavligit, G., Burgess, M. A., McCredie, K. B., Hunter, C., Freireich, E. J., and Hersh, E. M. 1974. Immunodiagnosis of acute leukemia: detection of residual disease. *J. Natl. Cancer Inst.* 53: 389–392.

93. Gutterman, J. U., Mavligit, G., McCredie, K. B., Bodey, Sr., G. P., Freireich, E. J., and Hersh, E. M. 1972. Antigen solubilized from human leukemia: lymphocyte stimulation. *Science* 177: 1114–1115.

94. Gutterman, J. U., Mavligit, G., Rossen, R., Butler, W. T., McBride, C. M., McCredie, K. B., Freireich, E. J., and Hersh, E. M. 1975. Tumor immunity in human acute leukemia and solid tumors: a multifaceted study of cell-mediated and humoral response to autologous tumor cells and soluble tumor antigen and the correlation with prognosis, in *Immunological Aspects of Neoplasia*. Williams and Wilkins Co., Baltimore. p. 343–365.

95. Gutterman, J. Y., Rodriguez, V., Mavligit, G., Burgess, M. A., Gehan, E., Hersh, E. M., McCredie, K. B., Reed, R., Smith, T., Bodey, Sr., G. P., and Freireich, E. J. 1974. Chemoimmunotherapy of adult acute leukaemia. Prolongation of remission in myeloblastic leukaemia with BCG. *Lancet* 2: 1405–1409.

96. Gutterman, J. U., Rossen, R. D., Butler, W. T., McCredie, K. B., Bodey, G.

P., Freireich, E. J., and Hersh, E. M. 1973. Immunoglobulin on tumor cells and tumor-induced lymphocyte blastogenesis in human acute leukemia. *N. Engl. J. Med.* 288: 169–172.

97. Guyer, R. J., and Crowther, D. 1969. Active immunotherapy in treatment of acute leukaemia. *Brit. Med. J.* 406–407.

98. Haegert, D. G., Cawley, J. C., Karpas, A., and Goldstone, A. H. 1974. Combined T and B cell acute lymphoblastic leukaemia. *Brit. Med. J.* 4: 79–82.

99. Halterman, R. H., and Leventhal, B. G. 1971. Enhanced immune response to leukemia. *Lancet* 2: 704.

100. Halterman, R. H., and Leventhal, B. G. 1972. Mixed leucocyte culture (MLC) reactivity to leukemic cells in patients, their twins and HL-A identical siblings. *Proc. Am. Assoc. Cancer Res.* 13: 6.

101. Halterman, R., Leventhal, B. G., and Mann, D. L. 1972. An acute leukemia antigen: correlation with clinical status. *N. Engl. J. Med.* 287: 1272–1274.

102. Han, T., and Wang, J. 1972. 'Antigenic' disparity between leukaemic lymphoblasts and normal lymphocytes in identical twins. *Clin. Exp. Immunol.* 12: 171–175.

103. Hanna, M. G., Ihle, J. N., and Lee, J. C. 1976. Autogenous immunity to endogenous RNA tumor virus: humoral immune response to virus envelope antigens. *Cancer Research* 36: 608–614.

104. Harris, R. 1973. Leukemia antigens and immunity in man. *Nature* 241: 95–100.

105. Hehlmann, R., Kufe, D., and Spiegelman, S. 1972. RNA in human leukemic cells related to the RNA of a mouse leukemia virus. *Proc. Natl. Acad. Sci.* 69: 435–439.

106. Heiniger, H., Chen, H. W., Applegate, Jr., O. L., Schacter, L. P., Schacter, B. Z., and Anderson, P. N. 1976. Elevated synthesis of cholesterol in human leukemic cells. *J. Molec. Med.* 1: 109–116.

107. Hellstrom, I., and Hellstrom, K. E. 1974. Cell-mediated immune reactions to tumor antigens with particular emphasis on immunity to human neoplasms. *Cancer* 34, No. 4 (supplement), 1461–1468.

108. Henle, G., Henle, W., and Horwitz, C. A. 1974. Antibodies to Epstein-Barr virus-associated nuclear antigen in infectious mononucleosis. *J. Inf. Dis.* 130: 231–239.

109. Henle, G., Henle, W., and Klein, G. 1971. Demonstration of two distinct components of the early complex of Epstein-Barr virus infected cells. *Int. J. Cancer* 8: 272–282.

110. Henle, W., Ho, H. C., Henle, G., and Kwan, H. C. 1973. Antibodies to Epstein-Barr virus related antigens in nasopharyngeal carcinoma. Comparison of active cases with long term survivors. *J. Natl. Cancer Inst.* 51: 361–369.

111. Herberman, R. B. 1973. *In vivo* and *in vitro* assays of cellular immunity to human tumor antigens. *Fed. Proc.* 32: 160–164.

112. Herberman, R. B. 1973. Cellular immunity to human tumor-associated antigens. *Israel J. Med. Sci.* 9: 300–307.

113. Herberman, R. B. 1974. Cellular immune reactions in human acute leukemia, in R. Barth, R. C. Gallo, S. Spiegelman, and F. Stohlman, Jr. (eds.), *Modern Trends in Human Leukemia*, Grune and Stratton, Inc. New York.

114. Herberman, R. B., Holden, H. T., Ting, C. C., Lavrin, D. L., and Kirchner, H. 1976. Cell-mediated immunity to leukemia virus- and tumor-associated antigens in mice. *Cancer Res.* 36: 615–621.

115. Herberman, R. B., Kirchner, H., Holden, H. T., Glaser, M., Haskill, S., and Bonnard, G. D. 1976. Cell-mediated immunity in murine virus tumor systems, in R. L. Crowell, H. Friedman, and J. E. Prier (eds.), *Tumor Virus Infections and Immunity*, Univ. Park Press, Baltimore, pp. 147–164.

116. Hersh, E. M., Gutterman, J. U., Mavligit, G., McCredie, K. B., Burgess, M. A., Mathews, A., and Freireich, E. J. 1974. Serial studies of immunocompetence of patients undergoing chemotherapy for acute leukemia. *J. Clin. Invest.* 54: 401–408.

117. Hersh, E. M., Whitecar, J. P., McCredie, K. B., Bodey, G. P., and Freireich, E. J. 1971. Chemotherapy, immunocompetence, immunosuppression, and prognosis in acute leukemia. *N. Engl. J. Med.* 285: 1211–1216.

118. Heyn, R. M., Joo, P., Karon, M., Nesbit, M., Shore, N., Breslow, N., Weiner, J., Reid, A., and Hammond, D. 1975. BCG in the treatment of acute lymphatic leukemia. *Blood* 46: 431–442.

119. Hilberg, R. W., Balcerzak, S. P., and LoBuglio, A. F. 1973. A migration inhibition-factor assay for tumor immunity in man. *Cell Immunol.* 7: 152–158.

120. Hilleman, M. R. 1974. Human cancer virus vaccines, and the pursuit of the practical. *Cancer* 34, No. 4 (supplement), 1439–1445.

121. Hino, S., Stephenson, J. R., and Aaronson, S. A. 1976. Radioimmunoassays for the 70,000 molecular weight glycoproteins of the endogenous mouse type C viruses: viral antigen expression in normal mouse tissues and sera. *J. Virol.* 18: 933–941.

122. Hirata, A. A., and Terasaki, P. I. 1970. Cross-reactions between streptoccal M-proteins and human transplantation antigens. *Science* 168: 1095–1096.

123. Hirsch, M. E., Kelley, A. P., Proffitt, M. R., and Black. P. H. 1975. Cell-mediated immunity to antigens associated with endogenous murine C-type leukemia viruses. *Science* 187: 959–961.

124. Hollinshead, A. C., Chretien, P. B., Lee, O., Tarpley, J. L., Kerney, S., Silverman, N. A., and Alexander, J. C. 1976. *In vivo* and *in vitro* measurements of the relationship of human squamous carcinomas to herpes simplex virus tumor associated antigens. *Cancer Res.* 36: 821–828.

125. Huebner, R. J., Kelloff, G. J., Sarma, P. S., Lane, W. T., Turner, A. C., Gildm, R. V., Oroszlan, S., Merer, H., Myers, D. B., and Peters, R. L. 1970. Group specific antigen expression during embryogenesis of the genome of the C-type RNA tumor virus: implications for ontogenesis and oncogenesis. *Proc. Natl. Acad. Sci.* 67: 366–376.

126. Huebner, R. J., and Todaro, G. J. 1969. Oncogenes of RNA tumor viruses as determinants of cancer. *Proc. Natl. Acad. Sci.* 64: 1087.

127. Hyde, R. M., Garb, S., and Bennett, A. J. 1967. Demonstration by immunoelectrophoresis of antigen in human myelogenous leukemia. *J. Natl. Cancer Inst.* 38: 909–919.

128. Ionnides, A. K., Rosner, F., Brenner, G., and Lee, S. L. 1968. Immunofluorescent studies of human leukemic cells with antiserum to a murine leukemic virus (Rauscher strain). *Blood* 31: 381–387.

129. Janossy, G., Roberts, M., and Greaves, M. F. 1976. Target cells in chronic myeloid leukaemia and its relationship to acute lymphoid leukemia. *Lancet* 2: 1058–1060.

130. Jeannet, M., and Magnin, C. 1971. HL-A antigens in malignant diseases. *Transplant Proc.* 3: 1301–1303.

131. Jeannet, M., and Magnin, C. 1971. HL-A antigens in haematological malignant diseases. *Eur. J. Clin. Invest.* 2: 39–42.

132. Johnson, A. H., Ward, F. E., Amos, D. B., Leikin, S, and Rogentine, N. 1976. HLA and acute lymphocytic leukemia. *Proceedings of 1st International Symposium on HLA and Disease*, INSERM, Paris, 227.

133. Jondal, M., Wigzell, H., and Aiuti, F. 1973. Human lymphocyte subpopulations: classification according to surface markers and/or functional characteristics. *Transplant. Rev.* 16: 163–195.

134. Karp, J. E., and Burke, P. J. 1976. Influence of humoral regulators on proliferation and maturation of normal and leukemic cells. *Cancer Res.* 36: 1674–1679.

135. Kassalke, J. T., Stutman, O., and Yunis, E. J. 1971. Blood group isoantigens in leukemic cells: reversibility of isoantigenic changes by neuraminidase. *J. Natl. Cancer Inst.* 46: 1201–1208.

136. Kennel, S. J., DelVillano, B. C., Levy, R. L., and Lerner, R. A. 1973. Properties of an oncornavirus glycoprotein: evidence for its presence on the surface of virim and infected cells. *Virology* 55: 464–475.

137. Kennel, S. J., and Feldman, J. D. 1976. Distribution of viral glycoprotein gp 69/71 on cell surfaces of producer and non-producer cells. *Cancer Res.* 36: 200–208.

138. Klein, D. L., Anderson, P. N., and Santos, G. W. 1975. Lymphocyte cytotoxicity to leukemic blast cells by normal individuals. *Proc. Amer. Assoc. Cancer Res.* 16: 149.

139. Klein, G. 1975. Epstein-Barr virus and neoplasia. *N. Engl. J. Med.* 293: 1353–1357.

140. Klein, G., Clifford, P., and Klein, E. 1967. Membrane immunofluorescence reactions of Burkitts' lymphoma cells from biopsy specimens and tissue culture. *J. Natl. Cancer Inst.* 39: 1027–1044.

141. Klein, G., Pearson, G., Henle, G., Henle, W., Diehl, V., and Niederman, J. C. 1968. II. Comparison of cells and sera from patients with Burkitts' lymphoma and infectious mononucleosis. *J. Exp. Med.* 128: 1021–1030.

142. Klein, G., Pearson, G., Henle, G., Henle, W., Goldstein, G., and Clifford, P. 1969. III. Comparison of blocking of direct membrane immunofluorescence and anti-EBV reactivities of different sera. *J. Exp. Med.* 129: 697–705.

143. Klein, G., Pearson, G., Nadkarni, J. S., Nadkarni, J. J., Klein, E., Henle, G., Henle, W., and Clifford, P. 1969. Relation between Epstein-Barr viral and cell membrane immunofluorescence in Burkitt tumor cells. I. Dependence of cell membrane immunofluorescence on presence of EBV virus. *J. Exp. Med.* 128: 1011–1020.

144. Klein, G., Svedmyr, E., Jondal, M., and Person, P. O. 1976. EBV-determined nuclear antigen (EBNA)—positive cells in the peripheral blood of infectious mononucleosis patients. *Int. J. Cancer* 17: 21–26.

145. Klouda, P. T., Lawler, S. D., Till, M. M., and Hardisty, R. M. 1974. Acute lymphoblastic leukaemia and HL-A: a prospective study. *Tissue Antigens* 4: 262–265.

146. Kourilsky, F. M., Dausset, J., and Bernard, J. 1968. A qualitative study of normal leukocyte antigens of human leukemic leukoblasts. *Cancer Res.* 28: 372–377.

147. Kourilsky, F. M., Daussct, J., Feingold, N., Dupuy, J. M., and Bernard, J. 1968. Leukocyte groups and acute leukemia. *J. Natl. Cancer Inst.* 41: 81–87.

148. Korngold, L., Van Leeuwen, G., and Miller, D. G. 1961. The antigens of human leukocytes II. The specificity of leukocyte antigens. *J. Natl. Cancer Inst.* 26: 557–567.

149. Kuntz, M. M., Innes, J. B., and Weksler, M. E. 1976. Lymphocyte transformation induced by autologous cells. *J. Exp. Med.* 143: 1042–1054.

150. Lapin, B. A., Yakovleva, L. A., Indzhlla, L. V., Agrba, V. Z., Tsiripova, G. S., Voevodia, A. F., Ivanov, M. T., and Diatcheuko, A. G. 1975. Transmission of human leukaemia to non-human primates. *Proc. Roy. Soc. Med.* 68: 141–145.

151. Lawler, S. D., Klouda, P. T., Smith, P. G., Till, M. M., and Hardisty, R. M. 1974. Survival and the HL-A system in acute lymphoblastic leukaemia. *Brit. Med. J.* 1: 547–548.

152. Lerner, R. A., Wilson, C. B., DelVillano, B. C., McConahey, P. J., and Dixon, F. J. 1976. Endogenous oncornaviral gene expression in adult and fetal mice: quantitative, histologic, and physiologic studies of the major viral glycoprotein gp70. *J. Exp. Med.* 143: 151–166.

153. Leventhal, B. G., Cohen, P., and Triem, S. C. 1974. Effect of chemotherapy on the immune response in acute leukemia.

154. Leventhal, B. G., Halterman, R. H., Rosenberg, E. B., and Herberman, R. B. 1972. Immune reactivity of leukemia patients to autologous blast cells. *Cancer Res.* 32: 1820–1825.

155. Leventhal, B. G., LePourheit, A., Halterman, R. H., Henderson, E., and Herberman, R. B. 1973. Immunotherapy in previously treated acute lymphatic leukemia. *Natl. Cancer Inst. Monogr.* 39: 177–187.

156. Levine, P. H., Herberman, R. B., Rosenberg, E. B., McClure, P. D., Roland, R., Peinta, R. J., and Ting, R. C. Y. 1972. Acute leukemia in identical twins: search for viral and leukemia associated antigens. *J. Natl. Cancer Inst.* 49: 943–952.

157. LoBuglio, A. F., and Neidhart, J. A. 1974. A review of transfer factor immunotherapy in cancer. *Cancer* 32, No. 4 (supplement), 1563–1570.

158. Lotem, J., and Sachs, L. 1974. Different blocks in the differentiation of myeloid leukemic cells. *Proc. Natl. Acad. Sci.* 71: 3507–3511.

159. Mak, T. W., Manaster, J., Howatson, A. F., McCullouch, E. A., and Till, J. E. 1974. Particles with characteristics of leukoviruses in cultures of marrow cells from leukemic patients in remission and relapse. *Proc. Natl. Acad. Sci.* 71: 4336–4340.

160. Mann, D. L., Abelson, L., Harris, S., and Amos, D. B. 1976. Second genetic locus in the HLA region for human B-cell alloantigens. *Nature* 259: 145–146.

161. Mann, D. L., Abelson, L., Henkart, P., Harris, S. D., and Amos, D. B. 1975. Specific human B lymphocyte alloantigens linked to HL-A. *Proc. Natl. Acad. Sci.* 72: 5103–5106.

162. Mann, D. L., Halterman, R., and Leventhal, B. G. 1973. Cross reactive antigens in human cells infected with Rauscher leukemia virus and on human acute leukemia cells. *Proc. Natl. Acad. Sci.* 70: 495–497.

163. Mann, D. L., Rogentine, G. N., Halterman, P., and Leventhal, B. 1971. Detection of an antigen associated with acute leukemia. *Science* 172: 1136–1137.

164. Mastrangelo, M. J., Berd, D., and Bellet, R. E. 1976. Critical review of previously reported clinical trials of cancer immunotherapy with non-specific immunostimulants. *Ann. N.Y. Acad. Sci.* 277: 94–122.

165. Mathé, G. 1975. Active immunotherapy as a treatment for minimum residual disease left by chemoradiotherapy in acute lymphoid leukemia, in *Immunological Aspects of Neoplasia.* William and Wilkins Co., Baltimore, pp. 633–667.

166. Mathé, G., Amiel, J. L., Schwarzanberg, L., Schneider, M., Caltan, A., Schlumberger, J. R., Hayat, M., and deVassal, F. 1969. Active immunotherapy for acute lymphoblastic leukemia. *Lancet* 1: 697–699.

167. Mathé, G., deVassal, F., Delgado, M., Pouillart, P., Belpomme, D., Joseph, R., Schwarzenberg, L., Amiel, J. L., Schneider, M., Cattan, A., Musset, M., Misset, J. L., and Jasmin, C. 1976. 1975 current results of the first 100 cytologically typed acute lymphoid leukemia submitted to BCG active immunotherapy. *Cancer Immunol. Immunother.* 1: 77–86.

168. Mathé, G., Pouillart, P., and Lapeyraque, F. 1969. Active immunotherapy of L1210 leukaemia applied after the graft of tumour cells. *Brit. J. Cancer* 23: 814–824.

169. Mathé, G., Schwarzenberg, L., Amiel, J. L., Pouillart, P., Hayat, M., de-Vassal, F., Rosenfeld, C., and Jasmin, C. 1975. New experimental and clinical data on leukaemia immunotherapy. *Proc. Royal Soc. Med.* 68 (4): 211–216.

170. McCoy, J. L., Herberman, R. B., Rosenberg, E. B., Donnelly, F. C., Levine, P. H., and Alford, C. 1973. [51]Chromium-release assay for cell-mediated cytotoxicity of human leukemia and lymphoid tissue culture cells. *Nat. Cancer Inst. Monogr.* 37: 59–67.

171. Medical Research Council. 1971. Treatment of acute lymphoblastic leukemia. Comparison of immunotherapy (BCG), intermittent methotrexate and no therapy after a five month intensive cytotoxic regimen (Concord Trial). *Brit. Med. J.* 4: 189–194.

172. Mellors, R. C., and Mellors, J. W. 1976. Antigen related to mammalian type-C RNA viral p30 proteins is located in renal glomeruli in human systemic lupus erythematosus. *Proc. Natl. Acad. Sci.* 73: 233–237.

173. Melnik, L., Courtney, R. J., Powell, K. L., Schaffer, P. A., Benyesh-Melnik, M., Dressman, G. R., Anzar, T., and Adam, E. 1976. Studies on herpes simplex virus and cancer. *Cancer Res.* 36: 845–856.

174. Messineo, L. 1961. Immunological differences of deoxyribonocleoproteins from white blood cells of normal and leukemic human beings. *Nature* 190: 1122–1123.

175. Metzgar, R. S., Mohanakumar, T., and Bolognesi, D. P. 1976. Antigenic relationships between murine, feline and primate RNA tumor viruses and membrane antigens of human leukemic cells. *Bibl. Haemat.* 43: 549–554.

176. Metzgar, R. S., Mohanakumar, T., and Bolognesi, D. P. 1976. Relationships between membrane antigens of human leukemic cells and oncogenic RNA virus structural components. *J. Exp. Med.* 143: 47–63.

177. Metzgar, R. S., Mohanakumar, T., Green, R. W., Miller, D. S., and Bolognesi, D. P. 1974. Human leukemia antigens: partial isolation and characterization. *J. Natl. Cancer Inst.* 52: 1445–1453.

178. Metzgar, R. S., Mohanakumar, T., and Miller, D. S. 1972. Antigens specific for human lymphocytic and myeloid leukemia cells: detection by non-human primate antiserums. *Science* 178: 986–988.

179. Mills, B., Sen, L., and Borella, L. 1976. Reactivity of anti-human thymocyte serum with acute leukemic blasts. *J. Int. Immunol.* 115: 1038–1044.

180. Mintz, U., and Sachs, L. 1975. Changes in the surface membrane of lymphocytes from patients with chronic lymphocytic leukemia and Hodgkin's disease. *Int. J. Cancer* 15: 253–259.

181. Mitchell, M. S. 1976. Role of "suppressor" T lymphocytes in antibody induced inhibition of cytophilic antibody receptors. *Ann. N.Y. Acad. Sci.* 276: 229–241.

182. Mitchell, M. S., Mokyr, M. B., Aspnes, G. T., and McIntosh, S. 1973. Cytophilic antibodies in man. *Ann. Int. Med.* 79: 333.

183. Mohanakumar, T., Metzgar, R. S., and Miller, D. S. 1974. Human leukemia cell antigens: serologic characterization with zenoantisera. *J. Natl. Cancer Inst.* 52: 1435–1444.

184. Nadkarni, J. S., Nadkarni, J. J., Klein, G., Henle, W., Henle, G., and Clifford, P. 1970. EB viral antigens in Burkitts' tumor biopsies and early cultures. *Int. J. Cancer* 6: 10–17.

185. Narang, H. K. 1973. Surface particles on leukemic lymphocytes in humans. *Cancer Res.* 33: 3216–3221.

186. Neidhart, J. A., and LoBuglio, A. F. 1974. Transfer factor therapy of malignancy. *Seminars Oncol.* 1: 379–385.

187. Obata, Y., Ikeda, H., Stockert, E., and Boyse, E. A. 1975. Relation of G_{IX} antigen of thymocytes to envelope glycoprotein of murine leukemia virus. *J. Exp. Med.* 141: 188–197.

188. O'Donnell, P. V., and Stockert, E. 1976. Induction of G_{IX} antigen and Gross cell surface antigen after infection by ecotropic and xenotropic murine leukemia viruses *in vitro*. *J. Virol.* 20: 545–554.

189. Old, L. J., Boyse, E. A., Geering, G., and Oettgen, H. 1968. Serologic approaches to the study of cancer in animals and in man. *Cancer Res.* 28: 1288–1297.

190. Old, L. J., Boyse, E. A., and Stockert, E. 1963. Antigenic properties of experimental leukemias. J. Serological studies *in vitro* with spontaneous and radiation induced leukemias. *J. Natl. Cancer Inst.* 31: 977–995.

191. Old, L. J., Stockert, E., Boyse, E. A., and Kim, J. H. 1968. Loss of TL antigen from cells exposed to TL antibody, study of the phenomenon in vitro. *J. Exp. Med.* 127: 523.

192. Oliver, R. T. D., Klouda, P., and Lawler, S. 1976. HL-A associated resistance factors and myelogenous leukaemia. *Proceedings of 1st International Symposium of HLA and Disease*, INSERM, Paris, 231.

193. Oren, M. E., and Herberman, R. B. 1971. Delayed cutaneous hypersensitivity reactions to membrane extracts of human tumour cells. *Clin. Exp. Immunol.* 9: 45–56.

194. Pearson, G., Klein, G., Henle, G., Henle, W., and Clifford, P. 1969. IV. Differentiation between Epstein-Barr viral and cell membrane immunofluorescence in Burkitt tumor cells. *J. Exp. Med.* 129: 707–718.

195. Pendergrass, T. W., Stoller, R. G., Mann, D. L., Halterman, R. H., and Fawmeni, J. F., Jr. 1975. Acute myelocytic leukemia and leukemia associated antigens in sisters. *Lancet* 2: 429–431.

196. Peto, R., and Galton, D. A. G. 1975. Chemoimmunotherapy of adult leukemia. *Lancet* 2: 454.

197. Powles, R. 1974. Active specific immunotherapy for acute myelogenous leukemia, in R. F. Beer, Jr., R. C. Tilghman, and E. G. Bassett (eds.). *The Role of Immunological Factors in Viral and Oncogenic Processes*, Johns Hopkins University Press, Baltimore, pp. 333–340.

198. Powles, R. 1974. Immunotherapy for acute myelogenous leukemia using irradiated and unirradiated leukemia cells. *Cancer* 32: No. 4 (supplement) 1558–1562.

199. Powles, R. L. 1974. Tumor associated antigens in acute leukemia, in F. J. Cleton, D. Crowther, and J. S. Matpas (eds.), *Advances in Acute Leukemia*, Chapter 5. North Holland Publishing Co. Amsterdam, Oxford.

200. Powles, R. L., Balchin, L. A., Hamilton-Fairley, G., and Alexander, P. 1971. Recognition of leukemia cells as foreign before and after autoimmunization. *Brit. Med. J.* 1: 486–489.

201. Powles, R. L., Crowther, D., Bateman, C. J. T., Beard, M. E. J., McElwain, T. J., Russell, J., Lister, T. A., Whitehouse, J. M. A., Wrigley, P. F. M., Pike, M., Alexander, P., and Hamilton-Fairley, G. 1973. Immunotherapy for acute myelogenous leukemia. *Brit. J. Cancer* 28: 365–376.

202. Ramachandar, K., Baker, M. A., and Taub, R. N. 1975. Antibody responses to leukemia-associated antigens during immunotherapy of chronic myelocytic leukemia. *Blood* 46: 845–854.

203. Rapin, A. M. C., and Burger, M. M. 1974. Tumor cell surfaces: general alterations detected by agglutinins. *Adv. Cancer Res.* 20: 1–91.

204. Rapp, F. 1974. Herpesvirus and cancer. *Adv. Cancer Res.* 19: 265–302.

205. Rappaport, F. 1974. Cross-reactive antigens, cancer, and transplantation. *Transplant. Proc.* 6: 39–43.

206. Reedman, B. M., Klein, G. M., Pope, J. H., Walters, M. K., Hilgers, J., Singh, S., and Johansson, B. 1974. Epstein-Barr virus-associated complement-fixing and nuclear antigens in Burkitt lymphoma biopsies. *Int. J. Cancer Res.* 13: 755–763.

207. Reitz, M. S., Miller, N. R., Wong-Staal, F., Gallagher, R. E., Gallo, R. C., and Gillespie, D. H. 1976. Primate Type-C virus nucleic acid sequences (wooly monkey and baboon types) in tissues from a patient with acute myelogenous leukemia and in virus isolated from cultured cells of some of the same patient.

Proc. Natl. Acad. Sci. 73: 2113–2117.

208. Rifkin, D. B., Compans, R. W., and Reich, E. 1972. A specific labeling procedure for proteins on the outer surface of membranes. *J. Biol. Chem.* 247: 6432–6437.

209. Rogentine, G. N., Trapani, R. J., Yankee, R. A., and Henderson, E. S. 1973. HL-A antigens and acute lymphocytic leukemia: the nature of the HL-A2 association. *Tissue Antigens* 3: 470–476.

210. Rogentine, G. N., Yankee, R. A., Gart, J. J., Nam, J., and Trapani, R. J. 1972. HL-A antigens and disease. *J. Clin. Invest.* 51: 2420–2428.

211. Rosenberg, E. B., Herberman, R. B., Halterman, R., McCoy, J. L., Levine, P. H., and Wunderlich, J. R. 1972. Lymphocyte cytotoxicity reactions to leukemia associated antigens in identical twins. *Int. J. Cancer* 9: 648–658.

212. Rudolph, R. H., Mickelson, E., and Thomas, E. D. 1970. A study by mixed leucocyte culture of leukemia twins, *in* J. E. Harris (ed.), *Proceedings of the Fifth Leukocyte Culture Conference*, pp. 319. Academic Press, New York.

213. Russell, J. A., Chapuis, B., and Powles, R. L. 1976. Various uses of BCG and allogeneic acute leukemia cells to treat patients with acute myelogenous leukemia. *Cancer Immunol. Immunother.* 1: 87–91.

214. Sahasrabudhe, M. B., Madyastha, K. R., Orema, S., Lele, R. D., Gollerkeri, M. P., and Rao, S. S. 1971. Induction of specific autoimmune response to leukaemic cells in human leukaemia patient by chemically tagged normal "O" group white blood cells. *Nature* 232: 198–199.

215. Sahasrabudhe, M. B., Prema, S., Madyastha, K. R., Gollerkeri, M. P., and Rao, S. S. 1971. Development of a specific anti-leukaemic serum for the treatment of leukaemia in clinics. *Nature* 232: 197–198.

216. Sanderson, A. R., Mahour, G. H., Jaffe, N., and Das, L. 1973. Incidence of HL-A antigens in acute lymphocytic leukemia. *Transplantation* 16: 672–673.

217. Santos, G. W., Mullins, G. M., Bias, W. B., Anderson, P. N., Graziano, K. D., Klein, D. L., and Burke, P. J. 1973. Immunological studies in acute leukemia. *Natl. Cancer Inst. Monogr.* 37: 69–75.

218. Santos, G. W., Sensenbrenner, L. L., Anderson, P. N., Burke, P. J., Klein, D. L., Slavin, R. E., Schacter, B. Z., and Borgaonkar, D. S. 1976. HL-A identical marrow transplants in aplastic anemia, acute leukemia, and lymphosarcoma using cyclophosphamide. *Transplant. Proc.* 8: 607–610.

219. Santos, G. W., Sensenbrenner, L. L., Burke, P. J., Mullins, G. M., Anderson, P. N., Tutschka, P. J., Braine, H. G., Davis, T. E., Humphrey, R. L., Abeloff, M. D., Bias, W. M., Borgaonkar, D. S., and Slavin, R. E. 1974. Allogeneic marrow grafts using cyclophosphamide. *Transplant. Proc.* 6 (No. 4): 345–348.

220. Sato, H., Boyse, E. A., Aoki, T., Iritani, C., and Old, L. J. 1973. Leukemia-associated transplantation antigens related to murine leukemia virus. The X.1 system: immune response controlled by a locus linked to H-2. *J. Exp. Med.* 138: 593–606.

221. Schacter, B., and Bias, W. B. 1974. Human sera cytotoxic to human leukemia cells. *Fed. Proc.* 33: 791.

222. Schacter, B., Bias, W. B., and Humphrey, R. L. 197. Normal human sera cytotoxic to cells of human acute leukemia. *Tissue Antigens* 8: 289–298.

223. Schacter, L. P., and Burke, P. J. 1976. Demonstration and characteriza-

tion of humoral regulators of cell proliferation in humans. *Proc. Amer. Assoc. Cancer Res.* 17: 70.

224. Schafer, W., Lange, J., Fischinger, P. J., Fromk, H., Bolognesi, D. P., and Pister, L. 1972. Properties of mouse leukemia viruses. II. Isolation of viral components. *Virology* 47: 210–217.

225. Schecter, G. P., Soehlen, F., and MacFarland, W. 1972. Lymphocyte response to blood transfusions in man. *N. Engl. J. Med.* 287: 1169–1173.

226. Schiffer, C. A., Lichtenfeld, J. L., Wiernick, P. H., Mardiney, Jr., M.R., and Joseph, J. M. 1976. Antibody responses in patients with acute non-lymphocytic leukemia. *Cancer* 37: 2177–2182.

227. Schlossman, S. L., Chess, L., Humphreys, R. E., and Strominger, J. L. 1976. Distribution of Ia like molecules on the surface of normal and leukemic human cells. *Proc. Natl. Acad. Sci.* 73: 1288–1292.

228. Schweitzer, M., Melief, C. J. M., and Eijsvoogel, V. P. 1973. Failure to demonstrate immunity to leukemia associated antigens by lymphocyte transformation *in vitro. Int. J. Cancer* 11: 11–18.

229. Sen, L., and Borella, L. 1975. Clinical importance of lymphoblasts with T markers in childhood acute leukemia. *N. Engl. J. Med.* 292: 828–832.

230. Sherr, C. J., and Todaro, G. J. 1975. Primate Type C virus p30 antigens in cells from humans with acute leukemia. *Science* 187: 855–857.

231. Shevach, E. M., Jaffe, E. S., and Greene, I. 1973. Receptors for complement and immunoglobulin on human and animal lymphoid cells. *Transplant. Rev.* 16: 3–28.

232. Shreffler, D. C., and David, C. S. 1975. The H-2 major histocompatibility complex and the I immune response region: genetic bariation function and organization. In: F. J. Dixon and H. J. Kunkel (eds.), *Advances in Immunology* 20: 125–195. Academic Press. New York.

233. Snell, G. D., and Cherry, M. 1972. Genetic factors in leukemia: loci determining cell surface alloantigens, in P. Emmelot and P. Bentvelzens (eds.), *RNA Viruses and Host Genome in Oncogenesis.* North Holland Publishing Co. Amsterdam and London, pp. 221–228.

234. Sokal, J. E., and Aungst, G. W. 1975. Immunotherapy with cultured human cells and BCG. *Transplant. Proc.* 7: 317–321.

235. Stephenson, J. R., and Aaronson, S. A. 1976. Search for antigens and antibodies cross-reactive with Type-C viruses of the woolly monkey and gibbon ape in animal models and in humans. *Proc. Natl. Acad. Sci.* 73: 1725–1729.

236. Stewart, T. H. M. 1969. The presence of delayed hypersensitivity reactions in patients toward cellular extracts of their malignant tumors. I. The role of tissue antigen, non-specific reactions of nuclear material, and bacterial antigen as a cause for this phenomenon. *Cancer* 23: 1368–1379.

237. Stockert, E., Boyse, E. A., Obata, Y., Ikeda, H., Sarkar, N. H., and Hoffman, H. A. 1975. New mutant and congenic mouse stocks expressing the murine leukemia virus-associated thymocyte surface antigen G_{IX}. *J. Exp. Med.* 142: 512–517.

238. Stockert, E., Boyse, E. A., Sato, H., and Itakura, K. 1976. Heredity of the G_{IX} thymocyte antigen associated with murine leukemia virus: segregation data simulating genetic linkage. *Proc. Natl. Acad. Sci.* 73: 2077–2081.

239. Stockert, E., Old, L. J., and Boyse, E. A. 1971. The G_{IX} system. A cell surface alloantigen associated with murine leukemia virus: implications regarding chromosomal integration of the viral genome. *J. Exp. Med.* 133: 1334–1355.

240. Strand, M., and August, J. T. 1973. Structural proteins of oncogenic ribonucleic acid viruses. Interspecies II: a new interspecies antigen. *J. Biol. Chem.* 248: 5627–5633.

241. Strand, M., and August, J. T. 1974. Structural proteins of RNA tumor viruses as probes for viral gene expression. *Cold Spring Harbor Symposium on Quantitative Biology* 39: 1109–1116.

242. Strand, M., and August, J. T. 1974. Type-C RNA virus gene expression in human tissue. *J. Virol.* 14: 1584–1596.

243. Strand, M., Lilly, F., and August, J. T. 1974. Host-control of endogenous murine leukemia virus gene expression—concentrations of viral proteins in high and low leukemia mouse strains. *Proc. Natl. Acad. Sci.* 71: 3682–3686.

244. Tejada, F., Bias, W. B., Santos, G. W., and Zieve, P. D. 1973. Immunologic response of patients with acute leukemia to platelet transfusions. *Blood* 42: 405–412.

245. Thiry, L. 1976. Herpes simplex virus and carcinoma of the cervix. *Eur. J. Cancer.* 12: 851–858.

246. Thomas, E. D., Bryant, J. I., Buckner, C. D., Clift, A., Fefer, A., Johnson, F. L., Nciman, P., Ramberg, R. E., and Storb, R. 1972. Leukemic transformation of engrafted human marrow cells *in vivo*. *Lancet* 1: 1310–1313.

247. Todaro, G. J., Benveniste, R. E., Collahan, R., Lieber, M. M., and Sherr, C. J. 1974. Endogenous primate and feline type C viruses. *Cold Spring Harbor Symp. Quant. Biol.* 39: 1159–1168.

248. Tung, J., Fleissner, E., Vitetta, E., and Boyse, E. A. 1975. Expression of murine leukemia virus envelope glycoprotein gp 69/71 on mouse thymocytes. Evidence for two structural variants distinguished by presence vs. absence of G_{IX} antigen. *J. Exp. Med.* 142: 518–523.

249. Tung, J. S., Vitetta, E. S., Fleissner, E., and Boyse, E. A. 1975. Biochemical evidence linking the G_{IX} thymocyte surface antigen to the gp 69/71 envelope glycoprotein of murine leukemia virus. *J. Exp. Med.* 141: 198–205.

250. Tung, J. S., Shen, F. W., Fleissner, E., and Boyse, E. A. 1976. X-gp70: a third molecular species of the envelope protein gp70 of murine leukemia virus, expressed on mouse lymphoid cells. *J. Exp. Med.* 143: 969–974.

251. Tyzzer, E. E. 1916. Tumor immunity. *J. Cancer Res.* 1: 125–156.

252. VanBeek, W. P., Smets, L. A., and Emmelot, P. 1975. Changes surface glycoprotein as a marker of malignancy in human leukemic cells. *Nature* 253: 457–460.

253. Viola, M. V., Frazier, M., Weirnick, P. H., McCredie, K. B., and Spiegelman, S. 1976. Reverse transcriptase in leucocytes of leukemic patients in remission. *N. Engl. J. Med.* 294: 75–80.

254. Viza, D. C., Bernardi-Degani, O., Bernard, C., and Harris, R. 1969. Leukaemia antigens. *Lancet* 2: 493–494.

255. Viza, D., Davies, D. A. L., and Harris, R. 1970. Solubilization and partial purification of human leukemic specific antigens. *Nature* 227: 1249–1251.

256. Vlodavsky, I., and Sachs, L. 1944. Difference in the cellular cholesterol

to phospholipid ratio in normal lymphocytes and lymphocytic leukemic cells. *Nature* 250: 67–68.

257. Vogeler, W. R., and Chan, Y. K. 1974. Prolonging remission in myeloblastic leukemic by Tice-Strain Bacillus Calmette Guerin. *Lancet* 2: 128–131.

258. Walford, R. L., Gossett, T., Smith, G. S., Zeller, E., and Wilkinson, J. 1975. A new alloantigenic system on human lymphocytes. *Tissue Antigens* 5: 196–204.

259. Walford, R. L., Waters, H., Smith, G. S., and Sturgeon, P. 1973. Anomalous reactivity of certain HL-A typing sera with leukemic lymphocytes. *Tissue Antigens* 3: 222–234.

260. Walford, R. L., Zeller, E., Combs, L., and Konrad, P. 1971. HL-A specificities in acute and chronic lymphatic leukemia. *Transplant. Proc.* 3: 1297–1300.

261. Walters, M. K., and Pope, J. H. 1971. Studies on the EB virus-related antigens of human leukocyte cell lines. *Int. J. Cancer* 8: 32–40.

262. Weiss, D. W., Stupp, Y., Many, N., and Izak, G. 1975. Treatment of acute myelocytic leukemia (AML) patients with the MER Tubercle Bacillus fraction: a preliminary report. *Transplant. Proc.* 7 (supplement): 545–552.

263. Yata, J., Klein, G., Kobayashi, N., Furukawa, T., and Yanagisawa, M. 1970. Human thymus-lymphoid tissue antigen and its presence in leukaemia and lymphoma. *Clin. Exp. Immunol.* 7: 781–792.

264. Yohn, D. S., Horoszewicz, J. S., Ellison, R. R., Mittelman, A., Chai, L. S., and Grace, Jr., J. T. 1968. Immunofluorescent studies in human leukemia. *Cancer Res.* 28: 1692–1702.

265. Yoshida, T. O., and Imai, K. 1970. Auto-antibody to human leukemic cell membrane as detected by immune adherence. *Rev. Europ. Etudes Clin. Biol.* 15: 61–65.

266. Zech, L., Haglund, U., Nilsonn, K., and Klein, G. 1976. Characteristic chromosomal abnormalities in biopsies and lymphoid-cell lines from patients with Burkitt and non-Burkitt lymphoma. *Int. J. Cancer* 17: 47–56.

CHAPTER 4

IMMUNO-COMPETENCE IN CHILDHOOD ACUTE LYMPHOCYTIC LEUKEMIA

Luis Borella
and James T. Casper

Midwest Childhood Cancer Center
Department of Pediatrics
The Medical College of Wisconsin
and Milwaukee Children's Hospital
1700 West Wisconsin Avenue
Milwaukee, Wisconsin 53233

Overt impairment of lymphocyte function does not precede the development of acute lymphocytic leukemia. Bacterial infections during active disease are usually secondary to neutropenia, whereas nonbacterial infections during remission are related to depression of lymphocytes by chemotherapy. Certain drug combinations preferentially suppress B lymphocytes. Termination of therapy leads to immunologic rebound, characterized by lymphocytosis, antibody production without extrinsic antigenic stimulation, and enhanced lymphocyte blastogenic responses. Bone marrow lymphocytosis may be misinterpreted as early leukemic relapse. Assessment of T and B markers on bone marrow cells does not distinguish between these two conditions. There is no evidence that either immune impairment or immunologic rebound correlates with the prognosis of childhood ALL.

Initiation, growth, and regression of neoplasia are in part regulated by immunologic mechanisms. Certain tumors develop more frequently in immunosuppressed patients (71) and impairment of immune responses appears to influence the prognosis of some human neoplasias (40, 43, 45). It is unlikely, however, that the same regulatory factors, whether immunologic, hormonal, or genetic, would affect all types of cancer to the same degree. This emphasizes the need for in-depth studies of particular neoplasias in order to understand basic differences between various forms of cancer and the mechanisms responsible for these differences.

Acute lymphoblastic leukemia (ALL) has special features which make this disease a prime candidate to study possible correlations between immunocompetence and cancer. By definition this neoplasm arises from the malignant transformation of immunocompetent cells, i.e., lymphocytes. Its development or expression is age-related, with a higher incidence in early childhood, between 2 and 6 years of age. Patients with ALL are treated for 2 ½ years to 3 years with a combination of immunosuppressive agents, but their treatment is then stopped, allowing the immunoevaluation of these patients independent of immune impairment due to drugs. Finally, marked improvement in prognosis of ALL during recent years has permitted the separation and comparison between patients who achieve long term remissions and those who develop early relapses.

Immunoevaluation and immunocompetence are vague terms with little meaning unless they signify a multivariant analysis of well-defined immunologic parameters which are determined at various stages of the disease. In cancer patients they should include a general evaluation of immunocompetence and, whenever possible, a simultaneous assay of immune responses to tumor-associated antigens. The sparcity of reports fulfilling these criteria emphasizes the problems encountered in this type of clinical study. These difficulties, which are inherent to the evaluation of patients with any form of cancer, are magnified in the study of childhood ALL. Therefore, in the first part of this review we will discuss some general pitfalls and problems related to the immunoevaluation of children, and particularly of children with ALL, before presenting current knowledge of their immunocompetence at various stages of their clinical course.

A. PROBLEMS IN THE EVALUATION OF IMMUNOCOMPETENCE IN CHILDHOOD ALL

1. Clinical and Biologic Heterogeneity of Childhood ALL

ALL can no longer be considered a homogenous disease, but rather several clinical entities with different target cells and pathogenesis. This concept has largely evolved from immunological studies on ALL phenotypes (12, 15, 18, 35, 80). These phenotypes have been identified by the presence on leukemic cells of surface markers and differentiation antigens which are expressed on normal, thymus-dependent (T) and thymus-independent (B) lymphocytes.

ALL is currently subclassified into T cell ALL, B cell ALL, and Non-T, Non-B, (or "common") ALL. T cell ALL represents 20 to 30% of childhood ALL. It is primarily a lymphatic disease and in most patients the target organ appears to be the thymus (80). In children, T cell ALL predominates in older boys, suggesting the possibility of genetic and hormonal influences. Some of the clinical manifestations of T cell ALL, such as early lymphatic spread and late blockade of erythropoiesis, are related to its extramedullary origin (16). This form of ALL has an aggressive course, reflected by a high initial WBC, high labeling and mitotic indices (S. Murphy, personal communication) and a poor response to therapy (16, 80). However, bone marrow replacement by leukemic cells appears to be a secondary phenomenon. T cell ALL is identified by the presence on bone marrow blasts of receptors for sheep erythrocytes (E^+ ALL) and thymus-associated antigens (12, 15, 18, 35, 80).

B cell ALL is a rare form of childhood ALL, representing only 2 to 3% of ALL. It also appears to run a very aggressive course, with a very poor response to current chemotherapy. This type of ALL is identified by the presence of monoclonal Ig on the membrane of leukemic lymphoblasts (18).

The third and more frequent ALL is the "common," or non-T, non-B ALL (70–80%). In contrast to the other two forms, this type of ALL has a good prognosis. Non-T, non-B ALL is primarily a bone marrow disease with secondary involvement of the lymphatic system. It has a peak incidence between 2 and 5 years of age, and has no sex predilection. Approximately one half of these patients present with a low WBC. Anemia is another common presenting symptom (16). This type of ALL is identified by the absence of T or B lymphocyte markers on bone marrow blasts. Additionally, these cells possess other cell surface antigens which are demonstrable using heteroantisera prepared against non-E rosette forming ALL blasts (E⁻ ALL) (15). Other reports also suggest that "common" ALL blasts express antigens present during early B-cell differentiation (57, 88).

Most of the studies concerned with immunocompetence of children with ALL reviewed in this chapter were performed prior to the knowledge that ALL is a heterogenous disease. Therefore, the interpretation of these results is complicated by an unknown variable, i.e., the phenotypic characterization of the patients studied. Even more important, future studies should aim to establish whether the immunocompetence of the host may be affected to different degrees, depending on the origin of the leukemic cells.

2. Age

There are normal variations in immunologic parameters during childhood, which are related to age and which should also be considered in the study of children with neoplasia. These differences express the normal maturation of the immune system. This process is influenced by the cumulative experience of the host to multiple antigenic challenges and is reflected by multiple changes in humoral and cell-mediated immune responses, ranging from levels of serum immunoglobulins (Ig) to patterns of delayed hypersensitivity.

Many investigators have utilized serum Ig as a parameter of immunocompetence in children with ALL (17, 22, 33, 34, 38, 58, 67, 74). The advantages are that the assay can be repeated in sequential serum samples and is relatively easy to perform. The main problem in the evaluation of results is the extreme variation of Ig levels in children of different ages and even between individuals of the same age (19). This is particularly critical in the first 3 years of life (19, 85). In the absence of intrauterine infection the newborn does not synthesize appreciable amounts of IgA and IgM, while levels of IgG, which is transferred transplacentally, are similar to those of the maternal serum. In the first months of life the catabolism of maternal IgG, leads to physiologic hypogamma-globulinemia, which usually reaches its nadir at 4 to 6 months. However, this phase is variable and may extend up to 3 years of age. Concomitantly, there is an increased synthesis of IgM and IgA. Another problem is that serum Ig may remain within normal limits in a severely immunosuppressed patient. This discrepancy might be explained by the following: 1) serum Ig reflects the summation of responses to multiple antigenic challenges which have occurred during the whole life span, and 2) there is a significant delay between the cessation of IgG synthesis at cellular level and an appreciable reduction of serum IgG levels due to the relatively long half life of IgG.

Contrasting with these age-dependent variations in Ig, the quality and quantity of antibody synthesized does not differ in children of various ages. The absence or low titers of the so called "natural antibodies," such as isohemagglutinins, in younger children is related to duration of antigenic exposure rather than to inability to produce these antibodies.

Similarly, lack of natural antigenic stimulation is the main limiting factor in the evaluation of anamnestic cell-mediated immunity in children. Candida, SK SD, mumps, Trichophyton, and PPD are antigens most frequently used to assay recall cell-mediated responses, both in vivo and in vitro. However, while 90% of adults develop a positive response to one or more of these antigens, normal children may not respond to any of them (85). Skin testing of diptheria and tetanus toxoid, antigens to which all children should have been exposed at an earlier age, might overcome this problem (32).

Other parameters of cell mediated immunity are primary delayed hypersensitivity to keyhole limpet hemocyanin and to dinitrochlorobenzene (DNCB), skin reactivity to PHA, and measurement of skin allograft rejection. There is no evidence that these responses differ in children of various ages. The magnitude of in vitro blastogenesis by normal lymphocytes upon stimulation with specific and non specific mitogens is also independent of age.

In contrast to these findings, the relative and absolute numbers of T and B lymphocytes vary with age. In a recent study comparing the number of E rosettes (T lymphocytes) and EAC rosettes (B lymphocytes) in infants, older children and adults, the percentage of T lymphocytes was lower in infants, intermediate in older children and higher in adults. However, because of the normal lymphocytosis of infants, the absolute number of T lymphocytes was higher in this age group (31). Conversely, the relative and absolute numbers of EAC-rosette-forming lymphocytes was increased in infants, slightly lower in older children and lowest in adults. It is unknown whether these differences are limited to the circulating pool or are also present in other lymphoid organs.

Another area in which the age of the patient must be taken into consideration is the differentiation of B lymphocytes into plasma cells after in vitro stimulation with pokeweed mitogen (PWM). Although newborns have increased number of B lymphocytes there are age related qualitative and quantitative differences in the ability of these cells to differentiate into plasma cells when stimulated with PWM (89). In newborns, fewer cells differentiate and most of the differentiated cells possess cytoplasmic IgM, whereas in the adult population, cells with IgG are more prevalent. Because of the small number of children studied and the variation among individual responses the exact age at which B-lymphocyte response reaches adult levels is not known.

3. Immunosuppression Secondary to Malnutrition

The growth of the tumor may profoundly affect the nutritional status of the host. Similarly, the toxic effects of antineoplastic drugs are not limited to lympho-hematopoietic cells, but includes multiple organ systems. Thus, most treatments produce gastrointestinal toxicity which may lead to protein-calorie deprivation of the host. It is important, but frequently difficult, to distinguish immunosuppression primarily due to disease or drugs from the secondary effects of malnutrition upon immunocompetent cells.

Malnutrition per se might impair both cell-mediated and humoral immune responses (21, 27, 29, 30, 62). Protein-deficient children have normal or elevated Ig, but antibody production is depressed (29). These patients may also present with a reduction in the relative and absolute number of circulating T lymphocytes (30). These defects are correctable by dietary protein. A recent study demonstrates that both the efferent and afferent limb of cell-mediated skin responses are affected in children with protein-calorie malnutrition (27). Following improvement in their diet, these immune functions returned to normal in one to two months. Other investigators have reported similar findings in attempting to sensitize malnourished children with BCG or DNCB (21).

At the time of diagnosis most children with ALL are well nourished. There are, however, variations in the initial nutritional status of individual patients and in the effects of drugs upon intake and metabolism of essential nutrients. Therefore, in the immuno-evaluation of patients with cancer one should also ascertain their nutritional status, at diagnosis and throughout their clinical illness. Abnormal immune parameters in a child with leukemia or lymphoma might be secondary to malnutrition and not as a result of the primary disease or direct immunosuppression by the treatment.

4. Limited Immunoevaluation

Evaluation of cancer patients is usually limited to a few tests which provide only a partial picture of the complex cell-to-cell interactions occurring during immune responses. Authors tend to forget these limitations and the data are frequently either erroneously or over interpreted. Examples of excessive extrapolation are frequently found in the cancer literature and could be simplistically summarized into three capital sins. The first is to assume that a single test accurately reflects the complexity of a particular type of immune response. The second is to directly extrapolate in vitro data to the in vivo phenomenon. The third is to apply information derived from a single physical compartment, such as peripheral blood, to deduce what may or may not occur in other lymphoid organs. In this list one should also include lack of knowledge of the distribution of various cell types in the samples used for any particular assay. This problem is discussed in more detail in the next section.

5. Source and Identification of Cells Used for in vitro Assays

In vitro tests are frequently used in the immunologic classification of ALL and in studies of immune function during diagnosis and treatment. The main source of cells for these assays is peripheral blood. It should be emphasized, however, that a reduction in number or function of circulating cells may not be related to suppression, but to an excessive migration of these cells into other organs. Antileukemia agents can affect the migratory patterns of normal lymphoid cells. T cells were found to be increased in the bone marrow and spleen of mice treated with cortisone and cyclophosphamide, respectively (23, 73). This effect was demonstrated by the enhanced response of bone marrow cells to in vitro stimulation with PHA and by their ability to mount a graft-vs.-host response and to act as helper cells in antibody production (23, 24). A similar phenomenon has been shown in man; T cells were sequestered in the bone marrow of children with ALL in remission undergoing immunosuppressive-antileukemic therapy. Bone marrow cells from these children had an augmented in vitro blastogenic response to PHA (10) and a high number of E rosette-forming lymphocytes (13). Thus, caution should be exercised in the interpretation of T cell function in peripheral blood, since it may not necessarily correlate with T cell function in other lymphoid compartments.

Another frequent mistake is to incorrectly assume that the sample tested contains a homogenous population of either neoplastic or normal cells. Many reports do not even include a differential count of the cells assayed. It is well known that leukemic cells and normal lymphocytes coexist in the peripheral blood of most children with untreated ALL. Although the interactions between these two cell populations are poorly understood, it has been shown that lymphocytes in the blood of some of these patients are capable of responding to mitogenic stimulation and carry normal differentiation markers (2, 13, 59).

Negligence in recognizing that normal cells might be present in the sample tested may lead to erroneous interpretation of data. An example is to be found in the immunological classification of ALL. As mentioned above, this disease is currently subclassified into T ALL, B ALL, and non-T, non-B ALL. In the course of these studies, some investigators have used cells from the initial bone marrow aspirate, while others determined phenotype markers on peripheral blood cells. The differing sources of cells may partially explain several discrepancies between the reports. There are three interrelated problems in the study of leukemic cell phenotypes in the peripheral blood of children with ALL: (1) About one third of children with ALL present with WBC lower than $10 \times 10^9/l$, (2) blood with a low absolute number of white cells contains a relatively high proportion of normal lymphocytes, and (3) cytomorphologic differentiation between normal lymphocytes and leukemic blasts is not always accurate. This is illustrated in Figure 1. The data are from a simultaneous evaluation of phenotype markers in the blood and bone marrow from a child with untreated ALL, who presented with an initial low WBC. In this assay, we tested T cell phenotype by E rosette formation (12, 80) and also by the presence of T-cell-associated antigens (68, 81). These antigens were identified with antisera prepared against normal human thymus (anti-T) and E-rosette-forming ALL blasts (anti-E^+ ALL) (15). The results show the marked discrepancy that can arise between blood and bone marrow.

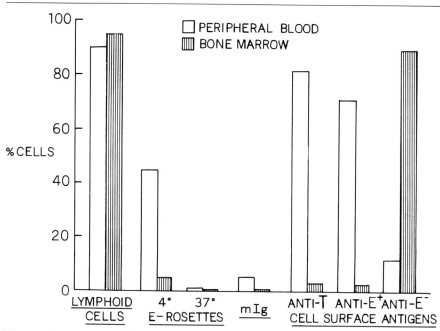

Fig. 1. Comparison of lymphoid cell phenotypes between peripheral blood and bone marrow in a child with untreated ALL. Note that in both compartments 90% of the cells were lymphoid cells.

Assay of circulating cells may have suggested that this child had T or E^+ ALL (45% E rosettes, 82% and 71% cells positive with anti-T and anti-E^+ ALL sera). However, the data from the bone marrow clearly indicate that this child had, in fact, non-T, non-B ALL and the circulating T cells in the peripheral blood were part of the large residual population of normal T lymphocytes. In contrast, the bone marrow had a significantly higher proportion of leukemic blasts which were identified with the anti E^- ALL serum (15).

6. Variations in Treatment

This is an obvious problem and specific examples will be presented in the following sections. Suffice it to say that immunological data from patients with ALL would be uninterpretable without knowing whether the patients were studied before or during treatment, and the details regarding schedule, doses, and drug combinations used in the chemotherapeutic regimens.

B. IMMUNOCOMPETENCE OF CHILDREN WITH ALL AT VARIOUS STAGES OF THE DISEASE

1. Immunocompetence at Diagnosis

The main criterion for the diagnosis of ALL is cytomorphology. On this basis, it is assumed that ALL is a malignant transformation of normal lymphocytes. Therefore, one would expect that the replacement of immunocompetent cells by neoplastic lymphoid cells should result in impairment of lymphocyte functions. Immunological studies performed in patients with ALL at the time of diagnosis suggest that this may not always be true.

At the time of diagnosis, most patients with ALL have normal or above normal serum Ig (22, 33, 34, 38, 58, 67, 74). In 28 children with ALL before initiation of therapy, IgG and IgM were normal, while IgA levels were low-normal (67). However, the control values used were those obtained from adults and consequently some of these values might actually have been elevated if compared with age-matched controls. Other reports have also demonstrated essentially normal Ig levels in untreated patients (33, 34, 38, 58, 74). Deviations from mean values were quite high, suggesting great interindividual differences among these children (22, 33). Results from a recent evaluation of Ig in 109 children with ALL prior to treatment are presented in Figure 2. The data indicates that most of these

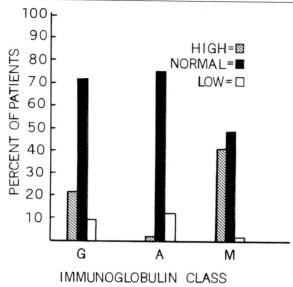

Fig. 2. Distribution of serum Ig in children with ALL at time of diagnosis. These values were compared to age-matched controls. (Data adapted from Ref. 38.)

patients had increased or normal IgG and IgM. There was, however, a significant proportion with low IgA (38). Information on antibody synthesis by children with untreated ALL is scarce. A few reports are available on patients studied before the development of effective antileukemia therapy. In more recent studies it is difficult to dissociate the effects of the disease from those of the treatment because chemotherapy is initiated immediately after diagnosis. More than two decades ago a group of patients with untreated acute leukemia were tested with capsular polysaccharides from pneumococci and found to have normal antibody titers (61). The type of leukemia was not mentioned. In another report, 4 children with ALL responded to immunization with mumps virus, diphtheria, and tetanus toxoid and typhus-paratyphoid vaccines (82). Normal antibody titers were demonstrated in 10 patients with ALL who were immunized with influenza virus vaccine (41). The age distribution was not specified. A more recent study in a larger group of patients which included children and adults with ALL, indicated that about half of these patients synthesized antibodies during the first weeks of treatment (26). Though limited, these data suggest that development of ALL may not necessarily lead to impairment of antibody production.

It is not clear to what degree cell-mediated immunity is affected by the leukemic process. There are, however, at least three lines of evidence suggesting that T lymphocytes are not significantly altered in most children with untreated ALL: (1) Some patients have a normal or slightly reduced delayed hypersensitivity (26). (2) Their peripheral blood lymphocytes are stimulated in vitro by PHA (2, 59). (3) Cytomorphologically normal lymphocytes with T markers are present in their peripheral blood (13) (see also Fig. 1). In contrast, others have reported depression of cell mediated responses in patients with untreated leukemia (28, 45). These data are difficult to evaluate because ALL and AML are considered under the same heading of acute leukemia and patients of different ages are grouped together. Moreover, depression of delayed hypersensitivity may be related to absence of nonlymphoid cells participating in the inflammatory response rather than to lymphocyte impairment. No information is available concerning the production of MIF or other soluble mediators of delayed hypersensitivity by lymphocytes from untreated patients. Although the serum from children with ALL, particularly those with WBC greater than $50 \times 10^9/l$, inhibits the mitogenic response of normal lymphocytes to PHA (54), this effect is related to the binding of macromolecules present in the serum to PHA and not to direct inhibition of lymphocytes by serum components (52).

Neutropenia is the primary factor in the development of severe bacterial infections among children with active ALL (9) and is due to bone marrow replacement by leukemic cells. Additionally, the function and metabolism of the residual granulocyte population can be depressed (51, 87). Bactericidal, phagocytic, and enzymatic activity of blood leukocytes was lower in children with acute leukemia in relapse than in those in remission (87). The main criticism of this report is that the data were not corrected for the absolute number of granulocytes. Thus, the results can be explained simply on the basis of granulocyte dilution with blasts. This factor was considered in a subsequent study of 18 children with untreated or relapsing acute leukemia and 20 children in leukemic remission (51). Half of the patients in relapse had abnormal bactericidal and NBT-reductase activity whereas these activities were normal during remission. Although these studies indicate that granulocyte functions are impaired during active disease the mechanisms of this disturbance are still poorly understood.

Another area deserving further investigation concerns the effects of ALL upon the complement system. A wide range of serum complement levels has been demonstrated in children with ALL at time of exacerbation of the disease (90). It was not mentioned whether these children were studied at diagnosis or at relapse during chemotherapy. C5, C8, C1 and whole complement activity were found to be elevated in another group of patients with untreated acute leukemia, the ages ranging from 6 to 62 years (64). A recent report examined the alternative complement pathway in children with untreated ALL (56). The authors describe an inhibitor to the activation of C3-C9 via the alternative pathway. Concurrent with this observation, they demonstrated elevated levels of C3 and factor B, which they were unable to explain. Whether or not this inhibition of the alternative pathway is crucial in the pathogenesis of ALL is not known at this time. Further research is needed to elucidate the role of complement in the immunological regulation or control of ALL.

This brief review emphasizes the wide gaps in our current knowledge regarding immunocompetence of children with ALL. The fact that neutropenia per se can explain most severe infections in these patients might satisfy many empirical minds. However, other questions will have to be answered before the pathogenesis of ALL can be solved. Specifically, the clinical and immunological heterogeneity of this disease should be considered in future studies on the immunocompetence of untreated patients.

2. Immunocompetence During Treatment

Within recent years significant advances have been made in the treatment of ALL (5, 66, 72, 83). Although the use of combination chemotherapy and preventive treatment of central nervous system leukemia has resulted in a marked prolongation of disease-free survival, ALL still represents a formidable challenge for clinicians and researchers. Witness to our ignorance are those children who die after short-term remissions or as a consequence of immunosuppressive therapy. Recent knowledge of the heterogeneity of childhood ALL emphasizes the old axiom that treatments should be tailored to each individual patient rather than to an intellectually conceived disease. With current protocols some patients with ALL are overtreated, thus increasing morbidity and the risk of long-term side effects, while others receive less than optimum therapy. Thus, clinical pharmacological studies on the synergism of various drug combinations should also consider their selective effects upon normal host cells, particularly their role in carcinogenesis and immunosuppression.

As a general principle all antileukemia drugs are immunosuppressive. Their "in vivo" and "in vitro" effects on various parameters of immune functions have been the subject of a number of excellent reviews (8, 39, 42, 65) and will not be discussed here. Various agents interfere with different biochemical events; the end result is inhibition of proliferation of immunocompetent cells. Clinically, these cellular or subcellular events may lead to mild or severe immune impairment, depending on drug combinations, dosages, and schedules of administration. We need simpler tests and more accurate criteria to predict which patients might be at high risk for serious infectious complications secondary to drug-induced immunosuppression. Unfortunately, the complexities of cell to cell interaction required for full expression of immunocompetence might preclude the development of a single accurate test to measure immunocompetence. Further, the degree of *"in vivo"* immunosuppression and *"in vitro"* parameters of cell function may not necessarily correlate with each other.

In this section we will review the immunosuppressive effect of antileukemic treatment through the various phases of treatment: induction of remission, preventive CNS therapy and maintenance or continuation chemotherapy. This discussion will be primarily based on our own experience with "total therapy" studies conducted at St. Jude Children's Research Hospital during the last decade. Although there are certain differences between this treatment and protocols used in other institutions most treatments for ALL combine the same antileukemic drugs and are based on similar principles. Therefore, we will attempt to derive general conclusions and try to correlate our data with the experience of other investigators.

INDUCTION OF COMPLETE REMISSION. The aim of the initial phase of treatment is to rapidly destroy the leukemic tissue and change a sick patient into a normal child. The main two drugs used are vincristine and prednisone. Both induce fast blast lysis without interfering with bone marrow repopulation by normal cells. About 9 in every 10 children with ALL achieve a remission with this drug combination. The addition of asparaginase to these drugs has increased even further the remission induction rate. There are no systematic studies on the immunocompetence of children with ALL at various intervals during the phase of remission induction. Although vincristine prednisone and asparaginase have been shown to be immunosuppressive agents, infections during this period are related not to drug-induced immunosuppression, but to preexisting granulocytopenia. Children with ALL may be infected at time of diagnosis, but most of them respond satisfactorily to antibiotics. In a series of 472 children with ALL only 2.5% developed fatal infections, usually gram negative sepsis, during the induction phase of treatment (83). After 4 weeks of induction treatment most children achieve complete remission. At this time the absolute number of lymphocytes in blood and percentage of lymphocytes in bone marrow are essentially within normal values and the percentage of bone marrow lymphocytes does not correlate with duration of hematological remission (36). It is unknown, however, if the proportions of various lymphocyte subsets in initial remission bone marrows are similar to those reported for normal bone marrow (14) and whether the kinetics of bone marrow repopulation with normal lymphocytes differs in patients with T, B, and "common" ALL.

"PROPHYLACTIC CNS TREATMENT." For many years it has been recognized that even in the absence of hematological relapse the leukemic process may re-occur in the deep arachnoid areas of the CNS. With the development of better methods to control bone marrow disease, the relative incidence of this complication increased and it became clear that CNS leukemia was a major limiting factor in the permanent control of the disease. We know now that 2400-rad cranial irradiation and intrathecal methotrexate for spinal prophylaxis given early during remission markedly reduce the incidence of CNS leukemia and prolong the duration of continuous complete remission (5, 25, 66, 72, 83). Equally beneficial results are obtained with prophylactic craniospinal irradiation without intrathecal methotrexate (3). Other studies have compared the efficacy of intrathecal methotrexate alone vs. cranial irradiation in preventing CNS leukemia. Results to date suggest that meningeal irradiation is superior to MTX alone (72). The question of whether cranial irradiation plus intrathecal methotrexate adds to the immunosuppression induced by systemic chemotherapy has not been answered satisfactorily. There is both clinical and laboratory evidence indicating that the combination of cranial and spinal irradiation depresses granulocyte and lymphocyte functions.

Peripheral blood cells from children with ALL undergoing craniospinal irradiation have been assayed with regard to their phagocytic, metabolic, and bactericidal activity (6). These studies were performed using patients in remission before, during and after radiation. The killing of staph aureus, Ps. aeruginosa and D. pneumoniae by blood lymphocytes was markedly reduced during the irradiation phase. In contrast, phagocytes killed normally each species of bacteria before and after craniospinal irradiation despite concurrent chemotherapy. Suppression of bactericidal activity during craniospinal irradiation was detected in the absence of patient serum, i.e., the defect was intrinsic to the phagocytic cell, but it was not related to efficacy of phagocytosis, which was normal. Similarly, oxygen consumption, activity of the hexose monophosphate shunt and myeloperoxidase activity were not impaired by irradiation. There was, however, a defect in the iodination of zymosan, which is dependent upon the concerted delivery of myeloperoxidase and hydrogen peroxide with the halide ion within the phagocytic vesicle. Both the impairment of bactericidal activity and this selective metabolic defect were transitory and not demonstrable 2 to 4 weeks after irradiation or during irradiation in children receiving only cranial irradiation. In another comparative study it was found that the incidence of leukopenia below 2000 WBC/mm2 was approximately double in children receiving craniospinal irradiation when compared to those undergoing cranial irradiation plus intrathecal methotrexate (3). Thus, the effects of craniospinal irradiation upon granulocytes may be related to both, impairment of granulocyte production and function.

Lymphocytes are also affected by craniospinal irradiation (20). A comparative study of children with ALL in remission who had or had not received craniospinal irradiation demonstrated that peripheral blood lymphopenia was more severe in the irradiated group (20). However, another study found no difference in the proportion of bone marrow lymphocytes between irradiated and nonirradiated patients (36). This discrepancy might be explained by differences in chemotherapeutic regimens or by the fact that different lymphoid compartments were studied. It is possible that T lymphocytes might be more sensitive to suppression by craniospinal irradiation. The depression of lymphocyte blastogenic response to PHA demonstrated in children treated with craniospinal irradiation favors this explanation (20). Since patients included in the study were treated with different sources of energy, including supervoltage, 250 kv, and cobalt, it is likely that depression of PHA-induced blastogenesis was due to irradiation of thymic and nonthymic lymphoid tissue, partially included in the spinal field.

Cranial irradiation plus intrathecal methotrexate and craniospinal irradiation are equally effective in the prevention of CNS relapse. Three of 45 patients treated with cranial irradiation and 2 of 49 undergoing craniospinal irradiation developed CNS leukemia (3). Contrasting with the laboratory findings described above, the incidence of severe clinical infections was similar in both groups. Interruption of chemotherapy which is usually due to unexplained fever, infection and severe leukopenia is another parameter of clinical immune impairment. In this study the total interruptions, the median duration of each interruption, the total days, and percent of days of interrupted chemotherapy were significantly greater in the group that received craniospinal irradiation than in the group undergoing cranial irradiation plus intrathecal methotrexate (3). Thus, although both methods can control the development of CNS leukemia, laboratory and clinical data indicate that the risk of granulocyte and lymphocyte impairment is higher with craniospinal irradiation. Therefore, cranial irradiation plus intrathecal methotrexate is currently recommended to prevent CNS leukemia in children with ALL until another equally effective but less hazardous method is found.

CONTINUATION THERAPY. The purpose of this phase of treatment is to eliminate all residual leukemic cells, particularly those outside the central nervous system. Continuation therapy is started as soon as a remission is achieved and, within the limits of tolerance of each patient, it is continued throughout the phase of prophylactic cranial irradiation. There is no definitive data regarding the minimal duration of this phase and ideal drug combinations needed to completely eradicate the disease. It is known, however, that most children who receive chemotherapy and remain in remission for 3 years will stay in remission if chemotherapy is stopped at this point (4, 75). Also, there is general agreement that a combination of at least 2 drugs, preferably, mercaptopurine and methotrexate should be used in this phase (66, 83).

Some general principles can be derived from the analysis of various reports on the immunosuppressive effects of the continuation phase of treatment in childhood ALL. The reader should be aware, however, that the multiplicity of variables such as duration of treatment, intermittent versus continuous therapy, type, dose, and route of administration, and selection of patients precludes a direct comparison of data from these various studies.

Serum Ig in children with ALL undergoing antileukemia treatment has been extensively investigated (17, 22, 33, 34, 38, 74). As parameters of immunocompetence or predictive indexes of higher risk for infection these results are generally disappointing. Most children with ALL in remission had normal serum Ig (17, 22, 33, 34, 38, 74). However, during treatment some of them develop a transient or persistent reduction of one or several Ig classes. Serum IgG has been found to be more frequently depressed than IgM during maintainence chemotherapy (17, 34). These findings agree with experimental data and studies on antibody production and indicate that chemotherapy may block the pathways during cell differentiation from IgM to IgG (17, 76, 77). Depressed serum Ig did not correlate with a high susceptibility to infection or increased risk of relapse (34, 67). This lack of correlation may be partially explained by the experimental design of these studies and by the extreme range of normal values. A marked fall in serum Ig levels in a child with ALL who has been followed with serial Ig determinations should be considered significant and alert the physician to the possibility of this patient being at high risk for serious infections. Conversely, antibody production may be depressed in patients with normal Ig.

As a parameter of immunocompetence, the measurement of serum antibody has the distinct advantage over serum immunoglobulins in that it is more sensitive, reflects recent cellular events and is specific. Most studies on antibody production in acute leukemia include patients with ages ranging from 3 to 70 years (26, 41, 43, 61, 82) and frequently AML and ALL have been analyzed together. To this clinical heterogeneity we should add the diversity of drug treatment, which not only varies between reports, but also within a single study (26, 69). There are two points, however, that emerge from these confusing and sometimes conflicting data: 1) Primary humoral immune responses are more suppressed by chemotherapy than anamnestic antibody production. 2) After short courses of multiple agent chemotherapy there is usually a prompt recovery of antibody production within a week after cessation of drugs.

There is limited information on the effects of maintenance chemotherapy in antibody production by children with ALL in remission (17, 69). One of these studies was performed with patients who had received the same combination chemotherapy regimen consisting of mercaptopurine, methotrexate and cyclophosphamide plus cyclic courses of vincristine and prednisone for periods ranging from 8 to 28 months (17). Patients and controls were immunized with the Hong Kong influenza vaccine prior to the Hong Kong influenza virus epidemic. This permitted the assay of the primary antibody response to the new antigenic determinant of the virus, the hemagglutinin, and the secondary antibody response to the other determinant, the neuraminidase, which was identical with the neuraminidase antigen on the influenza viruses that were current in the preceeding years.

As shown in Table 1, this form of continuation chemotherapy inhibited both the primary and secondary responses, but the primary antibody response was more suppressed. It has been shown that animals treated with antimetabolites had a selective suppression of IgG antibodies with a prolongation of the IgM response (76). Similarly, in this study children receiving combination chemotherapy showed a preferential suppression of IgG antibodies with persistance of IgM antibodies, but only to the primary stimulation with the hemagglutinin antigen (17). Assay of antibody response to poliovirus in children with ALL undergoing various drug combinations confirmed the marked effect of antileukemia treatment upon primary antibody responses, but failed to demonstrate a preferential effect upon IgG antibodies (69). Thus, prolongation of the phase of IgM production with a delayed or aborted maturation of the humoral immune

Table 1. Primary and secondary antibody responses to antigenic determinants of influenza virus by children with all receiving maintenance chemotherapy

	Primary Response Hemagglutinin Antibodies (Mean Log$_2$ Titer)		Secondary Response Neuraminidase Antibodies (Mean Log$_2$ Titer)	
	All	Controls	All	Controls
Prevaccination	< 2	< 2	4.9	5.9
Postvaccination	4.4	8.2	7.0	9.3
Negative responders	25%	0%	10%	0%

Source: Data adapted from Ref. 17.

response from IgM to IgG antibodies may not only depend on optimal timing and drug dosage, but also in the nature of the antigen (39).

A different approach to the study of cells involved in antibody production is to determine the number and distribution of progenitors of antibody forming cells, i.e., B lymphocytes. These cells are identified by the presence of membrane immunoglobulins, usually demonstrable by direct immunofluorescence of viable lymphocytes using fluorescein-conjugated antibodies to human immunoglobulins.

One study has found that the proportion of B lymphocytes in the blood of children with ALL in remission who had received methotrexate and mercaptopurine for one year was similar to that of normal individuals (20). However, another study demonstrated a marked reduction in relative and absolute numbers of B lymphocytes in the blood of children with ALL who had received a combination of mercaptopurine, methotrexate, and cyclophosphamide for 3 years (68). Variation in laboratory techniques, duration of treatment and schedules of drug administration might explain this apparent discrepancy. However, the major difference between these two reports is that cyclophosphamide was added to the continuation treatment of children in the second study.

Under well defined experimental conditions cyclophosphamide induces a more severe and longer lasting effect on B cell, than on T cells (60, 63, 73, 86). Three day old chickens treated with cyclophosphamide failed to produce antibodies and had depressed IgM and IgG serum levels, but graft-vs.-host reactivity remained intact (63). Poulter and Turk demonstrated a proportional increase in theta-carrying lymphocytes in peripheral lymphoid tissue of mice treated with cyclophosphamide (73). In animals treated with this drug the *in vitro* blastogenic response to PWM was impaired while the response to PHA was not affected (86). Cyclophosphamide not only does not inhibit but also may potentiate T-cell-mediated immunity (1, 60). Although this effect seems to be due to a selective suppression of antibody production by the drug (60) recent data indicates that cyclophosphamide can augment delayed-type hypersensitivity without affecting antibody responses (1).

To clarify whether the discrepancy between reports was due to the addition of cyclophosphamide, a comparative study was performed in 3 groups of children with ALL who had been randomized to receive three different drug combinations at maximum tolerated doses (38). One group received methotrexate and mercaptopurine, another methotrexate and cyclophosphamide, and the last, methotrexate, mercaptopurine, cyclophosphamide, and cytosine arabinoside (Ara-C). All patients were in remission and on the continuation phase of treatment for at least 6, but no more than 12 months. All had received cranial irradiation plus intrathecal methotrexate. The number of B and T lymphocytes in peripheral blood was determined by direct immunofluorescence of membrane Ig and E-rosette formation, respectively. The data presented in Figure 3 demonstrates that addition of cyclophosphamide produced a marked reduction of B lymphocytes, which was further potentiated by Ara-C. There was no significant difference in the number of T lymphocytes between groups. This result confirms our initial hypothesis that the addition of cyclophosphamide leads to a marked suppression of B lymphocytes. The data also emphasize the difficulties in comparing immune responses in patients treated with different drug combinations. This study did not include a simultaneous evaluation of the incidence and severity of infection in those 3 groups. Thus, at the present time one can only speculate about the clinical significance of these findings. Although the incidence of varicella-zoster infections and *Pneumocystitis carinii* pneumonitis was lower in children treated with mercaptopurine and methotrexate and higher in those receiving the 2 drugs plus cyclophosphamide and Ara-C (47), the reduction of B lymphocytes may be only one of multiple factors that may explain this difference.

Interpretation of data on suppression of cell-mediated immunity by drugs is hampered by the same heterogenity of patients and treatments previously described. There is agreement, however, that newly acquired

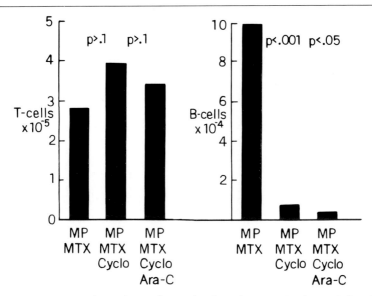

Fig. 3. Comparison of numbers of T and B lymphocytes in the peripheral blood of children with ALL in remission who were treated with 3 different drug combinations. The columns represent the mean number of cells per ml of blood. (Data adapted from Ref. 38.)

delayed hypersensitivity is more suppressed than established hypersensitivity (39). Delayed cutaneous hypersensitivity to Candida, SK-SD, tuberculin, and egg albumin was tested in a large group of patients with ALL undergoing chemotherapy (26). Their ages ranged from 4 to 81 years. The incidence of positive responders did not differ between leukemic patients (53%) and normal controls (66%), but the diameter of the skin reaction was significantly smaller in the leukemic group. In a recent study, 30 to 40% of children with ALL on maintenance therapy developed positive delayed hypersensitivity responses to primary sensitization with picryl chloride and dinitrofluorobenzene and to common recall antigens (70). The proportion of positive responders was higher in children receiving intermittent chemotherapy than in the group treated continuously with drugs (70). Two general principles emerge from these studies: (1) suppression of delayed cutaneous hypersensitivity by the same treatment varies markedly between individual patients, and (2) intermittent chemotherapy is less immunosuppressive than continuous intensive therapy.

Suppression of in vitro lymphocyte blastogenesis by short-term courses of chemotherapy has been amply documented (44, 53, 55). There are also a few studies on the effects of long term combination antileukemic therapy (7, 17, 37). Maintenance treatment of children with ALL in remission who were given mercaptopurine, methotrexate, and cyclophosphamide, either cyclically (7) or together in combination (17), did not significantly alter in vitro lymphocyte stimulation by PHA. All these patients had been treated for less than 3 years and most of them for less than one year. Contrasting with these results, lymphocyte response to PHA was significantly depressed in children who had been treated continuously with the same drug combination for 3 years (37). These data suggest that impairment of lymphocyte function may be cumulative and related to the duration of maintenance chemotherapy. In vitro blastogenic response to PHA may not be a very sensitive test, particularly if stimulation is not investigated as a function of PHA dose. Most children with ALL in remission who had not received craniospinal irradiation and were treated with mercaptopurine and methotrexate had lymphocytes that responded normally to PHA. However, antibody-dependent lymphocyte cytotoxicity was impaired in all patients (20).

Infectious diseases in children with cancer and particularly in childhood leukemia have been the subject of several excellent reports (46, 48, 84) and will not be discussed in detail here. It should be emphasized that the causes of severe, fatal infections are different in children with ALL in relapse and remission correlating with their different type of immunoimpairment. In patients with active disease an absolute neutrophil count of less than $500/mm^3$ is the herald of serious infections, and the most frequently encountered etiological agents in children who died in relapse are *Pseudomonas aeruginosa, Escherichia coli, Staphylococcus aureus,* and *Candida albicans* (46).

By contrast, death due to infections during remission of childhood ALL does not correlate with granulocytopenia and the primary causes of death are nonbacterial infections, including *Pneumocystis carinii,* herpesviruses, cytomegalovirus, and toxoplasmosis (84). Among these etiological factors, *Pneumocystis carinii* has been extensively investigated during recent years (47, 49, 50). This organism does not affect normal individuals, but induces a severe, bilateral alveolar pneumonitis in children with congenital immunological disorders, in patients receiving immunosuppressive therapy for malignancies or organ transplantation and in debilitated infants (49), (Fig. 4). The epidemiology of disease and factors that might predispose children with ALL in remission to *P. carinii* pneumonitis are poorly understood. Analysis of available data would suggest, that this disease occurs as a result of a severe combined immunodeficiency, involving both T and B lymphocytes, which is mediated by the direct effects of the immunosuppressive agents and by secondary protein-calorie malnutrition (38, 49, 50).

3. Immunocompetence After Cessation of Therapy

There is no evidence that prolonging the maintenance phase of therapy beyond 3 years would change the long term prognosis of childhood ALL. Thus, the treatment is currently stopped after 3 years of continuous complete remission (4, 75). Of 315 consecutive children with ALL

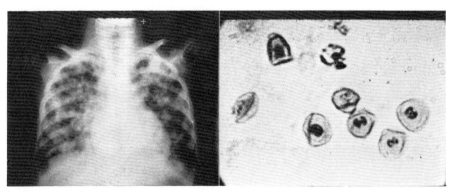

Fig. 4. Chest   roentgenogram   demonstrates   extensive   bilateral   alveolar pneumonitis in a child with ALL in remission. The right-hand side shows *Pneumocystitis carinii* organisms obtained from lung aspiration and stained with Gomori methenamine silver nitrate.

treated at a single institution 42% had their treatment stopped. Sixteen percent of this group have developed recurrent leukemia, mainly during their first year off therapy, i.e., 4 years after diagnosis (4, 75). Several immunological studies have been performed in these patients, before and at various intervals after cessation of therapy (11, 37, 78, 79). These studies had the following objectives: (1) to establish the kinetics of recovery of different immune cell compartments following 3 years of continuous immunosuppressive treatment, (2) to determine whether immunologic recovery correlates with the duration of leukemia-free survival, and (3) to investigate if alterations of lymphocyte function precede the hematological manifestations of leukemia relapse.

The bone marrow was the first lymphoid compartment to be repopulated after cessation of long term immunosuppressive therapy (11), while blood lymphocytes required 12 months off therapy before reaching normal values (38). Also there was roentgenographic evidence that the nasopharyngeal lymphoid tissue remained smaller than in normal controls, even one year after stopping chemotherapy. Marked bone marrow lymphocytosis develops within the first 4 weeks off treatment, but may persist for several months. This lymphoid population is usually heterogeneous. Although the predominant cells are small lymphocytes, larger and cytomorphologically more immature lymphoid cells are also present. In patients with bone marrow containing 40% or more lymphocytes, this phenomenon may be confused with an early leukemia relapse. Unfortunately, the assay of T and B cell markers is not useful to differentiate between normal lymphoid rebound and leukemia relapse. Seventy to eighty percent of normal bone marrow lymphocytes do not form E rosettes and do not possess mIg (14, 79), and in most children with ALL the leukemic cells have neither of these markers (18, 80). It is possible that in the future this differentiation might be possible by the identification of leukemia-associated antigens which are apparently not expressed by normal lymphoid cells (15, 18, 35).

Serum IgG and IgM rises following cessation of chemotherapy (11). Without immunization or evidence of infection these children also demonstrated a rise in antibody titers to Hong Kong influenza virus, to which they had been exposed during treatment (11). This should always be considered in the serological evaluation of infected children after chemotherapy is stopped. A rise in antibody titers following cessation of immunosuppressive drugs may reflect immunologic rebound to an "old" antigen and not necessarily be a consequence of an active infectious process. In addition, increased antibody titers to leukemia-associated antigens may be simply related to this general and nonspecific rebound of the B cell compartment.

In vitro lymphocyte function recovers promptly after short-term chemotherapy (39, 40, 61). A similar phenomenon was observed when long term maintenance therapy was stopped (37). The *in vitro* blastogenic responses to PHA and various antigens by blood lymphocytes from children with ALL in remission were investigated at various intervals after cessation of treatment (37). The data was analyzed in terms of the percentage of patients whose lymphocytes responded to stimulation and the magnitude of the observed response. The percentage of responders to all mitogens increased after therapy was stopped, but there were no significant changes in the magnitude of response to PHA between on and off-treatment periods. In contrast, the mean *in vitro* responses to KLH, *Candida*, and influenza antigens increased by 6 weeks following cessation of treatment and continued to increase through 13 to 36 weeks. Sequential assays of cells from individual patients demonstrated that the response to any of the mitogens and its variation with time after cessation of treatment was independent of the response to other mitogens. This study provided further information at the cellular level of the immunological rebound that follows cessation of long-term combination chemotherapy. It further emphasizes the need for controls in trials where immunotherapy is given after chemotherapy. Such controls are necessary before one can establish whether the observed responses are specific and secondary to adjuvants and/or tumor cells; or are a reflection of a general and nonspecific post-chemotherapy rebound.

This study on lymphocyte stimulation by mitogens also suggested that various lymphocyte subpopulations have different recovery kinetics. This concept was further substantiated by an analysis on the distribution of lymphocytes with T and B markers in blood and bone marrow (78, 79). During the first months after cessation of therapy there was a rise in bone marrow lymphocytes bearing IgM. However, no changes were detected in the proportion of lymphocytes with IgG or of rosette-forming lymphocytes (T cells) (79). This rise of bone marrow IgM lymphocytes preceded the rebound of B lymphocytes observed in peripheral blood (78). Within 2 to 4 months after cessation of therapy the intensity of fluorescence and the proportion of circulating lymphocytes bearing IgM and IgG increased significantly above normal levels. In contrast, the percentage of T lymphocytes decreased during the same period (78). Animal studies indicate that IgM bearing cells are the precursors of IgG and IgA lymphocytes. It is possible that similar patterns of differentiation are expressed by lymphoid cells during their recovery after prolonged immunosuppression.

In patients with solid tumors and myelogenous leukemia, the rebound that follows cessation of chemotherapy appears to correlate with prognosis (39, 40, 43). Patients who did not respond to chemotherapy failed to show the "rebound overshoot" phenomenon, suggesting that low immunological reactivity may be an indicator of poor prognosis. The data available to date does not permit the same conclusion with regard to childhood ALL. Patients at high risk for leukemia relapse could not be identified by the various parameters of immunologic rebound assayed (37, 78, 79). Moreover, in patients who relapsed there was no indication of lymphocyte impairment before or during bone marrow conversion. The number of patients who have been studied and had relapsed is, however, relatively small. Thus, larger numbers of children with ALL should be studied before one can conclusively establish whether recurrence of the disease may be preceeded by a phase of immune impairment.

SUMMARY

Evaluation of immunocompetence in childhood ALL is complicated by multiple variants and pitfalls. ALL is not a homogenous disease; it includes several clinical entities with different target cells and pathogenesis. Analysis of data should consider the wide range of normal values in childhood, which reflects the development of the immune system. Limited evaluation of a single lymphoid compartment neither provides a complete assessment of complex cell-to-cell interactions nor reflects lymphocyte function in other organs. Interpretation of data is further complicated by the diversity of treatments.

Despite these limitations several general conclusions can be derived from data currently available. Overt impairment of lymphocyte function does not precede the development of ALL. Bacterial infections during active disease are usually secondary to neutropenia whereas nonbacterial infections during remission are related to depression of lymphocytes by chemotherapy. Certain drug combinations preferentially suppress B lymphocytes. Termination of therapy leads to immunologic rebound, characterized by lymphocytosis, antibody production without extrinsic antigenic stimulation and enhanced lymphocyte blastogenic responses. Bone marrow lymphocytosis may be misinterpreted as early leukemic relapse. Assessment of T and B markers on bone marrow cells does not distinguish between these two conditions. There is no evidence that either immune impairment or immunologic rebound correlates with the prognosis of childhood ALL.

ACKNOWLEDGMENTS

The literature review for this chapter ended 15 October 1976 and was supported by Research Grant CA 18602 and Cancer Center Grant CA 17700, from the National Cancer Institute, by American Cancer Society Research Grant IM-100C and by the Faye McBeath Foundation. Leukemia-associated antigens and immunotherapy of childhood leukemia were not included in this review because these subjects are presented in another chapter of this book.

REFERENCES

1. Askenase, P. W., Hayden, B. J., and Gershon, R. K. 1975. Augmentation of delayed-type hypersensitivity by doses of cyclophosphamide which do not affect antibody responses. *J. Exp. Med.* 141: 697–702.

2. Astaldi, G., Massimo, L., Airo, R., and Mori, P. G. 1966. Phytohemagglutinin and lymphocytes from acute lymphocytic leukemia. *Lancet* 41: 1265–1266.

3. Aur, R. J. A., Hustu, H. O., Verzosa, M. J., Wood, A., and Simone, J. V. 1973. Comparison of two methods of preventing central nervous system leukemia. *Blood* 42: 349–357.

4. Aur, R. J. A., Simone, J. V., Hustu, H. O., Verzosa, M. J., and Pinkel, D. 1974. Cessation of therapy in childhood acute lymphocytic leukemia. *N. Engl. J. Med.* 291: 1230–1234.

5. Aur, R. J. A., Simone, J., Hustu, H. O., Walters, T., Borella, L., Pratt, C., and Pinkel, D. 1971. Central nervous system therapy and combination chemotherapy of childhood lymphocytic leukemia. *Blood* 37: 272–281.

6. Baehner, R. L., Neiburger, R. G., Johnson, D. E., and Murrmann, S. M. 1973. Transient bactericidal defect of peripheral blood phagocytes from children with acute lymphoblastic leukemia receiving craniospinal irradiation. *N. Engl. J. Med.* 289: 1209–1213.

7. Bakkeren, J. A. J. M., de Vaan, G. A. M., and Schretlen, E. D. A. M. 1972. Phytohaemagglutinin stimulation of peripheral lymphocytes in children with acute lymphoblastic leukaemia during remission. *Scan. J. Hemat.* 9: 36–42.

8. Berenbaum, M. D. 1965. Immunosuppressive agents. *Brit. Med. Bull.* 21: 140–146.

9. Bodey, G. P., Buckley, M., Sathe, Y. S. 1966. Quantitative relationships between circulating leucocytes and infection in patients with acute leukemia. *Ann. Intern. Med.* 64: 328–337.

10. Borella, L., and Green, A. A. 1972. Sequestration of PHA-responsive cells (T-lymphocytes) in the bone marrow of leukemic children undergoing long-term immunosuppressive therapy. *J. Immunol.* 109: 927–932.

11. Borella, L., Green, A. A., and Webster, R. G. 1972. Immunologic rebound after cessation of long-term chemotherapy in acute leukemia. *Blood* 40: 42–51.

12. Borella, L., and Sen, 1973. T cell surface markers on lymphoblasts from acute lymphocytic leukemia. *J. Immunol.* 111: 1257–1260.

13. Borella, L., and Sen, L. 1974. T- and B- lymphocytes and lymphoblasts in untreated acute lymphocytic leukemia. *Cancer* 34: 646–654.

14. Borella, L., and Sen, L. 1974. The distribution of lymphocytes with T- and B- cell surface markers in human bone marrow. *J. Immunol.* 112: 836–843.

15. Borella, L., Sen, L., and Casper, J. T. 1977. Acute lymphoblastic leukemia (ALL) antigens detected with antisera to E-rosette forming and non-E-rosette forming ALL blasts. *J. Immunol.* 118: 309–315.

16. Borella, L., Sen, L., Dow, L. W., and Casper, J. T. 1977. Cell differen-

tiation antigens versus tumor-related antigens in childhood acute lymphoblastic leukemia (ALL). Clinical significance of leukemia markers, in Recent Trends in the Immunological Diagnosis of Leukemias and Lymphomas. Eds., Thierfelder, S., Rodt, H., Thiel, E., (Springer-Verlag) pp. 77–85.

17. Borella, L., and Webster, R. G. 1971. The immunosuppressive effects of long-term continuation chemotherapy in children with acute leukemia in remission. Cancer Res. 31: 420–426.

18. Brouet, J. C., Valensi, F., Daniel, M. T., Flandrin, G., Preud'Homme, J. L., and Seligmann, M. 1976. Immunological classifications of acute lymphoblastic leukemias: Evaluation of its clinical significance in a hundred patients. Brit. J. Hemat. 33: 319–328.

19. Buckley, R. H., Dees, S. C., and O'Fallan, W. M. 1968. Serum Immunoglobulins. I. Levels in normal children and in uncomplicated childhood allergy. Pediatrics 41: 600–611.

20. Campbell, A. C., Hersey, P., Mac Lennan, I. C. M., Kay, H. E. M., and Pike, M. C. 1973. Immunosuppressive consequences of radiotherapy and chemotherapy in patients with acute lymphoblastic leukaemia. Brit. Med. J. 2: 385–388.

21. Chandra, R. K. 1972. Immunocompetence in undernutrition. J. Pediat. 81: 1194–1200.

22. Chandra, R. K. 1972. Serum immunoglobulin levels in children with acute lymphoblastic leukaemia and their mothers and siblings. Arch. Dis. Childhood 47: 618–624.

23. Cohen, J. J. 1972. Thymus derived lymphocytes sequestered in the bone marrow of hydrocortisone treated mice. J. Immunol. 108: 841–844.

24. Cohen, J. J., Fisbach, M., and Claman, H. N. 1970. Hydrocortisone resistance of graft vs. host activity in mouse thymus, spleen and bone marrow. J. Immunol. 105: 1146–1150.

25. Dritschilo, A., Cassady, J., Camitta, B., Jaffe, N., Paed, D., Furman, L., and Traggis, D. 1976. The role of irradiation in central nervous system and prophylaxis for acute lymphoblastic leukemia. Cancer 37: 2729–2735.

26. Dupuy, J. M., Kourilsky, F. M., Fradelizzi, D., Feingold, N., Jacquillat, C. L., Bernard, J., and Dausset, J. 1971. Depression of immunologic reactivity of patients with acute leukemia. Cancer 27: 323–331.

27. Edelman, R., Suskind, R., and Sirisinha, S. 1973. Mechanisms of defective delayed cutaneous hypersensitivity in children with protein-calorie malnutrition. Lancet 1: 506–509.

28. Epstein, W. L. 1958. Induction of allergic contact dermatitis in patients with the lymphoma-leukemic complex. J. Invest. Derm. 28: 39–42.

29. Faulk, W. P. 1974. Nutrition and immunity. Nature 250: 283–284.

30. Ferguson, A. C., Lawlor, G. J., Neuman, C. G., and Steihm, E. R. 1974. Decreased rosette forming lymphocytes in malnutrition and intrauterine growth retardation. J. Pediat. 85: 717–723.

31. Fleisher, T. A., Luckasen, J. R., Sabad, A., Gehrtz, R. C., and Kersey, J. H. 1975. T and B lymphocyte subpopulations in children. Pediat. 55: 162–165.

32. Franz, M. L., Carella, J. A., and Galant, S. P. 1976. Cutaneous delayed hypersensitivity in a healthy pediatric population: Diagnostic value of diptheria-tetanus toxoids. J. Pediat. 88: 975–977.

33. Freund, R., Rauer, U., and Hitzig, W. H. 1969. Quantitative immuno-globulin. Bestimmungen im laufe langdauernder cytostatischer therapie. *Mschr. Kinderheilk.* 117: 563–569.

34. Gooch, W. M., Fernbach, D. J. 1971. Immunoglobulins during the course of leukemia in children. Effects of various clinical factors. *Cancer* 28: 984–989.

35. Greaves, M. F., Brown, G., Rapson, N. T., and Lister, T. A. 1975. Antisera to acute lymphoblastic leukemia cells. *Clin. Immunol. Immunopath.* 4: 67–84.

36. Green, A. A. 1974. The prognostic value of bone marrow lymphocytes in acute lymphocytic leukemia of childhood. *Cancer* 34: 2009–2013.

37. Green, A. A., and Borella, L. 1973. Immunologic rebound after cessation of long-term chemotherapy in acute leukemia. II. *In vitro* response to phytohemagglutinin and antigens by peripheral blood and bone marrow lympho-cytes. *Blood* 42: 99–110.

38. Green, A. A., Sen, L., and Borella, L. 1975. Acute lymphocytic leukemia: a disease of lymphoid cells? *In* L. F. Sinks and J. O. Godden (eds.), *Conflicts in Childhood Cancer*, p. 69. Alan Liss, New York.

39. Harris, J., Sengar, D., Stewart, T., and Hyslop, D. 1976. The effect of immunosuppressive chemotherapy on immune function in patients with ma-lignant disease. *Cancer* 37: 1058–1069.

40. Harris, J. E., and Stewart, T. H. M. 1972. Recovery of mixed lymphocyte reactivity (MLR) following cancer chemotherapy in man, *in*, M. R. Schwarz (ed.), *Proceedings of the Sixth Leucocyte Culture Conference*, p. 555. Academic Press, New York.

41. Heath, R. B., Fairley, G. H., and Malpas, J. S. 1964. Production of an-tibodies against viruses in leukaemia and related diseases. *Brit. J. Haemat.* 10: 365–370.

42. Hersh, E. M. 1974. Immunosuppressive agents, *in* A. C. Sartorelli and D. G. Johns (eds.), *Handbook of Experimental Pharmacology XXXVIII. Antineoplas-tic and Immunosuppressive Agents*, pp. 577–617. Springer-Verlag, Berlin-Heidelberg, New York.

43. Hersh, E. M., Gutterman, J. U., Mavligit, G. M., Mountain, C. W., McBride, C. M., Burgess, M. A., Lurie, P. M., Zelen, M., Takita, H., and Vincent, R. G. 1976. Immunocompetence, immunodeficiency and prognosis in cancer, *in* H. F. Fried-man and C. Southam (eds.), *International Conference on Immunobiology of Cancer*, pp. 386. New York Academy of Sciences, New York.

44. Hersh, E. M., and Oppenheim, J. J. 1967. Inhibition of *in vitro* lymphocyte transformation during chemotherapy in man. *Cancer Res.* 27: 98–105.

45. Hersh, E. M., Whitecar, J. P., McCredie, K. B., Bodey, G. P., and Freireich, E. J. 1971. Chemotherapy, immunocompetence, immunosuppression and prog-nosis in acute leukemia. *N. Engl. J. Med.* 285: 1211–1216.

46. Hughes, W. T. 1971. Fatal infections in childhood leukemia. *Amer. J. Dis. Child.* 122: 283–287.

47. Hughes, W. T., Feldman, S., Aur, R. J. A., Verzosa, M. S., Hustu, H. O., and Simone, J. 1975. Intensity of immunosuppressive therapy and the incidence of pneumocystitis carinii pneumonitis. *Cancer* 36: 2004–2009.

48. Hughes, W. T., Feldman, S., and Cox, F. 1974. Infectious diseases in children with cancer. *Ped. Clin. N. Amer.* 21: 583–615.

49. Hughes, W. T., Price, R. A., Kim, H., Coburn, T. P., Grigsby, D., and Feldman, S. 1973. Pneumocystis carinii pneumonitis in children with malignancies. *J. Pediat.* 82: 404–415.

50. Hughes, W. T., Price, R. A., Sisko, F., Havron, W. S., Kafatos, A. G., Schonland, M., and Smythe, P. M. 1974. Protein-calorie malnutrition: A host determinant for *P. Carinii* infection. *Amer. J. Dis. Child.* 128: 44–52.

51. Humbert, J. R., Hutter, J. J., Thoren, C. H., and De Armey, P. A. 1976. Decreased neutrophil bactericidal activity in acute leukemia of childhood. *Cancer* 37: 2194–2200.

52. Humphrey, G. B., and Lankford, J. 1973. Inhibition of normal lymphocyte transformation by leukemic serum. *Exp. Hematol.* 1: 276–281.

53. Humphrey, G. B., Nesbit, Jr., M. E., Chary, K. K. V., Krivit, W. 1972. Impaired lymphocyte transformation in leukemic patients after intensive therapy. *Cancer* 29: 402–406.

54. Humphrey, G. B., Peterson, L., Whalen, M., Parker, D. E., Lankford, J., Krivitt, W., and Nesbit, M. 1975. Lymphocyte transformation in leukemic serum. *Cancer* 35: 1341–1345.

55. Jones, L. H., Hardisty, R. M., Wells, D. G., Kay, H. E. M. 1971. Lymphocyte transformation in patients with acute lymphoblastic leukemia. *Brit. Med. J.* 4: 329.

56. Kalwinsky, D. K., Urmson, J. R., Stitzel, A. E., and Spitzer, R. E. 1976. Activation of the alternative pathway of complement in childhood acute lymphoblastic leukemia. *Lab. Clin. Med.* 88: 745–756.

57. Kaplan, J., and Peterson, W. D. 1976. Null cell lymphoblastic leukemia is a malignancy of immature B lymphocytes. *Proc. Amer. Assoc. Cancer Res.* 17: 132.

58. Kiran, O., and Gross, S. 1969. The G-immunoglobulins in acute leukemia in children. *Blood* 33: 198–206.

59. Kourilsky, F. M., Lovric, L., and Levacher, A. 1966. Phytohemagglutinin and lymphocytes from acute leukemia. *Lancet* 2: 856–857.

60. LaGrange, P. H., Mackaness, G. B., and Miller, T. E. 1974. Potentiation of T-cell mediated immunity by selective suppression of antibody formation with cyclophosphamide. *J. Exp. Med.* 139: 1529–1535.

61. Larson, D. L., and Tomlinson, L. J. 1953. Quantitative antibody studies in man. III. Antibody response in leukemia and other malignant lymphomata. *J. Clin. Inv.* 32: 317–321.

62. Law, D. K., Dudrick, S. J., and Abdou, N. I. 1973. Immunocompetence of patients with protein-calorie malnutrition. *Ann. Intern. Med.* 79: 545–550.

63. Lerman, S. P., and Weidanz, W. P. 1970. The effect of cyclophosphamide on the ontogeny of the humoral immune response in children. *J. Immunol.* 105: 614–619.

64. Lichtenfeld, J. L., Wiernik, P. H., Mardiney, M. R., and Zarco, R. M. 1976. Abnormalities of complement and its components in patients with acute leukemia, Hodgkin's disease and sarcoma. *Cancer Res.* 36: 3678–3680.

65. Makinodan, T., Albright, J. F., Perkins, E. H., and Nettersheim, P. 1965. Suppression of immunologic responses. *Med. Clin. N. Amer.* 49: 1569–1596.

66. Mauer, A. M., and Simone, J. V. 1976. The current status of the treatment of childhood acute lymphoblastic leukemia. *Cancer Treat. Rev.* 3: 17–41.

67. McKelvey, E. M., and Carbone, P. P. 1965. Serum immune globulin concentrations in acute leukemia during intensive chemotherapy. *Cancer* 18: 1292–1296.

68. Mills, B., Sen, L., and Borella, L. 1975. Reactivity of anti-human thymocyte serum with acute leukemic blasts. *J. Immunol.* 115: 1038–1044.

69. Ogra, P. L., Sinks, L. F., and Karzon, D. T. 1971. Poliovirus antibody response in patients with acute leukemia. *J. Ped.* 79: 444–449.

70. Oldham, R. K., Weiner, R. S., Mathe, G., Breard, L., Simmler, M., Carde, P., and Herberman, R. B. 1976. Cell-mediated immune responsiveness of patients with acute lymphocytic leukemia in remission. *Int. J. Cancer* 17: 326–337.

71. Penn, J., and Starzl, T. E. 1972. Malignant tumors arising de-novo in immunosuppressed organ transplant recipients. *Transplantation* 14: 407–410.

72. Pinkel, D., Hustu, H. O., Aur, R. J. A., Smith, K., Borella, L., and Simone, J. 1977. Radiotherapy in leukemia and lymphoma of children. *Cancer* 39: 817–824.

73. Poulter, L. W., and Turk, J. L. 1972. Proportional increase in the θ carrying lymphocytes in peripheral lymphoid tissue following treatment with cyclophosphamide. *Nature New Biol.* 238: 17–18.

74. Ragab, A. H., Lindquist, K. J., Vietti, T. J., Choi, S. C., and Osterland, C. K. 1970. Immunoglobulin pattern in childhood leukemia. *Cancer* 26: 890–894.

75. Rivera, G., Pratt, C. B., Aur, R. J. A., Verzosa, M., and Hustu, H. O. 1976. Recurrent childhood lymphocytic leukemia following cessation of therapy. *Cancer* 37: 1679–1686.

76. Sahiar, K., and Schwartz, R. S. 1964. Inhibition of 19S antibody synthesis by 7S antibody. *Science* 145: 396–397.

77. Santos, G. W. 1967. Immunosuppressive drugs I. *Fed. Proc.* 26: 907–913.

78. Sen, L., and Borella, L. 1973. Expression of cell surface markers on T and B lymphocytes after long-term chemotherapy of acute leukemia. *Cell. Immunol.* 9: 84–95.

79. Sen, L., and Borella, L. 1974. Immunological rebound after cessation of long-term chemotherapy in acute lymphocytic leukemia: Changes in distribution of T and B cell populations in bone marrow and peripheral blood. *Brit. J. Haemat.* 27: 477–487.

80. Sen, L., and Borella, L. 1975. Clinical importance of lymphoblasts with T markers in childhood acute leukemia. *N. Engl. J. Med.* 292: 828–831.

81. Sen, L., Mills, B., and Borella, L. 1976. Erythrocyte receptors and thymus-associated antigens on human thymocytes, mitogen-induced blasts and acute leukemia blasts. *Cancer Res.* 36: 2436–2441.

82. Silver, R. T., Utz, J. P., Fakey, J., and Frei, E. 1960. Antibody response in patients with acute leukemia. *J. Lab. Clin. Med.* 56: 634–643.

83. Simone, J., Aur, R. J. A., Hustu, H. O., and Versoza, M. 1975. Acute lymphocytic leukemia in children. *Cancer* 36: 770–774.

84. Simone, J. V., Holland, E., and Johnson, W. 1972. Fatalities during remission in childhood leukemia. *Blood* 39: 759–770.

85. Steihm, E. R. 1973. Immunodeficiency disorders: general considerations, in *Immunologic Disorders in Infants and Children*, E. R. Steihm and V. A. Fulginiti, pp. 145–167. W. B. Saunders, Philadelphia.

86. Stockman, G. D., Heim, L. R., South, M. A., and Trentin, J. J. 1973. Differential effects of cyclophosphamide on the B and T cell compartments of adult mice. *J. Immunol.* 110: 277–282.

87. Strauss, R. B., Paul, B. B., Jacobs, A. A., Simmons, C., and Sbarra, A. J. 1970. The metabolic and phagocytic activities of leucocytes from children with acute leukemia. *Cancer Res.* 30: 480–488.

88. Tsubota, T., Minowada, J., Sinks, L. F., Han, T., and Pressman, D. 1976. Identification of surface marker system in lymphatic leukemias in man. *Proc. Amer. Assoc. Cancer Res.* 17: 73.

89. Wu, L. Y. F., Blanco, A., Cooper, M. D., and Lawton, A. R. 1976. Ontogeny of B- lymphocyte differentiation induced by pokeweed mitogen. *Clin. Immunol. Immunopath.* 5: 208–217.

90. Yoshikawa, S., Yamada, K., and Yoshida, T. 1969. Serum complement level in patients with leukemia. *Int. J. Cancer* 4: 845.

CHAPTER 5

IMMUNOLOGICAL ASPECTS OF CHILDHOOD LEUKEMIA

Martin J. Murphy, Jr.,
and Mahroo Haghbin

Memorial Sloan-Kettering
Cancer Center
New York, New York 10021

Although there is little doubt that some human acute leukemic cells have tumor-associated antigens, most of the antisera are neither specific nor are they characterized. The identification and complete characterization of specific leukemia antigens will be powerful tools to immunological classification of the leukemias.

Most patients with acute leukemia have relatively normal humoral and cell mediated immunity. With the introduction of chemotherapy, both B and T cell functions are suppressed, with B cells depressed to a greater extent. Continuous uninterrupted chemotherapy is more immunosuppressive than intermittent treatment. Neuroaxis irradiation also depresses immune functions. Correlation between immunocompetence and prognosis is still conjectured. After cessation of prolonged chemotherapy, there is an immune recovery period which extends up to twelve months, initially with a rise in bone marrow B lymphocytes.

INTRODUCTION

Acute leukemia, the most common neoplasm in children, has become a subject of increasing immunological investigation in recent years. This is because, during the past decade, the modern treatment of acute leukemia has resulted in a high proportion of children surviving continuously free of leukemia for five to ten years (42, 95). Since acute lymphoblastic leukemia is the predominant type of pediatric leukemia, most of this chapter will be devoted to the laboratory and clinical information concerning immunological aspects of childhood acute lymphoblastic leukemia. Our treatment of the accumulated information will be divided into three broad categories:

I. Immunological classification of acute lymphoblastic leukemia, including an analysis of immune competence prior to the institution of chemotherapy.
II. Effect of antileukemia therapy on immune responses.
III. Immunotherapy which mainly reviews studies utilizing *Bacillus Calmette Guerin* (BCG).

IMMUNOLOGICAL CLASSIFICATION OF ACUTE LYMPHOBLASTIC LEUKEMIA

Null Lymphoblastic and T Lymphoblastic Variants

The identification and differentiation of markers borne by lymphocytes, namely "T lymphocytes" (i.e., thymus-dependent) and "B lymphocytes" (i.e., thymus-independent), define the cell's origin. It has been speculated that the leukemias and lymphomas might be classifiable on the basis of their surface markers, and a reassessment of the pathogenesis of human lymphoproliferative neoplasia is progressing (1, 6, 11, 12, 16, 71, 89, 93). As noted in a recent editorial (34), acute lymphoblastic leukemia is a heterogeneous disease when evaluated on clinical presentation, responsivity to chemotherapy, and prognosis. Since Minowada et al. (75) observed that lymphoblasts from a cell line established from a patient with acute lymphoblastic leukemia had surface characteristics of T lymphocytes, investigators have attempted to determine whether all child-hood forms of this disease represent a malignant proliferation of T or B cells.

Most patients with this type of leukemia have lymphoblasts which are termed "null" cells since they neither express surface markers for B lym-phoblasts (1, 19, 24, 25, 33, 71, 93) nor T lymphoblasts (1, 6, 11, 12, 16, 19, 24, 25, 33, 59, 71, 93). Only very rarely have B lymphoblasts been iden-tified in acute lymphoblastic leukemia (33, 89). By contrast, approxi-mately 20% of all pediatric acute lymphoblastic leukemia patients have T lymphoblasts (14, 19, 59, 92, 98), which form heat-stable rosettes with sheep red blood cells and have two surface antigens characteristic of thymocytes (74).

Recently, Sen and Borella (92) have, on the basis of these observa-tions, proposed that there are two types of acute lymphoblastic leukemia in children and adolescents: (1) null cell and (2) T cell. Their thesis has, in the main, received support from other investigators (94, 98) and confirms and extends earlier observations (19, 59). Patients evidencing the T cell type usually present with a high white blood cell count, some with mas-sive leukemic infiltration, anterior mediastinal masses, and tend to be older. Sen and Borella (92) intimate that the "thymic" type of acute lym-phoblastic leukemia is more prevalent in boys, but this has been disputed (14). Although these patients initially respond to treatment, they fre-quently relapse within a year, with an overall unfavorable prognosis (44, 61, 92). Sen and Borella (92) suggest that lymphoblastic lymphoma and acute lymphoblastic leukemia with rosette-forming blast cells (i.e., the "thymic" or T lymphoblast variant) are similar diseases and that new developments in the treatment of one may also be efficacious to the other. The leukemic lymphoblasts of the remaining eighty percent of children with acute lymphoblastic leukemia do not have detectable cell surface immunological markers (i.e., the "null" cell variety). These patients are usually younger and present with an initially low white blood cell count and only rarely display a thymic shadow (i.e., a mediastinal or thymic mass). The sex ratio is equal. The majority of these patients remain leukemia-free after currently employed treatment.

In conclusion, acute lymphoblastic leukemia in children may be di-vided into (1) "thymic" or (2) "null cell" varieties, which are not only different in origin and possibly in pathogenesis, but moreover different with respect to their clinical features and prognosis. These cell surface immunological markers may be of more than mere descriptive value. One group of investigators has already indicated that a different approach to therapy should be considered for patients with the T lymphoblast variant at the time of diagnosis (98).

Leukemia Antigens

The evidence which indicates that human acute leukemic cells have tumor-associated antigens, and that patients may have humoral and cell-mediated immune reactions against these antigens, has already been extensively reviewed (45, 48, 82). Although studies on leukemias in experimental animals support the proposition that tumor cells may contain a complex variety of antigens, viral and virus-induced antigens, fetal antigens, tissue antigens, including tumor-associated transplantation and other cell surface antigens, differentiation antigens, and other normal antigens which may be expressed in higher quantities in tumor cells (47), it is not within the purview of this chapter to discuss these experimental model systems.

A number of leukemia-associated antigens in man, recognized by antibodies of normal human sera (7) or by heteroantisera raised in different species (3, 8, 14, 15, 22, 37, 65, 72, 73, 76), have been described. Since most of these antisera are neither specific nor are they characterized, the literature is also rife with contradictions. The identification and complete characterization of specific leukemic antigens are essential if these serological reagents are to meaningfully aid in immunological classification of the leukemias and if any rational immunotherapeutic measures are to be initiated in the treatment of leukemia.

There has been a steady advance toward a more complete utilization of various heteroantisera which potentially define leukemia-associated antigens (45, 82). The future usage of these heteroantisera as a routine screening procedure may prove of considerable diagnostic, if not prognostic, potential. Examples of such studies follow.

Grieves et al. (37) reported on the usage of antiserum to acute lymphoblastic leukemic cells that were produced by the inoculation of rabbits with acute lymphoblastic leukemic lymphoblasts coated in vitro with rabbit antibodies to normal lymphocytes. This serum did not react with normal lymphocytes and was able to differentiate a subgroup of acute lymphoblastic leukemic cases from other acute leukemias. The same authors recently have reported on further studies which claim definition of three distinct antigens on acute lymphoblastic leukemic cells, one of which is probably leukemia specific (15). Such a demonstration augers well for potential diagnostic value of such sera and the possibility of more accurate identification of rare leukemic cells in the marrow of patients considered in remission.

An antigen common to leukemic cells and normal thymus tissue has also been described (21, 22, 23, 56). The greatest amounts of this antigen, designated "HThy-L," were detected by immunodiffusion in normal thymocytes and the T lymphoblasts from acute lymphoblastic leukemic patients (22). HThy-L has not been found in extracts of normal peripheral blood nucleated cells. Recently, Chechik and Gelfand (22) reported that the HThy-L antigen was detected in sera from four patients with E-rosette-positive (i.e., T lymphoblastic) untreated acute lymphoblastic leukemia and one patient with previously treated acute myelogenous leukemia. Furthermore, there was a correlation between the HThy-L positivity and that of a poor prognosis. The salient feature of these studies was the disappearance of HThy-L antigenemia with treatment which was coincident with a decrease in the number of leukemia blast cells in the peripheral blood. Furthermore, the HThyl-L antigen was not detected in the sera of the remaining 22 patients with E-rosette-negative (i.e., null lymphoblastic) acute lymphoblastic leukemia and 7 patients with acute myelogenous leukemia. This exemplifies another one of the prospects whereby screening, monitoring, and even guiding of therapy might pivot about the fulcrum of leukemia antigen(s).

A recent study did not investigate cell-bound leukemia antigen but rather studied soluble immune complexes in the blood of children with untreated acute lymphoblastic leukemia. Jose et al. (56) acknowledged that the assessment of the immune capacity of patients with acute leukemia at diagnosis is technically compromised by the presence of peripheral blood blast cells leading to conflicting results. Attempts to define acellular leukemia-specific molecules (e.g., antibodies) or complexes has received attention. Doré et al. (27) detected antibodies to leukemia antigens in only 12 of 51 patients, while others have only seen demonstrable antibodies during remission (7, 26). Furthermore, serum from 8 of 19 newly diagnosed patients with acute myeloid leukemia and 1 of 5 patients with acute lymphoblastic leukemic blocked autologous blastogenesis to leukemic antigens, and this presence of blocking was indicative of a good prognosis (41).

In an attempt to extend the immunologic assessment of patients with acute leukemia at diagnosis and to then correlate the results of these investigations with the patients' own response to treatment, Jose et al. (56) analyzed lymphoid cell population and *soluble immune complexes* in the blood of 49 children with untreated acute lymphoblastic leukemia at diagnosis. The results of these immunologic investigations were correlated with the duration of first remission and survival (i.e., median follow-up time was 16 months, with a range of 10 to 37 months). The principal unfavorable findings at diagnosis were absolute numbers of T lymphoid cells outside the range of 850–2500/μl of peripheral blood (i.e., comparable to control values), an inability to respond *in vitro* to phytohemagglutinin, the presence of free leukemic blast cell membrane antigen in serum, and a low titer of complexed antibody. Of the 14 patients who showed two or more of the above itemized unfavorable findings at diagnosis, 11 have died, while only 4 of 35 with one or no immunologic abnormalities have died. Again, these criteria correlated with the clinical criteria for a poor prognosis (e.g., high white blood cell count at diagnosis). These results further bolster the contention that children who respond poorly to antileukemia therapy have profound immunologic abnormalities.

In summary, a revised classification of acute lymphoblastic leukemia based on enzymatic, antigenic, and immunologic serum soluble and cell surface marker difference may soon be in order. At the very least, we can say that the previously unrecognized cellular heterogeneity of acute lymphoblastic leukemia bears out the clinical heterogeneity of this disease (or these diseases?). At best we can speculate that the biological implications of this heterogeneity may be at the core of clonal neoplastic transformation and proliferation.

EFFECT OF ANTILEUKEMIA TREATMENT ON IMMUNE RESPONSES

Significant advances in the control of acute leukemia through the administration of multiple chemotherapeutic agents have led to an assessment of the immunologic status of patients undergoing chemotherapy. The interest stems from the fact that antileukemia drugs are potent immunosuppressive agents and that the number of fatal infections during remission has risen in recent years (96). In addition, abrogation of immunocompetence in patients with leukemia is an undesirable side effect, especially if tumor immunity plays a role in the nascent control of this disease (17, 97).

Immune status of pediatric leukemia patients has been evaluated during the phase of treatment as well as during the post-treatment recovery phase. To facilitate the analysis of these data, the two phases will be discussed separately.

Immune Status of Children with Acute Leukemia on Chemotherapy

The reader is referred to review articles describing the characteristic immunosuppressive properties of individual antileukemia agents (49, 62, 88). Many studies which will be discussed have been conducted in patients receiving multiple drug therapy and their analysis embraced both humoral and cellular immunity.

Humoral Immunity

Serum Immunoglobulin. Among the immunoglobulins, IgG, IgM, and IgA are those that have been measured in patients with acute leukemia. In a group of 6 adults and 28 children with acute lymphoblastic leukemia, McKelvey and Carbone (69) found that by the fourth week of induction therapy the mean serum IgG level dropped to 7.2 mg/ml from the normal range (i.e., 12 mg/ml) in the pretreatment phase. By the ninth week of induction therapy serum IgG levels moderately rose, and by the twentieth week the mean IgG value reached 9.5 mg/ml. Serum IgA levels did not change from the low initial value throughout the treatment course. Serum IgM levels were unaffected by the treatment and, if anything, the mean value tended to rise during the later weeks of therapy. Serum immunoglobulin levels were evaluated according to the chemotherapy regimen (i.e., methotrexate alone vs. combination of methotrexate, 6-mercaptopurine, prednisone, and vincristine for induction as well as maintenance). The fall in the level of serum IgG following induction therapy was similar for both regimes, but the group who were treated with methotrexate alone subsequently rose to a higher level.

Kiran and Gross (60) evaluated only the IgG values in 29 children with acute lymphoblastic leukemia at different phases of disease. The measurements were performed prior to and during remission induction, through the maintenance regimes and at the terminal stage of leukemia. In the seven newly diagnosed children who received prednisone and vincristine, there was a significant drop in the IgG levels after five weeks of treatment, compared to the values obtained at the outset ($P < 0.05$). In thirteen patients on continuous chemotherapy with one of the three drugs (i.e., methotrexate, 6-mercaptopurine, or cyclophosphamide) normal IgG levels persisted. Change of therapy was associated with a decline in the level of IgG. Six children were evaluated at the terminal stage of the disease, when their leukemia was no longer responsive to drug therapy and their serum IgG showed the lowest titer.

Ragab et al. (86) serially examined immunoglobulin determinations in children with acute lymphoblastic leukemia over a 16-month interval. In 12 children receiving initial therapy with prednisone and vincristine, there was a statistically significant decline in all three immunoglobulin titers at five weeks when compared to their pretreatment levels. Serum IgG declined lower than IgM and IgA, and the difference in IgG levels between pre- and post-treatment was significant at $P < 0.001$. The influence of disease status on immunoglobulin values was surveyed in two groups of children in this study. One group consisted of nineteen patients who were in continuous remission during the survey; the other was composed of forty who had at least one relapse during the same interval necessitating a change of therapy. In multiple determinations within both groups, the difference between IgG levels in continuous and short-term remission was significant. Serum IgG values were depressed in the short remission patients, but IgM and IgA levels were comparable to those in continuous remission. A change in the disease status from remission to relapse was not reflected in the immunoglobulin measurement, unless there was an alteration of the chemotherapy regime.

Gooch and Fernbach (35) examined the relationship between immunoglobulin values and clinical factors such as infection in the course of acute lymphoblastic leukemia. Serial determinations were performed in 19 children from the time of diagnosis to an average of 48 weeks. In 10/19 patients, Ig G fell to a mean of 43% below the pretreatment value during the first 4 weeks of chemotherapy. For the other two immunoglobulin classes studied, the depression was less frequent: IgA dropped in 7/19 and IgM declined in 4/19. Approximately half of the children whose immunoglobulin levels did not decline in the first 4 weeks of treatment also had infection at the time of diagnosis or within this interval, indicating an ability to mount an immunoglobulin response to infection. Of the 41 episodes of apparent infection during the course of study, 28 were associated with an increase in one or more immunoglobulin classes.

From these observations it can be concluded that in children with acute leukemia immunoglobulin levels are within the normal range at the time of diagnosis. Following induction chemotherapy, there is a temporary fall, most notably of IgG. During the maintenance regime, and while in continuous remission, immunoglobulin levels do not differ significantly from normal. Relapse does not alter the titers of the immunoglobulins, but a decline accompanies a change in chemotherapy. The ability to produce immunoglobulins in response to infection is retained in acute leukemia. The lowest immunoglobulin values throughout the course of the disease are seen in terminally ill patients whose leukemia is no longer sensitive to chemotherapy.

ANTIBODY RESPONSE   There are few studies concerning antibody response to viral or bacterial infections in children with acute leukemia. The earlier reports deal with groups in which children and adults were combined. Silver et al. (94) examined the antibody response of 10 patients composed of adults and children with either lymphoblastic or nonlymphoblastic leukemia.

The antigens given during the course of antimetabolite therapy were: typhoid, paratyphoid, influenza type A, mumps, diphtheria, and tetanus toxoid. Nine of the ten patients had a four-fold rise in antibody to at least one of the administered antigens, but the response was lower than the normal control subjects. Heath *et al.* (46) immunized 8 patients with acute leukemia receiving 6-mercaptopurine. The antibody rise to influenza A and B in this population was found to be comparable to that of normal subjects, contrary to an earlier study (94).

Hersh *et al.* (50) surveyed the suppression and recovery of the antibody response in patients with leukemia who were receiving intensive five day courses of either 6 mercaptopurine or methotrexate. Sixteen patients ranging in age from four to forty-five years (median: six years old) were evaluated; fifteen had lymphoblastic and one chronic granulocytic leukemia. Primary antibody response was measured after stimulation with three different antigens. When antigen was given twenty-four hours after the start of therapy, there was antibody rise in only 10/16. In contrast, 16/16 developed antibody in response to a different antigen, when it was administered 24 hours after the cessation of chemotherapy, but the median titers were lower than normal. Of the 14 patients who received a third antigen 72 hours following termination of therapy, ten reacted with a median antibody titer comparable to the normal controls.

Ogra *et al.* (78) examined the primary and secondary antibody responses to poliovirus vaccine (only type I poliovirus antibody was measured) in children with acute lymphoblastic leukemia who were receiving chemotherapy. Of the 10 who had primary immunization with inactivated polio virus, IgG antibodies were detected in low levels in 6, and none had IgA or IgM response. The preexisting antibodies were assayed in 13 children who had live polio vaccine 2 to 5 years prior to the diagnosis of leukemia. In this group, IgG poliovirus antibody was detectable only in four, and below the values of normal control children. In regard to the IgM antibody, no activity was found, and IgA was present in 1/13. After reimmunization, there was a three- to four-fold increase in the IgG antibody in those with pre-existing titers; an incremental increase similar to the control group of children.

There was no change in the IgA level, and in only one child a short-lived IgM antibody activity was detected. The investigation did not find any relationship between the disease status (i.e., remission or relapse) and antibody response. Dupuy *et al.* (28) examined the secondary response to the three strains of poliovirus vaccine administered at different stages of leukemia treatment. The study group consisted of both adult and pediatric cases having either lymphoblastic or nonlymphoblastic leukemia. During the induction phase the vaccine was given to 30 patients within the first 3 days of the initial therapy. Only 15/30 responded to any of the three strains, while in the control subjects, 24/26 showed antibody increase at least to one virus strain. Twelve patients who were on maintenance therapy and in remission for over a year were immunized. In this group, 10/12 had a significant antibody rise to at least one polio virus type. Eleven patients were given the vaccine on the first day of their reinduction course (which involved a change of chemotherapy drugs) during maintenance program. In this population (average remission duration of thirteen months), only 6/11 showed an increased antibody titer.

Borella and Webster (13) studied the primary and secondary antibody responses in children with acute lymphoblastic leukemia who were in continuous remission on long-term chemotherapy. Twenty patients receiving maintenance therapy for 8 to 28 months were investigated for their antibody titers to Hong Kong influenza virus. Antibodies to hemagglutinin antigen (primary response to Hong Kong virus) and neuraminidase antigen (secondary response, because of prior exposure to other types of influenza virus) were measured and compared with that of normal children. The control group responded to both antigenic determinants of the virus, while among the leukemia children 5 failed to produce antibodies to the hemagglutinin determinant and two did not produce antibody to the neuraminidase determinant.

At the peak of the antibody response, the mean hemagglutination inhibition titer of the leukemia children was at least ten-fold lower than that of the controls. The antibody response to the hemagglutinin antigenic determinant was more depressed than to the neuraminidase. Primary IgG antibody response was depressed to a greater extent than IgM in leukemic children, as was shown by inactivation with 2-mercaptoethanol. Secondary antibodies were mainly 2-mercaptoethanol resistant (IgG). The suppression of IgG antibody production during the course of chemotherapy has been observed with other antigens (87). In a group of children with acute lymphoblastic leukemia on drug therapy who were immunized with a lipopolysaccharide vaccine derived from seven immunotypes of *Pseudomonas aeruginosa,* the antibody production was mostly of IgM variety (43). From these studies, it can be concluded that patients with acute leukemia are capable of antibody production during their treatment course, but it differs in quantity and quality from that of the normal population. Primary antibody formation is not only lower but it is mainly of the IgM class; anamnestic antibody response shows less deviation from normal in both these respects. The quantity of antibody production is influenced by the timing of the antigenic stimulus in relation to the chemotherapy schedule.

Cell-Mediated Immunity

DELAYED HYPERSENSITIVITY REACTION.   Skin testing for the evaluation of cellular immune competence has been performed at different periods in the course of leukemia. Dupuy et al. (28) investigated the delayed hypersensitivity reaction to four recall antigens: Candida, tuberculin, streptokinase, and egg albumin in adults and children with lymphoblastic or nonlymphoblastic leukemia. Of the 50 patients who were tested prior to the treatment, 96% reacted to at least one antigen. However, the number of the positive skin tests observed for each antigen was smaller in the leukemic patients when compared to the normal controls ($P < 0.01$). The mean diameter of erythema for the positive reactions was also smaller in these patients than in the normal controls.

Thirty-two subjects were skin tested during the induction therapy; only three failed to respond, a rate which was similar to the pretreatment group, but the intensity of the reactions was less. Delayed hypersensitivity was abolished in patients who had bone marrow aplasia at the time of testing. Of the 31 who were aplastic as a result of chemotherapy, 8 were anergic, which was a reversal from positive to negative in 5/8. In 39 patients who were on a maintenance regime and in complete remission, the skin test reactivity was similar to the pretreatment group. Duration of remission did not influence the response to the delayed hypersensitivity, but skin testing shortly after institution of reinduction therapy in the maintenance program diminished the intensity of the reaction without changing the rate. Delayed cutaneous hypersensitivity reaction to the membrane extract of the leukemic cells has also been investigated in recent years (4, 63, 81).

Char et al. (20) studied the skin test responses to tumor-associated and common recall antigens in leukemia. The study group consisted of both children and adults afflicted with lymphoblastic (53 patients) and myelogenous (25 patients) leukemia. The patients were examined for reactivity to the membrane extracts of the autologous and allogeneic blasts and remission cells, in addition to the PPD, mumps, Candida, Trichophyton, and streptokinase-streptodornase antigens. Tests were performed between chemotherapy courses, usually 4 or more days following drug cessation. Among the patients with lymphoblastic leukemia 96% reacted to at least one of the recall antigens, the corresponding figure for the myelogenous group was 100%. No significant correlation between disease status, length of survival and skin test reactivity was found. Leukemic patients responded to PPD, mumps, and streptokinase-streptodornase in a similar manner as to the control subjects, but they were less reactive to Trichophyton and Candida antigens. Response to the autologous blast extract correlated with the disease status in both lymphoblastic and myelogenous leukemia, i.e., the reactivity was significantly less during relapse when compared to remission. The extract which was obtained from autologous cells in the course of remission failed to elicit any reactivity in both types of leukemia.

Delayed hypersensitivity response to the extract of allogeneic blast cells also correlated with the disease status. Of a battery of three or four allogeneic cells, marked difference in reactivity was observed with different extracts. Patients with lymphoblastic leukemia were not reactive to myelogenous blast cell preparation; allogeneic remission cell extracts also did not produce any skin reaction.

Cell-mediated immune responses have been also investigated in patients undergoing immunotherapy with BCG (*Mycobacterium bovis*). Leventhal *et al.* (64) studied 16 patients (median age: ten years) with acute lymphoblastic leukemia after remission induction. Nine were receiving BCG plus allogeneic leukemic cells, and seven methotrexate plus allogeneic cells. Both groups were skin tested with PPD, mumps, *Candida*, and streptokinase-streptodornase antigens, in addition to the extracts from autologous and allogeneic blast cells.

Assays for *in vitro* lymphocyte responses consisted of: mixed leukocyte culture, stimulation with phytohemagglutinin, PPD, streptolysin O reagent, smallpox vaccine, and *Candida* antigen. Skin testing revealed an increased reactivity to recall antigens for both groups, and 7/9 patients who had BCG acquired positive PPD reaction. The methotrexate group, which was treated at monthly intervals, showed a cyclic increase in the *in vitro* response of lymphocyte to antigens. The BCG group manifested an enhanced *in vitro* reactivity only to smallpox vaccine. Response to immunizing cells followed the same pattern *in vivo* and *in vitro* as did the response to recall antigens. Oldham *et al.* (80) investigated the cellular immune functions in patients with acute lymphoblastic leukemia during the course of continuous chemotherapy, intermittent chemotherapy, and immunotherapy. Patients ranged in age from 2 to 43 years and all were in remission at the time of study. The continuous chemotherapy group (28 patients) received 6-mercaptopurine plus methotrexate and was in remission for 2 to 3 months. The intermittent chemotherapy group (24 patients) received vincristine and methotrexate every 14 days, and was in remission for 8 to 9 months when tested just prior to the enrollment on immunotherapy. In the immunotherapy group, 6 patients had BCG and allogeneic blast cells for 60 days, 8 for 120 days, and 25 for 2 to 8 years. The tests for delayed hypersensitivity consisted of three recall antigens: PPD, mumps, and *Candida* in addition to 2,4-dinitrofluorobenzene and picryl chloride for primary sensitization. Skin tests with antigens derived from allogeneic lymphoblastoid cell lines were also carried out. *In vitro* lymphocyte stimulation was performed with phytohemagglutinin, pokeweed mitogen and PPD. Lymphocyte cytotoxicity assays were done with leukemic allogeneic blasts as target cells. In response to the recall antigens, 39% of the continuous chemotherapy and 92% of the intermittent chemotherapy group reacted. The corresponding figures for those receiving short-term immunotherapy and long-term immunotherapy were 93% and 100%, respectively. All patients on immunotherapy became responsive to PPD by day sixty, except one who did not react until day 120. Conversion from positive to negative skin tests was observed for mumps and Candida antigens in several patients receiving immunotherapy. Successful sensitization with 2,4-dinitrofluorobenzene was significantly greater in the group on intermittent chemotherapy than in the group on continuous regime. Sensitization with picryl chloride, which was done only in those on immunotherapy, was positive in 71% tested early, versus 33% who were tested later in the course of treatment. In response to the extracts derived from lymphoblastoid cell lines, patients on continuous chemotherapy and short-term immunotherapy failed to react. Those who had intermittent chemotherapy showed a low level of responsiveness, while the best response to these extracts was obtained in long-term immunotherapy groups. All the patients tested on immunotherapy gave a positive in vitro response to PPD. Mitogen stimulation with phytohemagglutinin and pokeweed was lower in both chemotherapy schedules when compared to the immunotherapy regime, and in the latter it did not differ significantly from that of the normal controls. Lymphocyte cytotoxicity toward leukemic blasts was more depressed during continuous chemotherapy than during intermittent chemotherapy while the immunotherapy group had a higher reaction rate compared to the other two groups.

IN VITRO LYMPHOCYTE TRANSFORMATION AND OTHER IMMUNE RESPONSES.

Lymphocyte transformation in response to mitogens has been shown to be depressed with the administration of chemotherapy in acute leukemia. Hersh and Oppenheim (52) studied the effect of high-dose 6-mercaptopurine and methotrexate combination with or without prednisone on lymphocyte transformation in response to phytohemagglutinin and smallpox vaccine. The drug combination was administered to the patients with acute leukemia for 5 to 7 days, and the assays were performed before, during, and after the chemotherapy course.

Lymphocyte transformation was completely abolished after 3 days of treatment, but a substantial recovery took place within three days after the end of treatment. The onset of recovery was prolonged to 25 days if the chemotherapeutic dose was high and the duration of treatment was 7 rather than 5 days. The degree of inhibition of lymphocyte transformation was not correlated with the absolute lymphocyte count except when the lymphocyte count was below 500/cu mm. Treatment with 6-mercaptopurine or methotrexate at doses which did not produce leukopenia took 2 to 5 weeks to cause maximum suppression of lymphocyte transformation. The effect of long-term chemotherapy was studied by Borella and Webster in twenty children with acute lymphoblastic leukemia in remission (13).

At the time of testing, these children were receiving maintenance chemotherapy of 6-mercaptopurine, methotrexate, cyclophosphamide, and periodic prednisone plus vincristine for 8 to 28 months. Lymphocyte transformation was found to be relatively unaffected by this regime. In another study, Borella and Green (9) assayed the response of bone marrow and peripheral blood lymphocytes to phytohemagglutinin in children with lymphoblastic leukemia who were receiving maintenance therapy for 18 to 36 months.

It was found that bone marrow cells in some children had a greater response to phytohemagglutinin than did peripheral blood. This observations may reflect a sequestration of the phytohemagglutinin-responsive cells within the bone marrow during the course of chemotherapy. Bakkeren et al. (5) investigated fourteen children with lymphoblastic leukemia at two different phases of their maintenance regime. Lymphocyte stimulation with phytohemagglutinin was unimpaired while patients were receiving 6-mercaptopurine, methotrexate, and cyclophosphamide. A temporary suppression was observed during the one-week intensive treatment with prednisone, vincristine, and daunorubicin. The testing at this phase was done on the fourth day of therapy and both phytohemagglutinin response and lymphocyte count were low compared to the pre-intensive program.

Campbell et al. (18) studied 57 children with acute lymphoblastic leukemia who had either chemotherapy alone, or chemotherapy plus craniospinal irradiation. These two groups were compared with respect to their lymphocyte functions which were evaluated during the maintenance regime which was 18 months after the initiation of therapy. The lymphocyte counts in both groups were below normal compared to the controls, but those patients who had craniospinal irradiation had a greater depression (i.e., 1400/cu mm in nonirradiated vs. 600/cu mm in irradiated). The lymphocyte response to phytohemagglutinin stimulation was also significantly depressed in the irradiated patients. A higher percentage of lymphocytes had surface immunoglobulin in the irradiated patients than in the nonirradiated group, but there was no difference in the absolute number of stainable cells for immunoglobulins per ml of blood between these two groups. The assay for cytotoxic activity of lymphocytes against antibody sensitized target cells revealed a greater decrease in cytotoxic activity for those children who were receiving chemotherapy alone.

Immunosuppressive effect of craniospinal irradiation has also been demonstrated in other studies. Graham-Pole et al. (36) studied children with leukemia who had cranial or craniospinal irradiation and found that the lymphocytic proliferative response to phytohemagglutinin and pokeweed mitogen was lower for patients treated with craniospinal irradiation than for those in which irradiation was confined to the cranium.

Recently, T and B lymphocyte surface markers have been studied during the course of therapy in acute lymphoblastic leukemia. Esber et al. (32) examined peripheral blood lymphocytes in 28 children with acute lymphoblastic leukemia during different phases of treatment. The mean percent of T and B lymphocytes, which was low at diagnosis, rose during induction therapy. The mean percent of the B lymphocytes upon remission was greater than that of the normal children. This rise was followed by a decline after irradiation to the neuroaxis or other sanctuaries and no subsequent change was observed 3 months later. A fall in the total T lymphocyte count occurred upon remission and was accelerated after administration of radiation therapy; however no significant decrease in T lymphocytes six months after irradiation was noted. The total number of peripheral blood lymphocytes mirrored the pattern of decline and recovery just described for T lymphocytes. A comparison of the total number of the circulating T and B lymphocytes demonstrated a greater reduction of the B lymphocytes with therapy. Irradiation to the neuroaxis and other sanctuary areas caused a greater depression in the number of T and B lymphocytes than did cranial irradiation alone or no irradiation.

From these studies, it can be concluded that chemotherapy suppresses cell mediated immunity, but the effect is temporary and with intermittent chemotherapeutic regimens there is recovery of cell mediated immunity after drug cessation. Established delayed hypersensitivity is more resistant to drug suppression than are de novo reactions. Antileukemia treatment is also associated with a suppression of B lymphocytes which is more marked than T lymphocytes. Patients who receive irradiation to the neuroaxis are more immunosuppressed than those who receive cranial irradiation alone or no therapeutic radiation whatsoever. Neuroaxis irradiation not only affects lymphocyte function, but it also induces a transient bactericidal deficiency of the blood phagocytes in the treated patients (2).

Correlation of Cell-Mediated Immunity with Prognosis

There is suggestive evidence from studies of patients with solid tumors that cell-mediated immune reactivity correlates with prognosis (29, 77, 84). Studies have been conducted to establish whether such a relationship exists in acute leukemia. The results, however, are in conflict. Greene et al. (39) studied sixty-five adults and children with acute nonlymphoblastic leukemia for skin test reactivity to recall antigens as well as to de novo sensitization to dinitrochlorobenzene. Among the patients who reacted to at least one recall antigen, the remission rate was 33%, while in the antigenic nonresponsive group the remission rate was 38%. There was also no correlation in response to de novo hypersensitivity with the frequency of remission. Among those who reacted to the dinitrochlorobenzene, 47% remitted, while the remission rate for nonresponders was 50%. Duration of remission was not correlated to delayed type hypersensitivity responsiveness.

The results of this study (39) are at variance with an earlier report (53), which describe a positive correlation between immunocompetence and response to treatment. Hersh et al. (51) undertook serial studies examining the immunocompetence of 55 adults with acute lymphoblastic and myelogenous leukemia. Immunity was measured by the delayed type hypersensitivity reaction to recall antigens and in vitro lymphocyte blastogenic response to phytohemagglutinin and streptolysin O. There was a good correlation between immunocompetence at the outset of treatment and the attainment of remission. In those who remitted, their immunocompetence declined during the second through the fifth month of treatment and this was followed by partial recovery of immunocompetency by the sixth month. This immune incompetence was more pronounced for patients who had achieved remission but subsequently relapsed. A change from an immunocompetent to immunoincompetent status heralded relapse. The results of this study were particularly striking with regard to the delayed type hypersensitivity tests, and less striking in respect to in vitro lymphocyte blastogenic responsiveness.

Studies have been conducted to compare and, whenever possible to correlate, cell-mediated immune responses to tumor associated antigens with disease status and patient prognosis. Oren and Herberman (81) investigated the cutaneous response of patients with acute leukemia to autologous membrane extract derived from leukemic cells. The rate of positive response for patients with acute lymphoblastic leukemia was 47%, while for acute myelocytic it was 92%. Furthermore, positive intradermal reactivity appeared to correlate with a state of remission.

Leventhal et al. (63) tested the immune reactivity of adults and children with acute leukemia to autologous blast cells with three different assays: (1) mixed leukocyte culture, (2) lymphocyte cytotoxicity, and (3) intradermal inoculation. The results of these three tests were not concordant and only cutaneous reactivity seemed to correlate with the disease status. Char et al. (20) examined 55 patients with acute leukemia for their skin test response to autologous and allogeneic blast extracts. In lymphoblastic leukemia in remission, 20/44 patients with autologous cells were positive, while in myelogenous leukemia, 16/19 patients were positive while in remission. In relapse, the response rate for both types of leukemia was significantly lower. Reaction to autologous blast cells also changed with a change in disease status. The mean length of remission was slightly but not statistically significantly longer in skin-test-positive patients. Gutterman et al. (40) examined the cell-mediated and humoral responses to leukemia cells in adults with acute leukemia. Persistence of positive blastogenic response in remission, presence of immunoglobulin un leukemic cells, and the presence of a serum-inhibitory effect on blastogenic response correlated with a good prognosis. Baker et al. (4) however, did not find a relationship between disease status or attainment of remission in 34 patients with acute leukemia who were skin-tested with autologous blast cells.

Immunologic Recovery After Cessation of Chemotherapy

Lymphocyte functions in acute lymphoblastic leukemia following cessation of treatment have been studied in a number of children. Humphrey et al. (55) measured the lymphocyte response to pokeweed mitogen in 9 children with lymphoblastic leukemia who had completed intensive chemotherapy and central nervous system irradiation. The reactivity of these patients was compared between a group of leukemic children who had not received intensive therapy and a group of normal controls. The blastogenic response of lymphocytes of patients not intensively treated was similar to that of the controls, but in the intensively treated children lymphocyte transformation was impaired one month after the cessation of therapy. In those who had serial evaluations, impaired transformation persisted for 3 months or more. No direct correlation between suppressed response to mitogen and absolute lymphocyte count was found. Borella et al. (10) investigated the lymphocyte count, immunoglobulin values, and antibody production after cessation of treatment. Eighteen children with lymphoblastic leukemia who had chemotherapy for 2½–3 years were studied. Between 4 and 20 weeks after termination of therapy, there was a significant expansion of the lymphocyte compartment in the bone marrow and peripheral blood, the rise beginning earlier in the bone marrow. There was also an increase in the serum IgG and IgM values, the most significant rise being a threefold increase in IgG within 2 months after termination of therapy; IgA titers were unchanged. One-fourth of the children had an antibody elevation to Hong Kong influenza virus, an antigen to which they were exposed through vaccination during chemotherapy. This immunologic rebound was age dependent and it was significantly greater in children whose treatment began under the age of five years.

The functional recovery of lymphocytes in relation to chemotherapy was studied by Green and Borella (38). The *in vitro* blastogenic response of lymphocytes was evaluated, using phytohemagglutinin, Keyhole limpet hemocyanin, *Candida,* and influenza antigens. Forty-two children with lymphoblastic leukemia who had 2½–3 years of chemotherapy were examined before and after cessation of therapy. In the peripheral blood there was no significant change in the magnitude of response to phytohemagglutinin between on and off therapy periods.

In contrast, response to influenza antigens increased at six weeks following termination of treatment and continued to increase up to thirty-six weeks. Simultaneous assays of peripheral blood and bone marrow cells indicated a different pattern of lymphocyte response to phytohemagglutinin and antigens in these two compartments. Peripheral blood lymphocytes showed equal or greater stimulation with phytohemagglutinin when compared to bone marrow lymphocytes although, in 40% of the assays bone marrow lymphocytes were more responsive to antigens than were peripheral blood lymphocytes.

In another study, Sen and Borella (90) investigated the kinetics of lymphocytes bearing surface markers for T and B lymphocytes following cessation of chemotherapy. Rosette formation was used as a marker for T lymphocytes, and surface immunoglobulins as a marker for B lymphocytes. Forty-four children with lymphoblastic leukemia who had three years of chemotherapy were studied on the last day of treatment and at various intervals thereafter. On the last day of therapy, the B lymphocyte population was markedly reduced, but the percentage of T lymphocytes was within the normal ranges. During the first 3 months off therapy, there was an increase in the proportion of immunoglobulin bearing cells (i.e., B lymphocytes), ultimately attaining levels higher than normal controls.

The cellular constituents of this rebound were composed of lymphocytes bearing IgG and IgM but not IgA. A change in the proportion of the rosette-forming cells (i.e., T lymphocytes), as a function of time after treatment cessation, was inversely related to those observed for B lymphocytes: that is, the percentage of T lymphocytes decreased during the first 3 months off therapy. When the absolute numbers of B and T lymphocytes were compared, the authors observed that B lymphocyte numbers increased and then reached a plateau phase by 2 to 3 months, however the number of T lymphocytes continued to rise, only reaching normal levels at twelve months off therapy.

Lymphocyte subpopulations within the bone marrow and in the peripheral blood of children with lymphoblastic leukemia after 2½–3 years of chemotherapy were also studied (91). Surface immunoglobulin and sheep rosette formation were used as markers for identification of B and T lymphocytes. The proportion of IgM- and IgG-bearing cells in the peripheral blood was significantly higher by 2 to 4 months than during the first month or 12 months after chemotherapy, the values at 12 months being similar to those of normal controls. No substantial change was observed during the recovery phase for the proportion of IgA bearing lymphocytes, their percentage being similar to the normal controls. Bone marrow lymphocytes, in contrast to peripheral blood lymphocytes, had a higher percentage of IgM-bearing cells during the first month than at 2 and 12 months after chemotherapy. The percentage of IgM bearing cells was essentially the same in the 2- and 12-month samples. The mean value of bone marrow IgG-bearing cells was significantly lower than the IgM-bearing lymphocytes.

The results suggest that within a month after stopping therapy there is a rebound of bone marrow B lymphocytes bearing IgM which precedes the appearance of IgG-bearing cells in the peripheral blood. Study of the rosette-forming cells in the peripheral blood and bone marrow indicated that the proportion of T lymphocytes in the peripheral blood was lower than the B lymphocytes during the two to four months post-therapy period. The proportion of T lymphocytes was higher in peripheral blood than in bone marrow in all the assays conducted after treatment cessation. No significant change was found in the proportion of T lymphocytes in the bone marrow at different intervals off chemotherapy. The study did not disclose any difference in the B lymphocyte rebound between those children who relapsed and those who continued in complete remission.

From these rather comprehensive studies it can be concluded that there is a recovery of immunocompetence after the cessation of long-term chemotherapy. The recovery is associated with a significant change in the distribution of lymphocyte subpopulations. The earliest change is the repopulation of the bone marrow with lymphoid cells which have a high proportion of IgM-bearing cells. Following the prompt rise of the bone marrow lymphocytes, there is a progressive expansion of the peripheral blood compartment of lymphocytes, reaching normal values approximately twelve months post-chemotherapy. During the 2- to 4-month interval after drug cessation, the increase in the peripheral blood lymphocytes is accompanied by a significant rise in the proportion of IgM- and IgG-bearing cells which exceed normal values. By 12 months, the proportion of B lymphocytes in the peripheral blood is similar to the normal controls. The proliferation of bone marrow lymphocytes with the presence of immature lymphoid cells can be mistaken for early leukemia relapse.

IMMUNOTHERAPY

Based on the experience with transplanted tumors in animals (68, 78), the first efficacious clinical immunotherapy in human leukemia was reported by Mathé et al. (66). Patients with acute lymphoblastic leukemia in remission were given Pasteur BCG by scarification and/or allogeneic blast cells following a course of chemotherapy. Twenty patients received immunotherapy, and ten no treatment after the initial chemotherapy course, as controls. All 10 controls relapsed within 130 days, while 8/20 patients treated with immunotherapy remained in remission up to 1,150 days.

Since 1969, the study has been expanded and recently the results of the treatment of one hundred patients with lymphoblastic leukemia were reported (67). After induction of remission and a course of chemotherapy and irradiation, patients were given Pasteur BCG by scarification technique and pooled, irradiated, allogeneic leukemic cells. During the more than twelve years since the beginning of these studies, no relapses were encountered beyond 3 years. The analysis of the 100 patients according to the cytological classification (e.g., microlymphoblastic, prolymphocytic, macrolymphoblastic, prolymphoblastic) disclosed that the best results of immunotherapy were obtained in the microlymphoblastic type, with an 85% survival at 5 years. In the entire group, no relapses were observed after 48 months. Immunologic monitoring of the patients showed a significant increase in null cells upon administration of immunotherapy (57).

Several attempts have been made to evaluate the efficacy of BCG treatment alone or in combination with administration of allogeneic blast cells for the prolongation of remission in acute lymphoblastic leukemia. In a study conducted by the Medical Research Council in Britain (70), the effect of Glaxo BCG given percutaneously after 5 months of chemotherapy was compared to twice weekly methotrexate for maintenance of remission. Those who received immunotherapy had a shorter length of remission than did the children who had the methotrexate regime.

The Children's Cancer Study Group in the United States (54) undertook an evaluation of immunotherapy with BCG (Research Foundation, Chicago) administered by an intradermal puncture device. Immunotherapy was started after chemotherapy remission induction and 2 or 10 months of continuation chemotherapy. Comparison between the children treated with immunotherapy with those who remained on chemotherapy did not show any benefit from BCG in prolonging the length of remission. Leventhal et al. (64) administered Pasteur BCG by scarification and allogeneic blast cells following chemotherapy-induced remission. Again, BCG failed to enhance the longevity of remission. Ekert et al. (30) used BCG intermittently with chemotherapy for remission maintenance of lymphoblastic leukemia in children. BCG therapy was not begun until at least 12 months after continuous chemotherapy. Follow-up immunologic evaluation indicated improvement in general immunity, but it was not clear whether this was due to interrupted chemotherapy program or immune stimulation from BCG.

The European Organization for Research on Treatment of Cancer also conducted an investigation on the efficacy of BCG in acute lymphoblastic leukemia (31). After one year of chemotherapy patients were randomized to continue chemotherapy or receive BCG scarification and allogeneic cells as immunotherapy. No significant difference in the duration of remission was found between these two groups, but the rate of remission fatalities in chemotherapy treated patients was 12% compared to none for immunotherapy.

Immunotherapy with BCG in acute myelogenous leukemia in adults has not shown convincing beneficial results in all the trials. The most significant benefit was the prolongation of survival in those patients who relapsed during immunotherapy (85).

From these studies it can be concluded that, as currently practiced, the role of immunotherapy in children with acute lymphoblastic leukemia is, at best, tenuous. At present, at least half of the children with lymphoblastic leukemia achieve a five year disease-free survival (95). If immunotherapy is going to make an impact in the treatment of this type of leukemia, it should be reflected in the salvage of those who fail the current chemotherapy regimes.

SUMMARY

Acute lymphoblastic leukemia in children may be divided into (1) "T-cell" or (2) "null-cell" varieties which are not only different in origin and possibly pathogenesis, but moreover different with respect to their clinical features and prognosis.

Although there is little doubt that some human acute leukemic cells have tumor-associated antigens, most of the antisera are neither specific nor are they characterized. The identification and complete characterization of specific leukemia antigens will be powerful tools to immunological classification of the leukemias.

Most patients with acute leukemia have relatively normal humoral and cell mediated immunity at the outset of treatment. With the introduction of chemotherapy, both B and T lymphocyte functions are suppressed with B cells depressed to a greater extent. Continuous uninterrupted chemotherapy is more immunosuppressive than intermittent treatment and neuroaxis irradiation also depresses immune functions. Correlation between immunocompetence and prognosis remains a matter of conjecture. After cessation of prolonged chemotherapy, there is an immune recovery period which extends up to twelve months, initially with a rise in bone marrow B lymphocytes. Further studies of immune responses in patients with acute leukemia should facilitate the design of therapeutic regimes with lesser immunosuppressive effects.

Although there is suggestive clinical evidence that the administration of BCG might prolong the duration of remission in acute lymphoblastic leukemia, the role of immunotherapy in the treatment of leukemia needs to be defined. Further work in tumor immunology should elucidate what immune responses must be stimulated for the destruction of leukemic cells, and when in the course of disease immunotherapy should be introduced.

ACKNOWLEDGMENTS

The literature review for this chapter ended 1 October 1976 and was supported by grants from the USPHS CA-17085, CA-05826, the Jean Shaland Fund, and the Gar Reichman Foundation.

REFERENCES

1. Aiuti, F., Lacava, V., Fiorilli, M., and Ciarla, M. V. 1973. Lymphocyte surface markers in lymphoproliferative disorders. *Acta Haematol. (Basel)* 50: 275–283.

2. Baehner, R. L., Neiburger, R. G., Johnson, D. E., and Murrmann, S. M. 1973. Transient bactericidal defect of peripheral blood phagocytes from children with acute lymphoblastic leukemia receiving craniospinal irradiation. *N. Engl. J. Med.* 289: 1209–1213.

3. Baker, M. A., Ramachandar, K., and Taub, R. N. 1974. Specificity of heteroantisera to human acute leukemia-associated antigens. *J. Clin. Invest.* 54: 1273–1278.

4. Baker, M. A., Taub, R. N., Brown, S. M., and Ramachandar, K. 1974. Delayed cutaneous hypersensitivity in leukaemic patients to autologous blast cells. *Brit. J. Haemat.* 27: 627–634.

5. Bakkeren, J. A. J. M., de Vaan, G. A. M., and Schretlen, E. D. A. M. 1972. Phytohaemagglutinin stimulation of peripheral lymphocytes in children with acute lymphoblastic leukaemia during remission. *Scand. J. Haemat.* 9: 36–42.

6. Belpomme, D., Dantchev, D., Du Rusquec, E., Grandon, D., Huchet, R., Pouillart, P., Schwarzenberg, L., Amiel, J. L., and Mathé, G. 1974. T and B lymphocyte markers on the neoplastic cell of 20 patients with chronic lymphoid leukemia. *Biomedicine* 20: 109–118.

7. Bias, W. B., Santos, G. W., Burke, P. J., Mullins, G. M., and Humphrey, R. L. 1972. Cytotoxic antibody in normal human serums reactive with tumor cells from acute lymphocytic leukemia. *Science* 178: 304–306.

8. Billing, R., and Terasaki, P. I. 1974. Human leukemia antigen. I. Production and characterization of antisera. *J. Natl. Cancer Inst.* 53: 1639–1643.

9. Borella, L., and Green, A. A. 1972. Sequestration of PHA-responsive cells (T-lymphocytes) in the bone marrow of leukemic children undergoing long-term immunosuppressive therapy. *J. Immunol.* 109: 927–932.

10. Borella, L., Green, A. A., and Webster, R. G. 1972. Immunologic rebound after cessation of long-term chemotherapy in acute leukemia. *Blood* 40: 42–51.

11. Borella, L., and Sen, L. 1973. T cell surface markers on lymphoblasts from acute lymphocytic leukemia. *J. Immunol.* 111: 1257–1260.

12. Borella, L., and Sen, L. 1974. T- and B-lymphocytes and lymphoblasts in untreated acute lymphocytic leukemia. *Cancer* 34: 646–654.

13. Borella, L., and Webster, R. G. 1971. The immunosuppressive effects of long-term combination chemotherapy in children with acute leukemia in remission. *Cancer Res.* 31: 420–426.

14. Brouet, J-C., Valensi, F., Daniel, M T., Flandrin, G., Preud'homme, J-L., and Seligmann, M. 1976. Immunological classification of acute lymphoblastic leukemias: Evaluation of its clinical significance in a hundred patients. *Brit. J. Haematol.* 33: 319–328.

15. Brown, G., Capellaro, D., and Greaves, M. F. 1975. Leukemia-associated antigens in man. *J. Natl. Cancer Inst.* 55: 1281–1289.

16. Brown, G., Greaves, M. F., Lister, T. A., Rapson, N., and Papamichael, M. 1974. Expression of human T and B lymphocyte cell surface markers on leukaemic cells. *Lancet* 2: 753–755.

17. Burnet, F. M. 1972. The concept of immunological surveilliance, *in* R. S. Schwartz (ed.), *Progress in Experimental Tumor Research*, Vol. B, pp. 1–27.

18. Campbell, A. C., Hersey, P., Mac Lennan, I. C. M., Kay, H. E. M., and Pike, M. C. 1973. Immunosuppressive consequences of radiotherapy and chemotherapy in patients with acute lymphoblastic leukaemia. *Brit. Med. J.* 2: 385–388.

19. Catovsky, D., Goldman, J. M., Okos, A., Frisch, B., and Galton, D. A. G. 1974. T-lymphoblastic leukaemia: A distinct variant of acute leukaemia. *Brit. Med. J.* 2: 643–646.

20. Char, D. H., Le Pourhiet, A., Leventhal, B. G., and Herberman, R. B. 1973. Cutaneous delayed hypersensitivity responses to tumor-associated and other antigens in acute leukemia. *Int. J. Cancer* 12: 409–419.

21. Chechik, B. E. 1968. O kharaktere serologichskoi blizosti gemotsitoblastov krovi bol'nykh ostrym leikozon i tkani vilochkooi zhelezy plodov cheloveka. *Biull. Eksp. Biol. Med.* 66: 85–88.

22. Chechik, B. E., and Gelfand, E. W. 1976. Leukaemia-associated antigen in serum of patients with acute lymphoblastic leukaemia. *Lancet* 1: 166–168.

23. Chechik, B. E., and Ramonova-Tskhovrebova, O. D. 1967. Analiz antigennoi struktury tkanei i leikotsitov cheloveka pri razlichnykh formakh leikoza i v norme. *Probl. Gemat.* 12: 3–10.

24. Chin, A. H., Saiki, J. H., Trujillo, J. M., and Williams, Jr., R. C. 1973. Peripheral blood T- and B-lymphocytes in patients with lymphoma and acute leukemia. *Clin. Immunol. Immunopathol.* 1: 499–510.

25. Collins, R. D., Smith, J. L., Clein, G. P., and Barker, C. R. 1974. Absence of B- and T-cell markers on acute lymphoblastic leukaemic cells and persistence of the T-cell marker on mitogen-transformed T-lymphocytes. *Brit. J. Haematol.* 26: 615–625.

26. De Carvalho, S. 1964. Identity of reaction of an autologous antibody in leukemic children in remission with a heterologous antibody produced antileukemic antigen. *Proc. Amer. Assoc. Cancer Res.* 5: 14 (Abstract).

27. Doré, J. F., Motta, R., Marholev, L., Hrsak, Y., Colas de la Nove, H., Seman, G., de Vassal, F., and Mathé, G. 1967. New antigens in human leukemic cells and antibody in the serum of leukemic patients. *Lancet* 2: 1396–1398.

28. Dupuy, J. M., Kourilsky, F. M., Fradelizzi, D., Feingold, N., Jacquillat, C. L., Bernard, J., and Dausset, J. 1971. Depression of immunologic reactivity of patients with acute leukemia. *Cancer* 27: 323-331.

29. Eilber, F. R., and Morton, D. L. 1970. Impaired immunologic reactivity and recurrence following cancer surgery. *Cancer* 25: 362-367.

30. Ekert, H., Jose, D. G., Wilson, F. C., Matthews, R. N., and Lay, H. 1975. Intermittent chemotherapy and immunotherapy with BCG in remission maintenance of children with acute lymphocytic leukemia: Effects upon immunological function. *Int. J. Cancer* 16: 103-112.

31. EORTC Hemopathies Working Party. 1976. Immunotherapy in acute lymphoblastic leukemia. *Proc. AACR, ASCO* 17: p. 217.

32. Esber, E., Di Nicola, W., Movassaghi, N., and Leikin, S. 1976. T and B lymphocytes in leukemia therapy. *Amer. J. Hemat.* 1: 211-218.

33. Gajl-Peczalska, K. J., Bloomfield, C. D., Nesbit, M. E., and Kersey, J. H. 1974. B-cell markers on lymphoblasts in acute lymphoblastic leukaemia. *Clin. Exp. Immunol.* 17: 561-569.

34. Gelfand, E. W., and Chechik, B. E. 1976. Unmasking the heterogeneity of acute lymphoblastic leukemia. *N. Engl. J. Med.* 294: 275-276.

35. Gooch, W. M., III, and Fernbach, D. J. 1971. Immunoglobulins during the course of acute leukemia in children. Effects of various clinical factors. *Cancer* 28: 984-989.

36. Graham-Pole, J., Willoughby, M. L. N., Aitken, S., and Ferguson, A. 1975. Immune status of children with and without severe infection during remission of malignant disease. *Brit. Med. J.* 2: 467-470.

37. Greaves, M. E., Brown, G., Rapson, R., and Lister, A. 1975. Antisera to acute lymphoblastic leukemia cells. *Clin. Immunol. Immunopathol.* 4: 67-84.

38. Green, A. A., and Borella, L. 1973. Immunologic rebound after cessation of long-term chemotherapy in acute leukemia. II. In vitro response to phytohemagglutinin and antigens by peripheral blood and bone marrow lymphocytes. *Blood* 42: 99-110.

39. Greene, W. H., Schimpff, S. C., and Wiernik, P. H. 1974. Cell-mediated immunity in acute nonlymphocytic leukemia. Relationship to host factors, therapy and prognosis. *Blood* 43: 1-14.

40. Gutterman, J. U., Hersh, E. M., Mavligit, G., Freireich, E. J., Rossen, R. D., Butler, W. T., McCredie, K. B., Bodey, Sr., G. P., and Rodriguez, V. 1974. Cell-mediated and humoral immune response to acute leukemic cells and soluble leukemia antigen—Relationship to immunocompetence and prognosis. *Recent Results in Cancer Research* 47: 97-112. Springer-Verlag, Heidelberg-Berlin.

41. Gutterman, J. U., Roseen, R. D., Butler, W. T., McCredie, K. B., Bodey, Sr., G. P., Freireich, E. J., and Hersh, E. M. 1973. Tumor induced blastogenesis in acute leukemia. *N. Eng. J. Med.* 288: 169-175.

42. Haghbin, M. 1976. Chemotherapy of acute lymphoblastic leukemia in children. *Amer. J. Hemat.* 1: 201-209.

43. Haghbin, M., Armstrong, D., and Murphy, M. L. 1973. Controlled prospective trial of *Pseudomonas aeruginosa* vaccine in children with acute leukemia. *Cancer* 32: 761-766.

44. Hardisty, R. M., and Till, M. M. 1968. Acute leukemia 1959–64: Factors affecting prognosis. *Arch. Dis. Child.* 43: 107–115.

45. Harris, R. 1973. Leukaemia antigens and immunity in man. *Nature* 241: 95–100.

46. Heath, R. B., Fairley, G. H., and Malpas, J. S. 1964. Production of antibodies against viruses in leukaemia and related diseases. *Brit. J. Haemat.* 10: 365–370.

47. Herberman, R. B. 1973. Immunologic reactions of experimental animals to tumor associated cell surface antigens, *in* L. L. Ioachin (ed.), *Pathobiology Annual*, Vol. 3, pp. 291–307. Appleton-Century-Crofts, New York.

48. Herberman, R. B., Lepourhiet, A., Hollinshead, A., Char, D., McCoy, J. L., and Leventhal, B. G. 1975. Humoral and cell-mediated immunity in human acute leukemia, *in 26th Annual Symposium of Fundamental Cancer Research: Immunological Aspects of Neoplasia*, pp. 423–438. Williams and Wilkins Co.

49. Hersh, E. M. 1974. Immunosuppressive agents, *in* A. C. Sartorelli and D. G. Johns (eds.), *Handbook of Experimental Pharmacology* XXXVIII. *Antineoplastic and Immunosuppressive Agents*, pp. 577–617. Springer-Verlag, Berlin-Heidelberg, New York.

50. Hersh, E. M., Carbone, P. P., and Freireich, E. J. 1966. Recovery of immune responsiveness after drug suppression in man. *J. Lab. Clin. Med.* 67: 566–572.

51. Hersh, E. M., Gutterman, J. U., Mavligit, G. M., McCredie, K. B., Burgess, M. A., Mathews, A., and Freireich, E. J. 1974. Serial studies of immunocompetence of patients undergoing chemotherapy for acute leukemia. *J. Clin. Invest.* 54: 401–408.

52. Hersh, E. M., and Oppenheim, J. J. 1967. Inhibition of in vitro lymphocyte transformation during chemotherapy in man. *Cancer Res.* 27: 98–105.

53. Hersh, E. M., Whitecar, Jr., J. P., McCredie, K. B., Dodey, Sr., G. P., and Freireich, E. J. 1971. Chemotherapy, immunocompetence, immunosuppression and prognosis in acute leukemia. *N. Engl. J. Med.* 285: 1211–1216.

54. Heyn, R. M., Joo, P., Karon, M., Nesbit, M., Shore, N., Breslow, N., Weiner, J., Reed, A., and Hammond, D. 1975. BCG in the treatment of acute lymphocytic leukemia. *Blood* 46: 431–442.

55. Humphrey, G. B., Nesbit, Jr., M. E., Chary, K. K. V., and Krivit, W. 1972. Impaired lymphocyte transformation in leukemia patients after intensive therapy. *Cancer* 29: 402–406.

56. Jose, D. G., Ekert, H., Colebatch, J., Waters, K., Wilson, F., and O'Keefe, D. 1976. Immune function at diagnosis in relation to responses to therapy in acute lymphocytic leukemia in childhood. *Blood* 47: 1011–1021.

57. Joseph, R. R., Belpomme, D., and Mathé, G. 1976. Increase in "null" cells in acute lymphocytic leukaemia in remission on long-term immunotherapy. *Brit. J. Cancer* 33: 567–570.

58. Kaplan, J., Mastrangelo, R., and Peterson, W. D. 1974. Childhood lymphoblastic lymphoma, a cancer of thymus-derived lymphocytes. *Cancer Res.* 34: 521–525.

59. Kersey, J. H., Sabad, A., Gajl-Peczalska, K., Hallgren, H. M., Yunis, E. J.,

and Nesbit, M. E. 1973. Acute lymphoblastic leukemia cells with T (thymus-derived) lymphocyte markers. *Science* 182: 1355–1356.

59a. Khalifa, A. S., Take, H., Cejka, J., and Zuelzer, V. W. 1974. Immuno-globulins in acute leukemia in children. *J. Podiatr.* 85: 788–791.

60. Kiran, O., and Gross, S. 1969. The G-immunoglobulins in acute leukemia in children. Hematologic and immunologic relationships. *Blood* 33: 198–206.

61. Lampkin, B. C., McWilliams, N. B., and Mauer, A. M. 1972. Treatment of acute leukemia. *Pediat. Clin. North Amer.* 19: 1123–1140.

62. Leventhal, B. G., Cohen, P., and Triem, S. C. 1974. Effect of chemotherapy on the immune response in acute leukemia. A review. *Israel J. Med. Sci.* 10: 866–887.

63. Leventhal, B. G., Halterman, R. H., Rosenberg, E. B., and Herberman, R. B. 1972. Immune reactivity of leukemia patients to autologous blast cells. *Cancer Res.* 32: 1820–1825.

64. Leventhal, B. G., LePourhiet, A., Halterman, R. H., Henderson, E. S., and Herberman, R. B. 1973. Immunotherapy in previously treated acute lymphatic leukemia. *Natl. Cancer Inst. Monogr.* 39: 177–187.

65. Mann, D. L., Rogentine, G. N., Halterman, R., and Leventhal, B. 1971. Detection of an antigen with acute leukemia. *Science* 174: 1136–1137.

66. Mathé, G., Amiel, J. L., Schwarzenberg, L., Schneider, M., Cattan, A., Schlumberger, J. R., Hayat, M., and de Vassal, F. 1969. Active immunotherapy for acute lymphoblastic leukaemia. *Lancet* 1: 697–699.

67. Mathé, G., de Vassal, F., Delgado, M., Pouillart, P., Belpomme, D., Joseph, R., Schwarzenberg, L., Amiel, J. L., Schneider, M., Cattan, A., Musset, M., Misset, J. L., and Jasmin, C. 1976. 1975 current results of the first 100 cytologically typed acute lymphoid leukemia submitted to BCG active immunotherapy. *Cancer Immunol. Immunotherapy* 1: 77–86.

68. Mathé, G., Pouillart, P., Lapeyraque, F. 1969. Active immunotherapy of L1210 leukaemia applied after the graft of tumour cells. *Brit. J. Cancer* 23: 814–824.

69. McKelvey, E., and Carbone, P. P. 1965. Serum immune globulin concentrations in acute leukemia during intensive chemotherapy. *Cancer* 18: 1292–1296.

70. Medical Research Council Report. 1971. Treatment of acute lymphoblastic leukaemia. Comparison of immunotherapy (B.C.G.), intermittant methotrexate, and no therapy after a five-month intensive cytotoxic regimen (Concord trial). *Brit. Med. J.* 4: 189–194.

71. Melief, C. J. M., Schweitzer, M., Zeylemaker, W. P., Verhagen, E. H., and Eijsvoogel, V. P. 1973. Some immunological properties of lymphoid cells from patients with acute lymphatic leukaemia (ALL). *Clin. Exp. Immunol.* 15: 131–143.

72. Metzgar, R. S., Mohanakumar, T., Green, R. W., Miller, D. S., and Bolognesi, D. P. 1974. Human Leukemia antigens: Partial isolation and characterization. *J. Natl. Cancer Inst.* 52: 1445–1453.

73. Metzgar, R. S., Mohanakumar, T., and Miller, D. S. 1972. Antigens specific for human lymphocytic and myeloid leukemia cells: Detection of nonhuman primate antiserums. *Science* 178: 986–988.

74. Mills, B., Sen, L., and Borella, L. 1975. Reactivity of anti-human thymocyte serum with acute leukemic blasts. *J. Immunol.* 115: 1038–1044.

75. Minowada, J., Ohnuma, T., and Moore, G. E. 1972. Rosette-forming human lymphoid cell lines. I. Establishment and evidence for origin of thymus-derived lymphocytes. *J. Natl. Cancer Inst.* 49: 891–895.

76. Mohanakumar, T., Metzgar, R. S., and Miller, D. S. 1974. Human leukemia cell antigens: Serologic characterization with xenoantisera. *J. Natl. Cancer Inst.* 52: 1435–1444.

77. Morton, D. L., Holmes, E. C., Eilber, F. R., and Wood, W. C. 1971. Immunological aspects of neoplasia. a rational basis for immunotherapy. *Ann. Intern. Med.* 74: 587–604.

78. Ogra, P. L., Sinks, L. F., and Karzon, D. T. 1971. Poliovirus antibody response in patients with acute leukemia. *J. Ped.* 79: 444–449.

79. Old, L. J., Clarke, D. A., and Benacerraf, B. 1959. Effect of Bacillus Calmette-Guerin infection on transplanted tumours of the mouse. *Nature* 184: 291–292.

80. Oldham, R. K., Weiner, R. S., Mathé, G., Breard, J., Simmler, M.-C., Carde, P., and Herberman, R. B. 1976. Cell-mediated immune responsiveness of patients with acute lymphocytic leukemia in remission. *Int. J. Cancer* 17: 326–337.

81. Oren, M. E., and Herberman, R. B. 1971. Delayed cutaneous hypersensitivity reactions to membrane extracts of human tumor cells. *Clin. Exp. Immunol.* 9: 45–56.

82. Pegrum, G. D. 1973. Leukaemic antigens. *Brit. J. Haematol.* 24: 1–6.

83. Pinkel, D. 1976. Treatment of acute leukemia. *Ped. Clin. North Amer.* 23: 117–130.

84. Pinsky, C. M., El Domeiri, A., Caron, A. S., Knapper, W. H., and Oettgen, H. F. 1974. Delayed hypersensitivity reactions in patients with cancer. Recent Results in Cancer Research 47: 37–41. Springer-Verlag, New York.

85. Powles, R. L. 1976. Immunotherapy in the management of acute leukaemia. *Brit. J. Haemat.* 32: 145–149.

86. Ragab, A. H., Lindquist, K. J., Vietti, T. J., Choi, S. C., and Osterland, C. K. 1970. Immunoglobulin pattern in childhood leukemia. *Cancer* 26: 890–894.

87. Santos, G. W. 1967. Immunosuppressive drugs I. *Fed. Proc.* 26: 907–913.

88. Santos, G. W. 1972. Chemical immunosuppression, in J. S. Najarian and R. L. Simmons (eds.), *Transplantation*, pp. 206–221. Lea & Febiger, Philadelphia.

89. Seligmann, M., Preud'homme, J.-L., and Brouet, J.-C. 1973. B and T cell markers in human proliferative blood diseases and primary immunodeficiencies, with special reference to membrane bound immunoglobulin. *Transplant. Rev.* 16: 83–113.

90. Sen, L., and Borella, L. 1973. Expression of cell surface markers on T and B lymphocytes after long-term chemotherapy of acute leukemia. *Cell. Immunol.* 9: 84–95.

91. Sen, L., and Borella, L. 1974. Immunological rebound after cessation of long-term chemotherapy in acute lymphocytic leukemia: Changes in distribution of T and B cell populations in bone marrow and peripheral blood. *Brit. J. Haemat.* 27: 477–487.

92. Sen, L., and Borella, L. 1975. Clinical importance of lymphoblasts with T markers in childhood acute leukemia. *N. Engl. J. Med.* 292: 828–831.

93. Shevach, E. M., Herberman, R., Frank, M. M., and Green, I. 1972. Recep-

tors for complement and immunoglobulin on human leukemic cells and human lymphoblastoid cell lines. *J. Clin. Invest.* 51: 1933–1938.

94. Silver, R. T., Utz, J. P., Fahey, J., and Frei, E., III. 1960. Antibody response in patients with leukemia. *J. Lab. Clin. Med.* 56: 634–643.

95. Simone, J. 1974. Acute lymphocytic leukemia in childhood. *Sem. Hematol.* 11: 25–39.

96. Simone, J. V., Holland, E., and Johnson, W. 1972. Fatalities during remission in childhood leukemia. *Blood* 39: 759–770.

97. Thomas, L. 1959. Discussion, *in* H. S. Lawrence (ed.), *Cellular and Humoral Aspects of the Hypersensitive States,* pp. 529–532. Hoeber-Harper, New York.

98. Tsukimoto, I., Wong, K. Y., and Lampkin, B. C. 1976. Surface markers and prognostic factors in acute lymphoblastic leukemia. *N. Engl. J. Med.* 294: 245–248.

Nothing is so firmly be-
lieved as what we least
know.
—Montaigne, *Essays.*

CHAPTER 6

IMMUNO-COMPETENCE IN RADIATION THERAPY PATIENTS

Nemetallah A. Ghossein
and Jay L. Bosworth

Department of Radiology
Section of Radiotherapy
The Albert Einstein
College of Medicine
Yeshiva University
Bronx, New York 10461

BACKGROUND

Soon after the discovery of X-rays by Conrad Roentgen, investigators began to notice the extreme radiosensitivity of certain organs. The first organs to attract their attention were the hematopoietic tissue and the male gonads. Senn, in 1903 (139), was the first to observe the reduction in the number of circulating leukocytes in irradiated leukemic patients. Since then, many authors have shown that the circulating lymphocytes and the lymphoid tissues throughout the body are exquisitely radiosensitive. The property of the lymphoid organs for rapid regeneration following irradiation was also noted. Heineke (76) in 1903 did a complete histological study of the effect of irradiation on lymphoid organs. He noticed that regeneration began soon after irradiation and complete repair occurred in 8 to 15 days. Pohle and Bunting (125), in 1936, found that the lymphoid cells of the spleen were sensitive to doses as low as 5 rads but that regeneration of the Malpighian corpuscles occurred within days following irradiation with doses as high as 1000 to 2000 rads. Ghossein et al., in 1963 (61), confirmed the findings of early workers that there was rapid destruction of the lymphoid cells of the thymus hours after irradiation, but complete regeneration of the thymus occurred within one month when doses as high as 3000 rads were given in a single exposure.

The effect of total body irradiation on the hematopoietic tissues and circulating white cells of both experimental animals and man has been extensively studied (5, 129). Animal experiments to study the changes associated with localized irradiation have been scanty. Radiotherapists throughout the years have noted that changes in leukocyte counts following localized irradiation depend on several factors, such as the dimension of the field of treatment, the area irradiated, the absorbed dose, and the number of fractions delivered. Usually, the larger the dimension of the irradiated field, the more drastic is the drop in leukocyte count. If the irradiated area includes bone marrow or large lymphoid aggregates, such as the spleen or Peyer's patches, the drop in count will be more significant than when the irradiated area is devoid of these elements. Finally, the larger the dose of irradiation and the fewer the number of fractions used to deliver this dose, the more pronounced is the drop in count.

Most of the early workers concerned themselves with changes in the morphology and number of the white blood cells following irradiation, rather than with changes in their functions. Certainly, decrease in the number of these cells, particularly the lymphocytes and macrophages, may be of significance. However, any drastic alterations of their capacity to perform their functions, which may be reflected clinically by decrease in the patient's defense mechanisms, should be of paramount importance. In the present chapter, the immune reactivity of patients undergoing radiotherapy will be explored.

I. EFFECT OF RADIATION ON THE WHITE CELLS

A. The Lymphocyte

As early as 1908, Russel (130) and Ehrlich (80) made the observation that lymphocytes and monocytes may play a role in tumor destruction. The effect of cellular immunity on tumors received an important impetus 40 years later, when Kidd and Toolan (95) in the early 1950s, noted that experimental tumors had a lymphocytic infiltrate a few days after transplantation and that there was morphological evidence to suggest direct killing of tumor cells by lymphocytes. Since then, in vivo (9) and in vitro (77) techniques have been developed for the study of tumor cell destruction by immune lymphocytes. Four stages are recognized in the killing of tumor cells by lymphocytes (3). In the first stage, there is active movement of the cells to bring their plasma membranes into contact. The second stage is characterized by the establishment of a firm adhesion between the lymphocyte and the tumor cell. The presence of Mg^{2+} is required. The third stage requires a living metabolizing lymphocyte to come into contact with the tumor cell for at least a few minutes in the presence of Ca^{2+}. The final stage of tumor lysis may occur in the absence of the lymphocyte. The membrane of the tumor cell becomes increasingly permeable to small molecules, leading to osmotic disequilibrium and cell burst. The fact that the lymphocyte plays an important role in tumor cell destruction has stimulated investigators to study the effect on cell-mediated immunity of agents known to produce lymphopenia, such as irradiation and cytotoxic drugs.

It is well established that following radiotherapy there is a diminution of the total number of circulating lymphocytes which may last for months or even years. Because of this decrease, many workers have hypothesized that radiotherapy may be detrimental to the host immune response and consequently may lead to a poor prognosis. Riesco (127) has correlated the pretherapy lymphocyte count with prognosis in patients treated by conventional methods, including radiotherapy, for a solid cancer. He found that there was a positive correlation between the 5-year survival and the pretherapy count. The same observation was made by Papatesta and Kark (121) in patients treated for breast cancer. They noted also an inverse correlation between the stage of the disease and the pretreatment number of lymphocytes. Others (30, 146) have speculated that radiotherapy may adversely affect prognosis because not only did it decrease the number of lymphocytes but it also altered the ratio between the thymus-derived (T cell) and bone-marrow-derived (B cell) lymphocytes. No proof has been presented to substantiate these speculations. In contrast to the prognostic significance of the pretreatment lymphocyte count, there is no clinical evidence to show that the prognosis is altered by the number of circulating lymphocytes present after radiotherapy and/or chemotherapy have been given. Clinically, these agents are known to be successful in the treatment of disease such as malignant lymphoma and testicular tumors, which require wide field irradiation or intensive chemotherapy; both are known to produce, consistently, a drop in count. The lymphopenia associated with these treatments does not seem to have altered the prognosis. In a recent randomized study (48) on patients treated by simple mastectomy and postoperative radiotherapy, which included part of the mediastinum, and patients treated by radical mastectomy alone, there was no significant difference in the incidence of metastases, again suggesting that the decrease in the number of circulating lymphocytes following irradiation has no deleterious effect on the course of the cancer.

T AND B CELLS.   Cellular immunity is known to be mediated, at least in part, by T lymphocytes. Emphasis has been placed on studies dealing with the effect of irradiation on these cells. Bartfeld (8) has found that 3 days following whole-body exposure of guinea pigs to 1000 rads, there was a 90% decrease in T lymphocytes obtained from lung alveolar washings. Using mouse lymphocytes, Anderson et al. (4) observed that no B cells survived an in vitro exposure dose of 300 rads, whereas the viability of T cells was reduced by 90%. B cell migration to the lymphoid organs was greatly reduced when compared to T cells. Although both T and B cells died very soon after irradiation, T lymphocytes were killed less rapidly.

Several investigators have found that following radiotherapy and regardless of the area irradiated, there was, in addition to a drop in the total lymphocyte count, an absolute decrease in the number of T cells leading to a reversal of the T/B lymphocyte ratio. Stjernsward et al. (147) studied 34 patients with cancer of the breast before and after postoperative radiotherapy. There was a drop in the number of T cells immediately following radiotherapy, and this drop persisted for at least one year; there was a corresponding rise in the number of B cells. The more marked the lymphopenia, the lower was the proportion of T cells. The decrease in number of T cells was attributed to inclusion of the thymus within the irradiated field. Elhilali *et al.* (43) examined 39 patients with urological cancers who had received radiotherapy one year previously. They found a decrease in T cell number as compared to the age matched control, and an absolute increase in the B cells. Stratton *et al.* (148) compared the effect of radiotherapy to the thymic area with pelvic irradiation. Regardless of the area treated there was a decrease in T and B cells although there was more depletion of T cells. Similar findings were reported by other investigators (20, 150). These investigations suggest that treatment of the thymic area does not appear to be selective in producing T cell depletion.

IN VITRO TESTS OF LYMPHOCYTE FUNCTION. The capacity of the lymphocytes to be stimulated by mitogens and to undergo blastic transformation *in vitro* has been used to assess the immunological competence of these cells. Specific mitogens such as PPD in tuberculin-positive individuals and nonspecific stimulants such as phytohemagglutinin (PHA) or pokeweed mitogen (PWM) have been commonly used. PHA is thought to stimulate the T cell whereas PWM is mostly a B cell mitogen, but may also stimulate T cells (104). A decreased capacity of lymphocytes to transform has been associated with a decrease in the general immunological responsiveness of the patient. Lack of activation of these cells has been found in patients with congenital thymic abnormalities (103), uremia (91), and certain chronic infections such as tuberculosis (152) and leprosy (32). It has also been reported that lymphocyte transformation is impaired in patients with advanced cancer (57).

The effect of radiotherapy on lymphocyte transformation has attracted a great deal of attention recently, particularly for patients receiving treatment to the thymic region. Stjernsward (146) found decreased transformation in breast cancer patients who received postoperative radiotherapy. Fifteen of nineteen had a decrease in PHA transformation, whereas only three had an increase when compared to those who did not receive postoperative treatment. Jenkins (88) found that there was a drop in PHA stimulation of between 15 and 39% following treatment. Thomas (151) and Braeman (15) have made the same observation and noted that recovery began one to two months following therapy; at 18 months, transformation was only 30% lower than the initial value (16). A decrease in transformation also occurred when radiotherapy was administered to sites other than the mediastinum. There was a lower reactivity in nine of ten patients following radiotherapy to the nasopharynx (164) or after pelvic irradiation (19).

Although many investigators demonstrated that the *in vitro* activation of lymphocytes decreased following radiotherapy, others have noted an increased reactivity after treatment. Blomgren (11) reported an increased responsiveness both to PHA and PWM following radiotherapy, when a small concentration of lymphocytes was used in the culture. Responsiveness decreased at higher cell concentration. He suggested that the optimal number of mitogen molecules necessary to induce DNA synthesis may not be the same for irradiated lymphocytes as it is for unirradiated cells. Radiation may cause either an increase in the proportion of lymphocytes requiring a higher concentration of the mitogen molecules or may cause alteration in the activation threshold of these cells. An increased proportion of the T lymphocytes in relation to the thymus independent cells was also noted. McCredie et al. (111) found a 50% increase in DNA synthesis following PHA stimulation in 152 patients irradiated for breast cancer and 101 patients treated for cancer of the cervix. The increase persisted for a year following radiotherapy. The predominant lymphocyte present following treatment was of the thymus-dependent type, and this cell persisted for quite some time after the peripheral count had returned to normal. Slater et al. (141) have found a depressed response to PHA and PWM that lasted for two months but observed a significantly higher response to these mitogens at six months following radiotherapy, suggesting an increased activity above the pretreatment value for both T and B lymphocytes. Einhorn et al. (42) reported an enhanced lymphocyte reactivity to the thyroglobulin following local irradiation of the thyroid gland in man. The enhancement lasted for at least three months.

Not only is there controversy regarding the inhibitory effect of radiotherapy on in vitro lymphocyte transformation, but the prognostic significance of this test in malignant disease has been questioned.

Ghossein et al. (62) determined PHA transformation before, after, and three to six months following radical radiotherapy given to 81 patients who had a variety of solid tumors. Their delayed hypersensitivity response was evaluated by skin reactivity to 2,4-dinitrochlorobenzene (DNCB). Although there was a significant decrease in lymphocyte transformation following treatment, there was no correlation between skin reactivity, which is known to have a prognostic significance, and PHA transformation either prior to or following treatment (Fig. 1). Levy and Kaplan (102) as well as Young et al. (170) found no correlation between lymphocyte transformation and survival or time of remission of patients with Hodgkin's disease. Braeman (15) and Thomas (151) failed to show a correlation between the lymphocyte transformation and survival of patients with lung cancer. T cell number and PHA transformation were measured in patients who were previously treated by radiotherapy alone or in combination with surgery for a laryngo-pharyngeal cancer. These patients had a significant depression of these in vitro tests despite the fact that they were cured of their cancer for from four to fifteen years (150).

O'Toole et al. (120) used an in vitro microcytotoxicity test to measure the specific destruction of a cultured bladder cancer cell line by the pa-

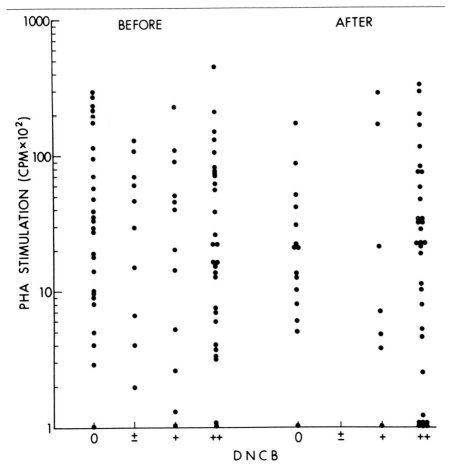

Fig. 1.   Relation between *in vitro* lymphocyte stimulation and degree of DNCB reaction before and 3 months following radiotherapy. (Reprinted with permission of J. B. Lippincott Co. from *Cancer* 35: p. 1619, 1975)

tient's peripheral lymphocytes. This test was used on patients treated with radiotherapy for a bladder cancer. Eighty-eight and forty-one percent of patients, with early and advanced cancer respectively, had lymphocyte cytotoxicity prior to treatment. During the course of radiotherapy, cytotoxicity was depressed in all patients. However, within 7 days of treatment 100% and 67% of patients with early and advanced cancer developed a positive response. Thus, there was an enhancement of cytotoxic activity of the lymphocytes after radiotherapy. One explanation offered by these authors is that soon after irradiation there is a release of a large amount of antigenic material from the irradiated tissues, which in-

Table 1. Viral plaque assay before and after radiotherapy

Ratio[a]	Before (18 pts.)	At Conclusion (18 pts.)	3 Months Later (12 pts.)
≤ 1	14/18 (78%)	12/18 (67%)	10/12 (83%)
> 1	4/18 (22%)	6/18 (33%)	2/12 (17%)

a. Ratio of virus plaques formed by stimulated lymphocytes of patients to virus plaques formed by stimulated lymphocytes of normal controls.

Source: A. Kadish, J. Bosworth, and N. A. Ghossein, unpublished data.

duces an immunologic response. In support of their theory, they have noted that the lymphocytes of patients who were free of disease from 1 to 10 years following treatment, and presumably had no available tumor antigen, had no cytotoxic activity. Following recurrence, a cytotoxic response appeared, indicating the presence of tumor-associated antigens.

In order to identify and enumerate antigen- and mitogen-activated lymphocytes, a virus plaque assay has been developed by Bloom and co-workers. They have shown that RNA viruses can replicate in activated T lymphocytes and that the virus plaque assay was a measurement of the number of activated cells (12, 89). They also observed a frequent disassociation between the ability of the lymphocyte to sustain virus replication and their ability to undergo a proliferative response. The disassociation in function may indicate that either a different subpopulation of T lymphocytes or different function or stage of development of the single population of T cells is being measured. The ability of the lymphocytes to undergo proliferation by mitogen which has been used as an *in vitro* correlate of cell mediated immunity may be only one aspect of T cell activities. The virus plaque assay was used by us to determine the effect of radiotherapy on the number of activated T cells[1]. Eighteen patients with a variety of localized solid cancers were studied before, immediately after, and 3 months following treatment. It should be noted that the patients had a lower number of virus plaques as compared to the unirradiated healthy controls. However, there was no statistical difference in the number of plaques formed before or following radiotherapy (see Table 1).

B. The Macrophage

Macrophages participate in all forms of inflammatory processes and are known to play an important role in the induction and expression of the immune response (110). Administered antigens can be found within the macrophage and on its surface (1). It has been shown that macrophages have surface receptors for IgG immunoglobulin (86) and for complement (155), and that antigen-antibody complexes have been found on their surface. These cells are known to have both nonspecific and specific cytotoxic effect on tumor cells (70, 46, 83) and it is also known that factors derived from macrophages can activate T and B lymphocytes (122). Because of their important role in cell-mediated immunity and tumor destruction, the effect of irradiation on the macrophages may be critical.

Although there are many studies showing that there is a change in the number of circulating lymphocytes and granulocytes following radiotherapy, there are few investigations dealing with alteration of the monocyte count and function following irradiation. Rotman et al. (128) determined the monocyte count in 29 patients undergoing radiotherapy for tumors located either in the pelvis or in the thorax. They found a significant rise in the number of monocytes from 290 to 411 per mm^3 3 weeks following initiation of therapy. The radiation induced monocytosis, according to these authors, may be due to proteins released from irradiated tissues which can act as antigens. Spier et al. (143) have noted an increase in monocytes and eosinophils in the peritoneal exudate following the injection of tetanus toxoid in immunized animals. Others have observed an increase in circulating monocytes shortly following injection of an antigen (169). Monocytosis is known to be associated with malignancy and may reflect a host response to tumor associated antigens (7, 115).

We have analyzed the differential counts of 80 patients undergoing radical radiotherapy for a variety of localized cancers (see Table 2). Although we could not document a monocytosis following irradiation there was no significant drop in the number of circulating monocytes, contrary to the drastic decrease in the lymphocyte count.

Table 2. Changes in peripheral white blood cell count following radiotherapy

	Before (Mean [±SE])	At Conclusion (Mean [±SE] % Change from pre-RT)		3 Months Later (Mean [±SE] % Change from pre-RT)	
WBC	7400 ± 261	5020 ± 158	−32	5843 ± 272	−21
Neutro.	4975 ± 238	3360 ± 140	−32	4223 ± 225	−15
Lymph.	1830 ± 80	873 ± 75	−52	1094 ± 86	−40
Eosin.	191 ± 16	345 ± 55	+81	140 ± 19	−27
Mono.	404 ± 28	440 ± 32	+10	385 ± 23	−5

Macrophages obtained from mice irradiated *in vivo* with 500 to 800 rads showed morphological changes which were not detectable by light microscopy but which could be detected by the scanning electron microscope. Following irradiation, the cell became rounded and/or elongated and had invaginations on its outer surface (59). The property of close apposition which is usually observed between normal unirradiated macrophages and lymphocytes was lost. It was speculated that the loss of this property may be reflected immunologically by the inability of irradiated macrophages to participate in antibody production against certain antigens (55). *In vivo* (56) radiation doses of up to 800 rads and *in vitro* (137) doses of up to 10,000 rads did not alter the capacity of these cells to phagocytize bacteria or particulate antigens. Irradiated macrophages appear to have a greater surface binding capacity for antigens and were more effective in inducing an immune response to these antigens than were normal macrophages. Alveolar macrophages obtained from rabbit lungs which were irradiated with 400 rads *in vivo* 10 or 11 days before removal, showed an increased level of hydrolytic enzymes compared to nonirradiated controls (112). It was suggested that irradiation may lead to activation of macrophages with respect to their capacity to process antigens and that there was an enhancement of the immunogenicity of antigens adherent to or associated with irradiated macrophages (58, 138). Vorbrodt *et al.* (160, 161) have shown by histochemical methods and by electron microscopy that radiation killed cancer cells from a basal carcinoma of the skin were phagocytosed by tissue macrophages. Cancer cells, which were altered but not killed by irradiation, may stimulate or activate macrophages to interact with them and to destroy them (162). Other studies dealing with the intracellular function of macrophages have demonstrated that there are no changes in DNA and RNA synthesis following irradiation (58).

Lysozyme appears to be continuously released from macrophages regardless of the state of phagocytosis or stimulation of these cells (67). This bacteriolytic enzyme may be an important mediator of the antineoplastic activity of the macrophage (119). Currie and Eccles (28) and Currie (27) have found that serum lysozyme activity may be a useful marker for macrophage-induced host response against tumors, both in experimental animals and in man. They have found that an increased infiltration of tumors by macrophages was associated with a high level of serum lysozyme. We have measured the lysozyme level[1] of patients before and after radical radiotherapy for a localized cancer. These data are shown in Table 3. It can be seen that, as in the monocyte count, there was no significant decrease in lysozyme level following treatment, indicating that this bacteriolytic enzyme, which is considered an important mediator of macrophage activity, is not altered after radiotherapy.

Table 3.   Levels of lysozyme before and after radiotherapy

	Number of Cases	Mean (±S.E.)
Before R.T.	175	6.9 ± 0.15 μg/ml
End of R.T.	122	6.8 ± 0.18 μg/ml
3 months after	68	6.12 ± 0.21 μg/ml

Source: H. Keiser, N. A. Ghossein, and J. Bosworth, unpublished data.

The effect of irradiation on macrophage migration inhibition has also been studied. This test is considered to represent, at least in part, an *in vitro* correlate of cell-mediated immunity. Migration inhibition was not altered by radiation doses which varied from 800 to 10,000 rads (158, 134, 159).

In summary, although there may be changes in the morphological appearance of the irradiated macrophage which can be detected by electron microscopy, there is no evidence to indicate that radiation doses in the therapeutic ranges do alter the multiple functions of the macrophage, as far as can be detected by present techniques.

C. Neutrophil Granulocytes

Since neutrophil granulocytes arise from hemopoietic stem cells, irradiation of areas containing bone marrow may result in a drop in circulating neutrophils. This drop is usually less precipitous and less pronounced than that of the circulating lymphocytes. It reaches its greatest level by the completion of therapy and recovery usually takes place within three to six months (129). In Table 2 is shown the mean drop in neutrophils following radical radiotherapy. There was approximately a 30% drop in the neutrophil count at the completion of irradiation and by 3 months the count was only 15% lower than that of the initial value.

It is well known that total body irradiation or irradiation of large areas can reduce the number of neutrophils by damaging the precursor cell in the bone marrow. This may result in an increased sensitivity to infection in both animal and man (6, 82). However, the neutrophil itself, being a nondividing cell, appears to be quite resistant to irradiation. Human leukocytes were irradiated *in vitro* with doses varying between 200 rads and 1 million rads. There was no significant change in the chemotactic, phagocytic, and bactericidal properties of these cells when doses up to 5000 rads were given. Doses of 50,000 rads and above had to be given to decrease the chemotactic and phagocytic properties by 50% (81). Hancock, Bruce, and Richmond (75) have studied the phagocytic and killing functions of peripheral neutrophils obtained from 62 patients with malignant lymphoma who were treated with radiotherapy and chemotherapy. They noted that although the number of circulating neutrophils was diminished, there was no alteration of their phagocytic and bactericidal functions.

The inflammatory reaction, the neutrophil and macrophage being its major component, may be an important part of the host defense mechanism. This certainly is a part of the efferent arm of cell mediated response. It has already been demonstrated by the skin window technique that there is a defect in macrophage migration in patients with cancer (35, 66). A defective inflammatory reaction has been suggested as the cause for an inadequate delayed hypersensitivity response in patients with cancer (90). In order to study the effect of radiotherapy on the inflammatory component of the immune response, we have skin tested patients with croton oil, as described previously (62). The results are shown in Table 4; 70% of 197 patients were reactive to croton oil before radiotherapy. Three months after treatment, 81% were reactive when rechallenged with this irritant. Over 50% of patients who had a negative inflammatory response became reactive following treatment. These data indicate that the inflammatory response was not inhibited by radical irradiation and, indeed, may have been improved after treatment. The reason for the improvement of the inflammatory response in some patients is not known. The same mechanisms may be involved as those responsible for enhancement of skin reactivity to DNCB following irradiation.

Table 4.   Croton oil reactivity before and 3–6 months after radiotherapy

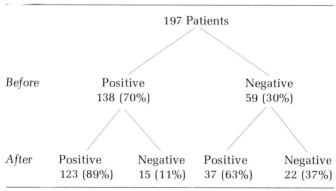

D. The Eosinophil

Several authors have reported the occurrence of eosinophilia during radiotherapy, particularly when the abdomen or pelvis are treated (63, 98, 116). Radiation related eosinophilia was reported as far back as 1924 (113). The etiology of the eosinophilic reaction, which can be demonstrated both in tissues within the field of irradiation (60) and in the peripheral blood is not known. There is evidence to indicate that the eosinophil is an integral part of the cell mediated immunity (144). This cell, in addition to its ability to phagocytose antigen-antibody complexes may mediate inflammatory reactions and modify the delayed hypersensitivity response (84). There is experimental evidence to show that T-cell participation is required for the production of an eosinophilic response and that this response cannot be elicited in the absence of the thymus. Thymus deprived mice (163) and patients with thymic aplasia (24) were unable to mount an eosinophilic response. Infection with the parasite Schistoma mansoni is known to produce eosinophilia in the tissues surrounding the egg of the parasite and in the peripheral blood. This reaction was absent in infected athymic mice, indicating that T cell participation is required (85). It has been mentioned previously that irradiation may cause antigenic alterations of cells, whether normal or malignant, in such a way that they may appear foreign to the host (2, 65). These antigens may stimulate a cell-mediated response which, in part, is reflected by eosinophilia and/or monocytosis. The increase in number of these cells may be an indication that a cell mediated response to altered antigens has been triggered. The occurrence of eosinophilia during radiotherapy has been considered to be a sign of a favorable prognosis (64). One might speculate that if local irradiation was inhibitory to the cell-mediated immunity, a decrease in the number of these cells might have occurred.

II. EFFECT OF IRRADIATION ON DELAYED HYPERSENSITIVITY AND CELLULAR IMMUNITY

A large body of evidence has accumulated in the past two decades to substantiate a relation between cell-mediated immunity and the course of neoplastic disease. As a natural consequence of this knowledge, investigators became concerned about the effect that certain treatment modalities, mainly irradiation and systemic chemotherapy, may have on the immune system. In spite of the clinical interest in the effect of radiotherapy on cellular immunity, little experimental work relevant for the clinician has been performed. Most of the experiments which have been done to study the effect of irradiation on immunity have been performed on animals which have received total body irradiation, often to lethal doses. The data thus obtained cannot be applied to clinical radiotherapy except, perhaps, in those rare instances when total body radiotherapy has been administered. Another reason for the reluctance in extrapolating data obtained from animal experiments to patients is that the time sequence between irradiation and antigen administration in animals is not comparable to that in humans. The sequence of exposure of the immunocompetent cells to antigens, be it *in vitro* or *in vivo*, and irradiation is of paramount importance. Several animal studies have shown that when irradiation is given before immunization, there is a marked depression of antibody formation and, also, but to a lesser extent, of the delayed hypersensitivity response. However, when antigen stimulation precedes irradiation by a few days to a few hours, the immunological response becomes highly radioresistant (149). The latter sequence of events reflects more closely the clinical condition since radiotherapy is given after the immunocompetent cells have been exposed to tumor associated antigens.

Salvin and Smith (135) irradiated guinea pigs with 300 rads total body, in one exposure, 18 hours either before or after intradermal injection of diphtheria toxoid in Freund's adjuvant. When irradiation was given before sensitization, there was no inhibition of delayed hypersensitivity but there was delay in the appearance of circulating antibodies and Arthus-type reaction. When it was administered after sensitization, delayed hypersensitivity, the time of appearance of antibody and Arthus reaction were similar to the unirradiated controls. Although there was a marked decrease in the number of circulating lymphocytes in the irradiated animals, there was no decrease in the hypersensitivity reaction. Guinea pigs irradiated with 200 rads whole body 48 hours after immunization with diphtheria toxoid or ovalbumin in Freund's adjuvant showed delayed hypersensitivity reaction similar to that of controls (154). Only a quarter of the animals irradiated 24 hours before immunization showed delayed reaction. Almost all animals irradiated before antigen injection had no circulating antibody, whereas almost all animals irradiated 48 hours after immunization formed antibody.

These findings confirmed those of Salvin and Smith that in spite of the fact that irradiated animals had severe leukopenia, their capacity to develop a delayed hypersensitivity reaction was not impaired. Rabbits irradiated with doses varying from 400 to 1100 rads total body and sensitized with Freund's adjuvant either at the same time or 28 days after irradiation had a decrease in skin reactivity and prolongation of skin graft rejection time from 8 to 12 days (17).

Maguire and Maibach (107) found that contact dermatitis to a challenge dose of DNCB was not attenuated in guinea pigs irradiated with 320 to 2500 rads total body, when irradiation was delivered 2 to 8 weeks after the sensitizing dose of DNCB had been administered. Visakorpi (158) noted that there is only a temporary suppression of delayed hypersensitivity in rats which received 800 rads total body 10 days after immunization with bovine serum albumin in complete Freund's adjuvant. Skin reaction to the antigen was suppressed for only 4 to 5 days and recovery occurred in spite of a persistent low leukocyte count. Animals that received only 400 rads did not have any suppression of delayed hypersensitivity. As an *in vitro* correlate of delayed hypersensitivity, the migration of macrophages was determined two days following irradiation at the time when the skin test was known to be negative. There was no difference in the migration inhibition between irradiated and nonirradiated animals, indicating that there can be discordance between *in vivo* and *in vitro* tests of cellular immunity.

Established immunity also appears to be highly radioresistant. Frankel and Wilson (54) using specific cellular immunity to *Besnoitia jellisoni*, a protozoan of the golden hamster, found that established immunity to the parasite was highly radioresistant, requiring 1800 rads total body to be suppressed.

Like the *in vivo* experiments, *in vitro* studies have shown that the radiosensitivity of the immunological response depends upon the sequence of exposure of the immunocompetent cells to the antigen and the administration of irradiation. When irradiation was delivered after lymphocytes have been stimulated *in vitro* by PHA, there was no reduction in the percent of cells stimulated, whereas there was marked inhibition of transformation when irradiation was given 10 hours or more before stimulation (136). Similar findings were reported by Vaughan-Smith and Ling (156), using another T cell mitogen, concanavallin A (Con A). There was increase in radioresistance of the lymphocytes when they were stimulated and subsequently irradiated. These data indicate that cell-mediated immunity, similar to antibody formation, is radioresistant if the immune system is exposed to the antigen before a radiation is given.

Skin reactivity as a test of delayed hypersensitivity has been found to be a prognostic indicator in the cancer patient. Several recall antigens such as PPD, mumps, *Candida,* and streptokinase-streptodornase (SKSD) have been used. A positive intradermal reaction to these antigens requires prior sensitization and therefore is a measure of the immunological memory. A de novo antigen such as DNCB evaluates the ability to develop cell mediated immunity, since most people have not been exposed to this substance. A positive correlation between delayed hypersensitivity and short term survival has been found in patients treated by surgery (37), chemotherapy (79), chemoimmunotherapy (72), and radiotherapy (14).

Skin tests have been used and found to be of prognostic value in patients with a variety of solid tumors such as head and neck cancers (108), melanoma (72), GI tumors (13), and even in patients with metastatic breast cancer (26). Eilber and Morton (37) as well as Lee and Sparkes (100) found that DNCB may be a better prognostic indicator than the recall antigens.

Enhancement as well as depression of skin reactivity has been reported following treatment with radiotherapy. Using various recall antigens, Slater (141) and Cosimi (25) have reported a decrease in reactivity following radiotherapy. Gross et al. (71) evaluated the skin reactivity to DNCB of 45 patients who had received radiotherapy for various tumors. They found that irradiation did not significantly alter the response of 85% of their patients. In 20% of them there was an enhancement of skin reactivity. Similar results were reported by Clement and Kramer (23), who used common recall antigens.

We have evaluated the delayed hypersensitivity of 686 patients referred for radical radiotherapy, by measuring the skin response to DNCB[2]. These patients did not have previous chemotherapy or known metastatic disease. 398 patients were sensitized with 2 mg and challenged with 100 mcg, 50 mcg and 25 mcg 2 weeks following sensitization. Another 288 patients were sensitized to only 0.5 mg, as part of a study to determine if reactivity to lower concentrations of the sensitizing dose may be a more discriminating prognostic indicator. In Table 5 is shown the reactivity to the 50-mcg challenge dose. Prior to treatment, almost 50% of patients were positive reactors regardless of the sensitizing dose. Three to six months following radiotherapy there was a significant rise in the incidence of positive reactors to the challenge dose.

One hundred and forty-two patients were skin tested both before and 3 months after treatment. Only 9% of the positive reactors became negative, whereas over 40% of the initially negative converted to positive. (See Table 6.) The effect of irradiation of the thymic area was also examined. Over 230 patients received irradiation to the region of the thorax. Approximately 50% were reactive prior to treatment. Following radiotherapy,

Table 5. Pre- and post-radiotherapy DNCB reactivity to 50-mcg challenge dose

Irradiation	Number Positive to 2-mg Sensitization		Number Positive to 0.5-mg Sensitization	
Before	187/398	47%	141/288	49%
3 months after	90/142	63%	65/92	70%

$P < 0.001$

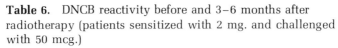

Table 6. DNCB reactivity before and 3–6 months after radiotherapy (patients sensitized with 2 mg. and challenged with 50 mcg.)

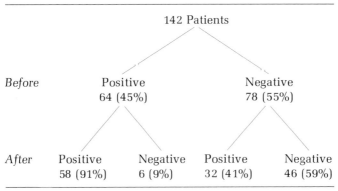

142 Patients

	Positive 64 (45%)		Negative 78 (55%)	
Before				
After	Positive 58 (91%)	Negative 6 (9%)	Positive 32 (41%)	Negative 46 (59%)

67% were positive. These data confirm the findings of others that there may be improvement in reactivity following radiotherapy. We have reported previously that those who became reactive following treatment had the same short-term prognosis as those patients who were DNCB positive prior to treatment.

The reason for the enhancement of the delayed hypersensitivity reaction following treatment is not understood. It was suggested that the conversion from negative to positive may be due to enhancement of the immunological response secondary to a decrease in the tumor burden (71, 72). This explanation may apply to patients with significant tumor masses. However, many of our patients who converted had minimal disease. Another explanation, which seems quite plausible, is that radiation may suppress B cell function. Enhancement of delayed hypersensitivity has been reported following the administration of cyclophosphamide (94, 153). This radiomimetic drug has a suppressor effect on certain selective functions of B cells, such as antibody production. Suppression of antibody has been shown to produce an increase in delayed hypersensitivity. Others have noted an enhancement of delayed hypersensitivity by depletion of suppressor T cells following cyclophosphamide administration (114). The same mechanisms may be at play following irradiation, leading to an enhancement of delayed hypersensitivity.

In order to determine the long-term effect of radiotherapy on the immune system, we evaluated 52 patients who had been treated by radiotherapy and cured of a gynecological malignancy for a period of at least 3 years. The incidence of positive reactors to DNCB in this group was 87%, almost similar to that of the normal population (73). Kun and

Johnson (97) found that there was no decrease in skin reaction of patients with Hodgkin's disease who had been free of tumor for at least 5 years following radiotherapy.

III. EFFECT OF IRRADIATION ON ANTIBODY FORMATION

A. Serum Immunoglobulins

Serum immunoglobulins, mainly IgG, IgA, and IgM, are known to be important in host defenses against infection, but their role in the defenses against tumor is not clear. The interaction between cell-mediated and humoral-mediated reactions, although often considered as two functionally separate responses, appears to be quite intricate. It has been mentioned above that macrophages possess surface receptors for IgG and that antigen-antibody complexes are bound to their surface. The cooperation between T and B cells has recently received a great deal of attention (92). T cells may act either to enhance immunoglobulin production or to suppress B cell function, the so-called "helper" and "suppressor" effect. Similarly, by producing antibodies B cells may alter T cell function.

Since humoral antibodies may play a role in tumor immunity, the effect of radiotherapy on the antibody response will be reviewed. For the past three decades, investigators (34, 96, 149) have stressed the importance in antibody response of the time sequence between antigen administration and irradiation. This response may be effectively suppressed, as has been mentioned previously, if the antigen is given after irradiation has been delivered, and may be unaltered or even enhanced if the antigen is administered before irradiation (33, 105). These data have been accumulated from animals given irradiation to large areas or total body irradiation. Similarly, local irradiation to the site of antigen injection may result in an increase in antibody production. Rabbits injected intracutaneously with sheep erythrocyte or diphtheria toxoid and then irradiated within one hour to the site of injection, have been found to have an enhanced antibody response in the serum and at the site of injection (68, 69). When irradiation was given before the antigen was injected, there was a marked depression of antibody formation.

It has been known for a long time that lymphocytes are among the most radiosensitive of the mammalian cells, having a D_0 of 75 to 100 rads. The resting lymphocyte is apparently unable to repair radiation induced damage. When radiation is given after the lymphocyte has been activated by an antigen, it acquires the ability to repair some radiation damage and this is reflected by an increase in radioresistance (145). Activated cells have been found to have a D_0 of greater than 7000 rads (93). Makinodan et *al.* (109) have studied the effect of irradiation on the secondary response of mouse spleen cells to sheep erythrocytes. When irradiation was given 4 days following antigenic stimulation, the antibody-producing cells had a D_0 of more than 10,000 rads. It was estimated that 19 S and 7 S antibody-producing cells have a D_0 of 6200 rads and 4250 rads respectively (131, 132). It becomes apparent, therefore, that when irradiation is given after antigen administration the antibody response will become progressively radioresistant, depending on the ratio of cells already committed to antibody production to cells in the proliferating or uncommitted state. As mentioned previously, it is assumed that radiotherapy is delivered after the immunocompetent cells have already been activated by tumor associated antigens. Therefore, it is unlikely that therapeutic doses of local irradiation can affect antibody-producing cells which are already committed to antibody synthesis.

In contrast to the well-documented decrease in cellular immunity in patients with malignant tumors, the ability of these patients to form humoral antibodies seem to be relatively well preserved. Serum proteins levels and the capacity to form humoral antibodies appear to be relatively normal, particularly in patients with malignancies other than lymphoproliferative diseases (99, 101). Patients who have advanced malignant disease may have a poor antibody response and the decrease in antibody formation may indicate a grave prognosis (87, 106). Plesnicar (124) analysed the immunoglobulins' levels (IgG, IgM, IgA) in patients who have cancer of the cervix. He found statistically significant high levels of IgG in patients with Stage I disease as compared to healthy controls and to patients with Stage III disease. IgM values were below that of the controls in patients with advanced disease but not in those with early cancer. He suggested that these changes may reflect the host immunological response to the extent of the cancer. There was no mention of the effect of treatment on immunoglobulins levels.

Wohl and Ghossein (166) have measured immunoglobulins levels before and after radical radiotherapy in 22 patients with a localized solid cancer. No significant differences in mean levels from normal controls could be detected following irradiation. A recent analysis of another 20 patients treated by radical radiotherapy gave the same results (Table 7).

If local radiotherapy does not appear to alter immunoglobulins levels, the effect of whole body irradiation in humans produces a significant depression in serum antibodies. This subject was reviewed recently by Chaskes *et al.* (21). Almost half of their patients who received therapeutic total body irradiation for a hematological malignancy had a decrease in immunoglobulins levels. The production of IgG appears to be the least sensitive, whereas IgA concentration was affected in most patients. The change in IgM was intermediate between IgG and IgA. Substantial recov-

Table 7. Mean immunoglobulins levels of 20 patients who received radical radiotherapy

	Pre-R.T. (±S.E.)	Post-R.T. (±S.E.)	3 Months Post-R.T. (±S.E.)
IgG	1686 ± 206	1613 ± 135	1415 ± 150
IgM	88.5 ± 9.8	81.5 ± 9	99.6 ± 18
IgA	189 ± 37	161 ± 22	178 ± 33

ery occurred for most patients by the seventh week following treatment. As expected, infections were not found in any of their patients who had low immunoglobulins without having a concomitant severe granulocytopenia.

B. Autoantibodies

Autoantibodies to a variety of cancers have been detected by cytotoxic and immunofluorescent techniques (142). Cancer cells may have antigens on their surface, either normal fetal or tumor-induced, which may react with the host immune system to form so-called tumor-specific autoantibodies. Farrow et al. (47) have suggested that the process of malignant transformation of a normal cell may lead to exposure of cellular antigens with the subsequent formation of autoantibodies. In theory at least, irradiation, by altering cells, may expose their cellular components to the immune mechanisms leading to the production of organ specific and non-organ specific antibodies (65). Thyroid irradiation may cause elevation of antibody titer against thyroglobulin (39) or cytoplasmic antigen (38, 118). Similarly, irradiation of the uterus may produce antibodies against its epithelial lining (40, 41). Agents other than radiation may also induce autoantibodies, presumably by altering the cell surface antigens (167).

Non-tumor specific or non-organ specific antibodies may occur in patients with cancer. A higher frequency of antinuclear antibodies (ANA) has been reported in patients with malignant disease (18, 172) and it was suggested that these autoantibodies may have prognostic significance (165).

We have previously reported the occurrence of non-organ-specific antibodies following radiotherapy (10). In a recent investigation we have examined the sera of 104 patients with a localized solid cancer for the presence of ANA by the indirect immunofluorescent test prior to receiving radical irradiation. Nine percent of the sera were positive, confirming the results of Burnham and Zeromski et al. (18, 172). However, 15% of the patients who were initially negative developed ANA within 6 months of completion of treatment. We have also measured the C^{3} component of the complement by the radical immunodiffusion technique in 54 patients. Five and a half percent of these patients had complement levels which were considered low (below 120 mg/100 ml). Following irradiation, 11% of those who had a normal level of complement developed a low titer.[1] These data are indicative that a nonspecific autoimmune response may be induced by irradiation. The clinical significance of these antibodies is not known. None of our patients who had abnormal serological findings developed evidence of autoimmune diseases.

IV. EFFECT OF RADIOTHERAPY ON THE BARRIER FUNCTION OF REGIONAL LYMPH NODES

The ability of the lymph node to act as a barrier which can filter and perhaps destroy cancer cells is one of the fundamental concepts of cancer management. Patients who have a cancer which has a propensity to metastisize through the lymphatics, theoretically should be cured if the malignant cells have not extended beyond the regional lymph nodes. These involved nodes can either be destroyed by irradiation or removed surgically. This concept is the basis for elective irradiation or surgical excision of regional nodes draining a curable primary cancer. If the normal lymph node acts as an efficient barrier to the spread of cancer cells, it should be of paramount importance to the clinician to know of the effect of radiotherapy on this function.

In 1860, Virchow (157) noted that the morphology of the node is such that it may act as a filter to particulate matter. The concept that the lymph node may trap cancer cells is an extension of this basic observation. There is evidence to suggest that the lymph node is an effective filter for certain particulate matter (36, 168). The argument for the existence of an efficient lymph node barrier to tumor cells began when Zeidman and Buss (171), using V_2 and Brown-Pearce carcinoma in rabbit found that there was no evidence of distant spread despite the fact that there was intranodal growth of the injected cancer cells. Engeset (44) as well as Saldeen (133) reached a similar conclusion. Fisher and Fisher (49), using erythrocytes as well as V_2 carcinoma cells found that the lymph nodes were inefficient in filtering tumor cells, whereas they were extremely efficient in retaining erythrocytes. They concluded that the properties of the cancer cell itself, as much as the biological and mechanical properties of the node, are a determinant in the spread of cancer beyond the node.

The reported effects of irradiation on the lymph node barrier function are contrary and confusing. Different materials of different sizes have been used experimentally to study alteration in function following irradiation. Substances varied between thoratrast particles of 250 Å to charcoal particles, having a diameter of 60 microns. The results of some of these experiments are shown in Table 8. It appears that the reported changes in the barrier function following irradiation may depend on the type and size of the material used. For example, Fisher and Fisher (50) found that local irradiation significantly reduced the barrier function to erythrocytes, but it failed to influence the already deficient barrier function of the nodes toward tumor cell dissemination. Dettman et al. (31) reported no change in the capacity of the lymph node to filter colloidal gold following relatively large doses of irradiation, whereas Sinha and Goldberg (140) noted a reduction in the filtration capacity after 1500 to 3000 rads. Radiation given in doses equivalent to the therapeutic ranges were found to have no effect on the filtering capacity to thorotrast. It was also noted that patients who received extensive pelvic irradiation for a cervical cancer had no visible change in the appearance or the size of the lymph nodes, as determined by lymphography (178).

Hall and Morris (74) examined the immunological responsiveness of the sheep lymph nodes following nodal irradiation with doses varying between 400 and 2000 rads. They found that the antibody response to Salmonella Typhi antigen and the composition of the lymph were not altered significantly by irradiation. They concluded that although there is depletion of the lymphoid elements following irradiation, repopulation occurred from entry of circulating lymphocytes which are derived from the body pool.

In spite of the controversial data, regarding the effect of irradiation on the nodal function, clinicians have used radiotherapy for a long time and with success to sterilize cancer deposits in nodes. Few oncologists will dispute the fact that there has been improvement in survival following radiotherapy to retroperitoneal lymph nodes in patients with cancer of the testicles, or following pelvic irradiation of patients with carcinoma of the cervix. Similarly, prophylactic irradiation of the lymphatics of the neck of patients at high risk of having occult metastasis from a head and neck cancer has markedly decreased local recurrence and increased survival (51). In the controversial area of breast cancer treatment, it has been shown that patients who received radical radiotherapy, as the primary mode of treatment for breast cancer, have had as long a survival and perhaps a lower incidence of distant metastasis as those patients who were treated by radical surgery only (123). Patients who had high doses of preoperative radiotherapy for a locally advanced breast cancer faired at 10 years as well as those patients who had surgery, even though those who received preoperative treatment had more advanced lesions (53). Post-

Table 8. Effect of lymph node irradiation on its barrier function

Authors	Animal	Substances Injected	Time of Injection After Radiotherapy	Radiation Dose	Barrier Function
Engesett (45)	Rat	Toad lymphocyte (15 μ)	22 wks	3000 r	Reduced
		Charcoal (60 μ)	20 wks	3000 r	No change
		Walker Ca 256 (17–18 μ)	12–17 wks	3000 r	? Reduced
		Human erythrocytes	1–2 wks	3000 r	Reduced
Dettman, et al. (31)	Dog	Colloidal gold Au^{198} (5–50 μ)	1 day to 1 month	2000, 6000, 10,000 r	No change
Fisher & Fisher (50)	Rabbit	Rabbit erythrocytes (7 μ)	1–25 days	1000, 2000, 4000 r	Reduced
		V$_2$ tumor cells (17 μ–18 μ)	1–28 days	1000, 2000, 4000 r	No change
Herman, et al. (78)	Dog	Thorotrast 250 Å	2 hr to 42 days	1000–3000 r	No change
Sinha & Goldberg (140)	Rat	Colloidal gold Au^{198} (5–50 μ)	2 wks	1500–3000 r	Reduced
O'Brien, et al. (117)	Rabbit	V$_2$ tumor cells (17 μ–18 μ)	10 days	1000–3000 r	Reduced

operative radiotherapy given to the chest wall and peripheral lymphatics of the breast is known to reduce the incidence of local recurrences (52). However, this treatment was incriminated in the production of an increase in the incidence of distant metastasis by lowering the host defenses (29). Chu and her colleagues (22), from the Breast Service of Memorial Hospital, New York City, reviewed the effect of postoperative radiotherapy. Patients who were given irradiation had more advanced local disease. There was a significant increase in survival for those patients who had massive involvement of the axilla and who had irradiation, as compared to those who did not receive postoperative treatment. The incidence of distant metastasis was the same in irradiated and nonirradiated patients.

It should be pointed out that the experience of clinicians over the years contradicts the theory that irradiation of the lymphatics, by impairing the local and general immunity, may lead to an increase of either local recurrence or distant metastases and that patients who receive radiotherapy have a lower survival rate than those who do not.

CONCLUSION

It has often been stated that radiotherapy and, by the same argument, chemotherapy have a harmful effect on the cancer patient by altering certain in vitro parameters of cell mediated immunity. Such an argument presupposes an ability of the host to deal with its own tumor by immunological mechanisms when an alteration of these mechanisms would be detrimental. The poor results obtained in untreated cancer patients would seem to be a proof against such reasoning. Certainly, no oncologist in his right mind would withhold treatment from patients with, for example, cancer of the cervix, or head and neck, or seminoma, or Hodgkin's disease, in the belief that radiotherapy may alter the number of T cells or because there is doubtful evidence of changes in lymph node barrier function following irradiation.

The discovery of an assay for the cancer patient, equivalent to the blood sugar test, is not seen on the horizon. Until such a test is developed to give accurate guidance in the choice of a therapeutic modality, clinicians will have to rely on their past experience in prescribing the appropriate treatment.

We have not touched upon the use of specific and nonspecific immunostimulants, so-called immunotherapy, in patients receiving radiation. The reported benefits in humans from the use of immunostimulation are dubious at best and have as yet failed to show clinical significance. Regardless of the disturbance in the immunological tests which are observed following treatment, the best immunostimulant must still be adequate treatment, whether by surgery, radiotherapy, or chemotherapy.

SUMMARY

Irradiated patients may have marked depletion of lymphocytes and alteration of T/B cell ratio. Some in vitro assays of lymphocyte function, such as transformation by mitogens, may be depressed for a long time. There is little alteration of macrophage number or function. Monocytosis and eosinophilia are observed following irradiation, which may indicate stimulation of cell-mediated immunity by radiation altered cellular antigens. Inflammatory and delayed hypersensitivity reactions are not significantly depressed and may be enhanced following treatment. Specific and nonspecific autoantibodies may be induced by irradiation. There is no experimental or clinical proof to demonstrate that radiotherapy decreases the barrier function of the lymph node against cancer cells.

NOTES AND ACKNOWLEDGMENTS

1. This research was supported in part by N.I.H. Grant No. CA 17251.
2. This investigation was supported by N.I.H. Grant No. CA 13806.

REFERENCES

1. Ada, G. L., Parish, C. R., Nossal, G. J. V., and Abbot, A. 1967. The tissue localization, immunogenic and tolerance-inducing properties of antigens and antigen-fragments. Cold Spring Harbor Symp. Quant. Biol. 32: 381–393.

2. Allegretti, N., Stankovic, V., Vlahovic, S., and Sestan, N. 1961. The sensitizing effect of whole body X-irradiation in guinea pigs. Int. J. Radiat. Biol. 3: 259–263.

3. Allison, A. C., and Ferluga, J. 1976. How lymphocytes kill tumor cells. Editorial, N. Engl. J. Med. 295: 165–167.

4. Anderson, R. E., Sprent, J., Miller, J. F. 1974. Radiosensitivity of T & B Lymphocytes. Effect of irradiation on cell migration. Eur. J. Immunol. 4: 199–203.

5. Andrews, J. R. 1968. The Radiobiology of Human Cancer, pp. 105–114. W. B. Saunders Co., Philadelphia.

6. Balish, E., Pearson, T. A., and Chaskes, S. 1973. Irradiated humans microbial flora, immunoglobulins, complement (C'_3), tranferring, agglutinins and bacteriocidins. Rad. Res. 43: 729–756.

7. Barrett, O. 1970. Monocytosis in Malignant Disease. Ann. Interm. Med. 73: 991–992.

8. Bartfeld, H. 1975. Cell-mediated immunity: its modulation by X-rays. Effect of X-irradiation of T-lymphocyte numbers and function. *Ann. N.Y. Acad. Sciences*: 1965. 342–351.

9. Bennett, B. 1965. Specific suppression of tumor growth by isolated peritoneal macrophages from immunized mice. *J. Immunol.* 95: 656–664.

10. Berger, P. S., Keiser, H. D., and Ghossein, N. A. 1975. The induction of non-organ specific autoimmune phenomena by radiotherapy. *Radiology* 116: 215–216.

11. Blomgren, H., Glas, U., Melen, B., and Wasserman, J. 1974. Blood lymphocytes after radiation therapy of mammary carcinoma. *Acta Radiol. (Ther.)* 13: 185–200.

12. Bloom, B. R., Jiminez, L., Marcus, P. D. 1970. A plaque assay for enumerating antigen. *J. Exp. Med.* 132: 16–30.

13. Bone, G., Appelton, D. R., and Venables, C. W. 1974. The prognostic value of the cutaneous delayed hypersensitivity response to 2,4-dinitrochlorobenzene in gastrointestinal cancers. *Brit. J. Cancer* 29: 403–406.

14. Bosworth, J. L., Ghossein, N. A., and Brooks, T. L. 1975. Delayed hypersensitivity in patients treated by curative radiotherapy—its relation to the tumor response and short term survival. *Cancer* 36: 353–358.

15. Braeman, J., and Deeley, T. J. 1972. Immunological studies in irradiation of lung cancer, *Ann. Clin. Res.* 4: 355–360.

16. Braeman, J., and Deeley, T. J. 1973. Radiotherapy and the immune response in cancer of the lung. *Brit. J. Radiol.* 46: 446–449.

17. Brooke, M. S. 1962. The effect of total body X-irradiation of the rabbit on the rejection of homologous skin grafts and on the immune response. *J. Immunol.* 88: 419–425.

18. Burnham, T. K. 1972. Anti-nuclear antibodies in patients with malignancies. *Lancet* 2: 436.

19. Byfield, P. E., Stratton, J. A., and Small, R. 1974. Lymphocyte response after radiotherapy. *Lancet* 1: 309.

20. Catalona, W. J., Potvin, C., and Chretien, P. B. 1974. Effect of radiation therapy for urologic cancer on circulating thymus derived lymphocytes. *J. Urol.* 112: 261–267.

21. Chaskes, S., Kingdon, G. C., and Balish, E. 1975. Serum immunoglobulin level in humans exposed to therapeutic total-body gamma irradiation. *Rad. Res.* 62: 145–158.

22. Chu, F. C. H., Lucas, J. D., Jr., Farrow, J. H., and Nickson, J. J. 1967. Does prophylactic radiation therapy for cancer of the breast predispose to metastasis? *Amer. J. Roentgenol.* 99: 987–994.

23. Clement, J. A., and Kramer, S. 1974. Immunocompetence in patients with solid tumors undergoing cobalt-60 irradiation. *Cancer* 34: 193–196.

24. Cleveland, W. W., Fogel, B. J., Brown, W. T., et al. 1968. Foetal thymic transplant in a case of DiGeorge's syndrome. *Lancet* 2: 1211–1214.

25. Cosimi, A. B., Brunstetter, F. H., Kemmerer, W. T., and Miller, B. N. 1973. Cellular Immune competence of breast cancer patients receiving radiotherapy. *Arch. Surg.* 107: 531–535.

26. Cunningham, T. J., Daut, D., Wolfgang, P. E., Mellyn, M., Maciolek, S.,

Sponzo, R. W., and Horton, J. 1976. A correlation of DNCB-induced delayed cutaneous hypersensitivity reactions and the course of disease in patients with recurrent breast cancer. Cancer 37: 1696–1700.

27. Currie, G. A. 1976. Serum lysozyme as a marker of host resistance. II. Patients with malignant melanoma, hypernephroma or breast carcinoma. Brit. J. Cancer 33: 593–599.

28. Currie, G. A., and Eccles, S. A. 1976. Serum lysozyme as a marker of host resistance. I. Production by macrophages resistant in rat sarcomata. Brit. J. Cancer 33: 51–59.

29. Dao, T. L., and Kovaric, J. P. 1962. Incidence of pulmonary and skin metastases in women with breast cancer who received post-operative irradiation. Surgery 52: 203–212.

30. Dellon, A. L., Potvin, C., and Chretien, P. G. 1975. Thymus dependent lymphocyte levels during radiation therapy for bronchogenic and esophageal carcinoma: correlations with clinical course in responders and non-responders. Amer. J. Roent. 123: 500–511.

31. Dettman, P. M., King, E. R., and Zimberg, Y. H. 1966. Evaluation of lymph node function following irradiation or surgery. Amer. J. Roent. 96: 711–718.

32. Dierks, R. E., and Shepard, C. D. 1968. Effect of phytohemagglutinin and various microbacterial antigens on lymphocyte cultures from leprosy patients. Proc. Soc. Exp. Biol. Med. 127: 391–398.

33. Dixon, F. J., and McConahey, P. J. 1963. Enhancement of antibody formation by whole-body X-irradiation. J. Exp. Med. 117: 5, 833–848.

34. Dixon, F. J., Talmage, D. W., and Maurer, P. M. 1952. Radiosensitive and radioresistant phases in antibody response. J. Immunol. 68: 693–700.

35. Dizon, O. S., and Southam, C. M. 1963. Abnormal cellular response to skin abrasion in cancer patients. Cancer 16: 1288–1292.

36. Drinker, C. K., Field, M. E., and Ward, H. K. 1934. The filtering capacity of lymph nodes. J. Exp. Med. 59: 393–405.

37. Eilber, F. R., and Morton, D. L. 1970. Impaired immunologic reactivity and recurrence following cancer surgery. Cancer 25: 362–367.

38. Einhorn, J., Fagraeus, A., and Jonsson, J. 1965. Thyroid antibodies after 131 treatments for hyperthyroidism. J. Clin. Endocrinol. 25: 1212–1224.

39. Einhorn, J., Fagraeus, A., and Jonsson, J. 1966. Thyroid antibodies in euthyroid subjects after iodine-131 therapy. Radiat. Res. 28: 296–301.

40. Einhorn, N., and Jonsson, J. 1972. Antibodies to a HeLa cell line in carcinoma of the cervix uteri. The effect of radiation therapy. Acta Radiol. (Ther.) 11: 83–89.

41. Einhorn, N., Jonsson, J., and Fagraeus, A. 1969. Immunological reactions after irradiation of the uterus. Radiat. Res. 40: 465–472.

42. Einhorn, N., Packalen, T., and Wasserman, J. 1971. Lymphocyte stimulation by thyroglobulin after local irradiation of thyroid gland in man. Acta Radiol. Ther. Phy. Biol. 10: 481–487.

43. Elhilali, M. M., Britton, S., Brosman, S., and Fahey, J. L. 1976. Critical evaluation of lymphocyte functions in urological cancer patients. Canc. Res. 36: 132–137.

44. Engeset, A. 1959. An experimental study of the lymph node barrier; injec-

tion of Walker carcinoma 256 in the lymph vessels. *Acta. Un. Int. Cancer* 15: 879–883.

45. Engeset, A. 1969. Irradiation of lymph nodes and vessels. Experiments in rats, with reference to cancer therapy. *Acta Radiol. Suppl.* 229: 5–125.

46. Evans, R., and Alexander, P. 1970. Cooperation of immune lymphoid cells with macrophages in tumor immunity. *Nature* 228: 620–622.

47. Farrow, L. J., Holborow, E. J., and Brighton, W. D. 1971. Reaction of human smooth muscle antibody with liver cells. *Nature New Biology* 232: 186–187.

48. Fisher, B. 1976. Trials of conservative operation in the United States: A report of NSABP efforts. *Breast Cancer: A Report to the Profession.*

49. Fisher, B., and Fisher, E. 1967. Barrier function of lymph node to tumor cells and erythrocyte. I. Normal Node. *Cancer* 20: 1907–1913.

50. Fisher, B., and Fisher, E. 1967. Barrier function of lymph node to tumor cells and erythrocyte. II. Effect of X-rays, inflammation, sensitization and tumor growth. *Cancer* 20: 1914–1919, 1967.

51. Fletcher, G. H. 1972. Elective irradiation of subclinical disease in cancers of the head and neck. *Cancer* 29: 1450–1454.

52. Fletcher, G. H. 1973. *Textbook of Radiotherapy* (2nd ed.), Chap. 6, pp. 457–493. Lea and Febiger, Philadelphia.

53. Fletcher, G. H., Montague, E. D., and White, E. C. 1970. Role of Radiation Therapy in the Primary Management of Breast Cancer, *in Progress in Clinical Cancer.*, pp. 242. Grune and Stratton, New York.

54. Frenkel, J. K., and Wilson, H. R. 1972. Effects of radiation on specific cellular immunities: Besnoitiosis and a Herpes virus infection of hamsters. *J. Inf. Dis.* 125: 216–230.

55. Gallily, R., and Ben-Ishay, Z. 1974. Interaction between normal or irradiated macrophage and lymphocytes in mice. *Cell. Immunol.* 2: 314–324, 1974.

56. Gallily, R., and Zylberlicht, D. 1975. Impairment of the bactericidal activity of murine macrophages following X-irradiation. *Immunochemistry* 12: 611–614.

57. Garrioch, D. B., Good, R. A., and Gatti, R. A. 1970. Lymphocyte response to PHA in patients with non-lymphoid tumors. *Lancet* 1: 618.

58. Geiger, B., and Gallily, R. 1974. Effect of X-irradiation on various functions of murine macrophages. *Clin. Exp. Immunol.* 16: 643–655.

59. Geiger, B., and Gallily, R. 1974. Surface morphology of irradiated macrophages. *J. Reticuloendothel. Soc.* 15: 274–281.

60. Gelfand, M. D., Tepper, M., Katz, L. A., Binder, H. J., Yesner, R., and Floch, M. H. 1968. Acute radiation proctitis in man. Development of eosinophilic cryptabscesses. *Gastroenterology* 54: 401–441.

61. Ghossein, N. A., Azar, H. A., and Williams, J. 1963. Local irradiation of the thymus. Histological changes with observations on circulation, lymphocytes and serum protein fractions in adult mice. *Amer. J. Path.* 43: 369–375.

62. Ghossein, N. A., Bosworth, J. L., and Bases, R. E. 1975. The effect of radical radiotherapy on delayed hypersensitivity and the inflammatory response. *Cancer* 35: 1616–1620.

63. Ghossein, N. A., Bosworth, J. L., Stacey, P., Muggia, F. M., and Krishnaswamy, V. 1975. Radiation-related eosinophilia. *Radiology* 117: 413–417.

64. Ghossein, N. A., and Stacey, P. 1973. The prognostic significance of radiation-related eosinophilia: A preliminary report. *Radiology* 107: 631–633.

65. Ghossein, N. A., and Tricoche, M. 1971. Synthesis of immunoglobulins by rat thymus after thymic irradiation. *Nature New Biology* 234: 16–17.

66. Goldsmith, H. S., Levin, A. G., and Southam, C. M. 1965. A study of cellular responses in cancer patients by qualitative and quantitative Rebuck tests. *Surg. Forum* 16: 102–104.

67. Gordon, S., Todd, S., and Cohn, Z. A. 1974. *In vitro* synthesis and secretion of lysozyme by mononuclear phagocytes. *J. Exp. Med.* 139: 1228–1248.

68. Graham, J. B., Graham, M., Neri, L., and Wright, K. D. 1956. Enhanced production of antibodies by local irradiation. 1. Measurement of circulating antibodies. *J. Immunol.* 76: 103–109.

69. Graham, J. R., and Leskowitz, S. 1956. Enhanced production of antibodies by local irradiation. 2. Measurement of local antibodies. *J. Immunol.* 76: 110–117, 1956.

70. Granger, G. A., and Weiser, R. S. 1964. Homograft target cells: specific destruction *in vitro* by contact interaction with immune macrophages. *Science* 145: 1427–1429.

71. Gross, L., Manfredi, O. L., and Protos, A. 1973. Effect of cobalt-60 irradiation upon cell-mediated immunity. *Radiology* 106: 653–655, 1973.

72. Gutterman, J. U., Mavligit, G., Gottlieb, J. A., Burgess, M. A., McBride, C. E., Einhorn, L., Freireich, E. J., and Hersh, E. M. 1974. Chemoimmunotherapy of disseminated malignant melanoma with dimethyltriazenocarboxamide and Bacillus Calmette-Guerin. *N. Engl. J. Med.* 291: 592–597.

73. Halili, M., Bosworth, J. L., Romney, S., Moukhtar, M., and Ghossein, N. A. 1976. The long term effect of radiotherapy on the immune status of patients cured of a gynecologic malignancy. *Cancer* 37: 2875–2878.

74. Hall, J. G., and Morris, B. 1964. Effect of X-irradiation of the popliteal lymph node on its output of lymphocytes in immunological responsiveness. *Lancet* 1: 1077–1080.

75. Hancock, B. W., Bruce, L., and Richmond, J. 1976. Neutrophil function in lymphoreticular malignancy. *Brit. J. Cancer* 33: 496–500.

76. Heineke, H. 1903. Über die Einwirkung der Röntgenstrahlen auf Tiere. *München. Med. Wochenschr.* 50: 2090–2092.

77. Hellström, K. E., and Hellström, I. 1970. Immunologic defenses against cancer, in R. A. Good and D. W. Fisher, (eds.), *Immunobiology* 1970, pp. 209–224. Sinaver Associates, Stamford, Conn.

78. Herman, P. G., Benninghoff, D. L., and Mellins, H. Z. 1968. Radiation effect and the barrier function of the lymph node. *Radiology* 91: 698–702.

79. Hersh, E. M., Whitecar, J. P., McCredie, K. B., Bodey, G. P., and Freireich, E. J. 1971. Chemotherapy, immunocompetence, immunosuppression and prognosis in acute leukemia. *N. Engl. J. Med.* 285: 1211–1216.

80. Himmelweit, F. (ed.). 1957. *The Collected Papers of Paul Ehrlich.* Pergamon Press, New York.

81. Holley, T. R., Van Epps, D. E., Harvey, R. L., Anderson, R. E., and Williams, R. C. 1974. Effect of high doses of radiation on human neutrophils, chemotaxis, phagocytosis and morphology. *Amer. J. Path.* 75: 61–72, 1974.

82. Hollingsworth, J. W., and Beeson, P. B. 1955. Experimental bacteremia in normal and irradiated rats. *Yale J. Biol. Med.* 28: 56–62.

83. Holtermann, O. A., Djerassi, I., Lisafeld, B. A., Elias, E. G., Papermaster, B. W., and Klein, E. 1974. *In vitro* destruction of tumor cells by human monocytes. *Proc. Soc. Exp. Biol. Med.* 1217: 456–459.

84. Honsinger, R. W., Jr., Silverstein, D., and Van Arsdel, P. O. 1972. The eosinophil and allergy: why? *J. Allergy Clin. Immunol.* 49: 142–155.

85. Hsu, C. K., and Hsu, S. H. 1976. Immunopathology of schistosomiasis in athymic mice. *Nature* 262: 397–399.

86. Huber, H., Douglas, S. D., and Fudenberg, M. H. 1969. The IgG receptor: an immunological marker for the characterizations of mononuclear cells. *Immunology* 17: 7–21.

87. Humphrey, L. J., Lincoln, D. M., and Griffin, W. O., Jr. 1968. Immunologic response in patients with disseminated cancer. *Ann. Surg.* 168: 374–381.

88. Jenkins, V. K., Olson, M. H., Ellis, H. N., and Cooley, R. N. 1975. Effect of therapeutic radiation on peripheral blood lymphocytes in patients with carcinoma of the breast. *Acta Radiol. Therapy Physics Biol.* 14: 385–395.

89. Jiminez, L., Bloom, B. R., Blume, M. R., and Oettger, H. F. 1971. On the number and nature of antigen-sensitive lymphocytes in the blood of delayed hypersensitive human donors. *J. Exp. Med.* 133: 740–751.

90. Johnson, M. W., Maibach, H. I., and Salmon, S. E. 1971. Skin reactivity in patients with cancer. *N. Engl. J. Med.* 22: 1255–1257.

91. Kasakura, S., and Lowenstein, L. 1967. The effect of uremic blood on mixed leukocyte reactions and on cultures of leukocytes with phytohemagglutinin. *Transplantation* 5: 283–289.

92. Katz, D. H., and Benacerraf, B. 1972. The regulatory influence of T-cells and B-cell responses to antigen. *Adv. Imm.* 15: 1–94.

93. Kennedy, J. C., Till, J. E., and Siminovitch, L., *et al.* 1965. Radiosensitivity of the immune response to Sheys red cells in the mouse, as measured by the hemolytic plaque method. *J. Immunol.* 94: 715–722.

94. Kerckhaert, J. A. 1974. Influence of cyclophosphamide on the delayed hypersensitivity in the mouse after intraperitoneal immunization. *Ann. Immunol.* 125: 559–568.

95. Kidd, J. G., and Toolan, M. W. 1950. The association of lymphocytes with cancer cells undergoing distinctive neurobiosis in resistant and immune hosts. *Amer. J. Path.* 26: 672–673.

96. Kohn, H. I. 1951. Effect of X-rays upon hemolysin production in the rat. *J. Immunol.* 66: 525–533.

97. Kun, E., and Johnson, E. 1975. Hematologic and immunologic status in Hodgkin's disease five years after radical radiotherapy. *Cancer* 36: 1912–1916.

98. Kurohara, S. S., Hempelmann, L. H., Englaner, C. L. S., *et al.* 1964. Eosinophilia after exposure to ionizing radiation. *Radiat. Res.* 23: 357–368.

99. Larson, D. L., and Tomlinson, L. J. 1953. Quantitative antibody studies in

man. III. Antibody response in leukemia and other malignant lymphoma. *J. Clin. Investigation* 32: 317–321.

100. Lee, Y. N., Sparkes, F. C., Eilber, F. R., and Morton, D. L. 1975. Delayed cutaneous hypersensitivity and peripheral lymphocyte counts in patients with advanced cancer. *Cancer* 35: 748–753.

101. Leskowitz, S., Phillipino, L., Hendrick, G., and Graham, J. B. 1957. Immune response in patients with cancer. *Cancer* 10: 1103–1105.

102. Levy, R., and Kaplan, H. S. 1974. Impaired lymphocyte function in untreated Hodgkin's disease. *N. Engl. J. Med.* 290: 181–186.

103. Lischner, H. W., Dacou, C., and DiGeogre, A. M. 1967. Normal lymphocyte transfer (NLT) test: Negative response in a patient with congenital absence of the thymus. *Transplantation* 5: 555–557.

104. Lischner, H. W., Valdes-Dapena, M. A., Biggin, J., Hann, S., and Amoni, N. 1973. In F. Daguillard (ed.), *Proceedings of the Seventh Leucocyte Culture Conference*, pp. 547–560. Academic Press, New York.

105. Loiseleur, J., Girard, O., and Petit, M. 1965. Augmentation du taux des anticorps tetanique et dyphterique consécutivement a l'action des rayons X. *C. R. Acad. Sc. Paris* 260: 3230–3231.

106. Lytton, B., Hughes, L. E., and Fulthorpe, A. J. 1964. Circulating antibody response in malignant disease. *Lancet* 1: 69–71.

107. MaGuire, H. C., and Maibach, H. I. 1963. Effect of X-ray lymphopenia on contact dermatitis. *Arch. Dem.* 88: 768–770.

108. Maisel, R. H., and Ogara, J. H. 1974. Abnormal dinitrochlorobenzene skin sensitization—a prognostic sign of survival in head and neck squamous cell carcinoma. *Laryngoscope* 84: 2012–2019.

109. Makinodan, T., Nettesheim, P., Morita, *et al.* 1967. Synthesis of antibody by spleen cells after exposure to kilo-roentgen doses of ionizing radiation. *J. Cell Physiol.* 69: 355–366.

110. McCluskey, R. T., and Cohen, S. (eds.). 1974. *Mechanisms of Cell Mediated Immunity*, pp. 61–96. John Wiley & Sons, New York.

111. McCredie, J. A., Inch, W. R., and Sutherland, R. M. 1972. Effect of postoperative radiotherapy on peripheral blood lymphocytes in patients with carcinoma of the breast. *Cancer* 29: 349–356.

112. Meyer, O. T., and Dannenberg, A. M.: Radiation, infection and macrophage function. II. Effect of whole body radiation on the number of pulmonary alveolar macrophages and their levels of hydrolytic enzymes. *J. Reticulendothel. Soc.* 7: 79–90, 1970.

113. Minot, G. R., and Spurling, R. G.: The effect on the blood of irradiation, especially short wave length roentgen-ray therapy. *Amer. J. Med. Sci.* 168: 215–241, 1924.

114. Mitsuoka, A., Baba, M., and Morikawa, S. 1976. Enhancement of delayed hypersensitivity by depletion of suppressor T-cells with cyclophosphamide in mice. *Nature* 262: 77–78.

115. Moldow, R. E.: Monocytosis in malignancy. *Ann. Int. Med.* 74: 449, 1971.

116. Muggia, F. M., Ghossein, N. A., and Wohl, H. 1973. Eosinophilia follow-

ing radiation therapy. *Oncology* 27: 118–127.

117. O'Brien, P. H., Moss, W. T., Ujiki, G. T., Pubong, O., and Towne, W.: Effect of irradiation on tumor infused lymph nodes. *Radiology* 94: 407–411, 1970.

118. O'Gorman, P., Staffurth, J. S., and Ballentyne, M. R. 1964. Antibody Response to Thyroid Irradiation. *J. Clin. Endocrinol.* 24: 1072–1075.

119. Osserman, E. F. 1975. Lysozyme. *N. Engl. J. Med.* 292: 424–425.

120. O'Toole, C., Perlmann, P., Unsgaard, B., Moberger, G., and Edsmyn, F. 1972. Cellular immunity to human urinary bladder carcinoma. I. Correlations to clinical stage and radiotherapy. *Int. J. Cancer* 10: 77–91.

121. Papatesta, A. E., and Kark, A. 1974. Peripheral lymphocyte counts in breast carcinoma. An index of immune competence. *Cancer* 34: 2014–2017.

122. Parker, C. W. 1976. Control of lymphocyte function. *N. Engl. J. Med.* 295: 1180–1186.

123. Peters, M. V. 1975. Cutting the "Gordian knot" in early breast cancer. *Ann. Royal Coll. Phys. Surgeons Can.* 186–192.

124. Plesnicar, S. 1972. Immunoglobulin in carcinoma of the uterine cervix. *Acta Radiol.* 11: 37–47.

125. Pohle, E. A., and Bunting, C. H. 1936. Histologische Untersuchungen an der Rattenmilz nach abgestuften Röntgenstrahlendosen. *Strahlentherapie* 57: 121–124.

126. Regaud, C., and Cremieu, R. 1912. Données relatives aux petetes cellules ou lymphocytes du parenchyme thymique d'après les résultats de Rontgenisation du thymus chez le chat. *Compt. Rend. Soc. Biol. Paris* 72: 253–254.

127. Reisco, A. 1970. Five year cancer cure: relation to total amount of peripheral lymphocytes and neutrophils. *Cancer* 25: 135–140.

128. Rotman, M., Ansley, H., Rogow, L., and Stowe, S. 1977. Monocytosis: A new observation during radiotherapy. *Int. J. Rad. Onc. Biol. Physics* 2: 117–121.

129. Rubin, P., and Casarett, G. W. 1968. *Clinical Radiation Pathology*, pp. 779–865. W. B. Saunders Co., Philadelphia.

130. Russell, B. R. G. 1908. *The Third Scientific Report of the Imperial Research Fund*, p. 34.

131. Sado, T. 1969. Functional and ultrastructural studies of antibody producing cells exposed to 10,000 rads in millipore diffusion chambers. *Int. J. Radiat. Biol.* 25: 1–22.

132. Sado, T., Kurotsut, and Kamisaku, M. 1971. Further studies on the radioresistance of antibody producing cells characterization of the survival. *Radiat. Res.* 48: 179–188.

133. Salden, T. 1963. Experimental studies on spread of Rous sarcoma in rats. *Acta Rath. Microbiol. Scan. Suppl.* 162: 1–87.

134. Salvin, S. B., and Nishio, J. 1972. Lymphoid cells in delayed hypersensitivity. III. The influence of X-irradiation on passive transfer and on in-vitro production of soluble mediators. *J. Exp. Med.* 135: 985–996.

135. Salvin, S. B., and Smith, R. F. 1959. Delayed hypersensitivity in the development of circulating antibodies. The effect of X-irradiation. *J. Exp. Med.* 109: 325–338.

136. Sato, C. 1970. Change in the type of radiation cell-killing on human

lymphocytes after blast transformation by phytohemagglutin. *Int. J. Radiol. Biol.* 18: 483–485.

137. Schmidtke, J. R., and Dixon, F. J. 1972. The functional capacity of X-irradiated macrophages. *J. Immunol.* 108: 1624–1630.

138. Schmidtke, J. R., and Dixon, F. J. 1973. The effect of *in-vivo* irradiation on macrophage function. *J. Immunol.* 110: 848–854.

139. Senn, N. 1903. Case of splenomedullary leukemia successfully treated by the use of the Roentgen rays. *Med. Rec.* 64: 281–283.

140. Sinha, B. K., and Goldenberg, G. J.: Effect of irradiation on lymph flow and filtration function of lymph node. *Cancer* 26: 1239–1245, 1970.

141. Slater, M., Ngo, E., and Lau, B. H. S.: Effect of therapeutic irradiation of the immune responses. *Amer. J. Roent.* 126: 313–320, 1976.

142. Southam, C. M. 1975. *In* M. Samter (ed.), *Immunological Disease*, Vol. 1, p. 743. Little Brown and Co., Boston.

143. Spiers, R. S., and Spiers, E. E. 1974. Quantitative Studies of Inflammation and Granuloma Formation, *in* C. G. VanArman (ed.), *White Cells in Inflammation.* Thomas, Springfield, Ill.

144. Spiers, R. S., Spiers, E. E., and Ponzio, N. M. 1974. Eosinophils in Humoral and Cell-Mediated Responses, *in* A. Gottlieb (ed.), *Developments in Lymphoid Cell Biology*, pp. 51–73, Chap. III. CRC Press, Cleveland.

145. Stewart, C. C., and Perez, C. 1976. Effect of irradiation on immune responses. *Radiol.* 118: 201–210, 1976.

146. Stjernsward, J. 1972. Immunological changes after radiotherapy to mammary carcinoma. *Ann. Inst. Pasteur* 122: 883–894.

147. Stjernsward, J., Vanky, F., Jondal, M., Wigzell, H., and Sealy, R. 1972. Lymphopenia and change in distribution of human B and T lymphocytes in peripheral blood induced by irradiation for mammary carcinoma. *Lancet:* 1352–1356.

148. Stratton, J. A., Byfield, P. E., Small, R. C., Byfield, J., and Pilch, Y. 1975. Acute effects of radiation therapy, including or excluding the thymus, on the lymphocyte subpopulations of cancer patients. *J. Clin. Invest.* 56 (1): 88–97.

149. Taliaferro, W. H., Taliaferro, L. G., and Jaroslow, B. N. 1964. *Radiation and the Immune Response.* Academic Press, New York.

150. Tarpley, J. L., Potvin, C., Chretien, P. B. 1975. Prolonged depression of cellular immunity in cured laryngopharyngeal cancer patients treated with radiation therapy. *Cancer* 35: 638–644.

151. Thomas, J. W., Coy, P., Lewis, H. S., and Yuen, A. 1971. Effect of therapeutic irradiation of lymphocyte transformation in lung cancer. *Cancer* 27: 1046–1050.

152. Thomas, J. W., Naiman, S. C., and Clements, D. 1967. Lymphocyte transformation by phytohemagglutinin: II. In the tuberculous patient. *Canad. Med. Assoc. J.* 97: 836–840.

153. Turk, J. L., Parker, D., and Poulter, L. W. 1972. Functional aspects of the selective depletion of lymphoid tissue by cyclophosphamide. *Immunology* 23: 493–501.

154. Uhr, J. W., and Scharff, M. 1962. Delayed hypersensitivity. V. The effects

of X-irradiation on the development of delayed hypersensitivity and antibody formation. *J. Exp. Med.* 112: 65–76.

155. Unanue, E. R., and Askonas, B. A. 1968. Persistence of immunogenicity of antigen after uptake by macrophage. *J. Exp. Med.* 127: 915–926.

156. Vaughan-Smith, S., and Ling, N. R. 1975. The effects of X-rays on the responses of porsine lymphocytes to the mitogenic stimulus of concanavallin A *in vitro. Int. J. Radiat. Biol.* 24: 73–85.

157. Virchow, R. 1860. *Cellular Pathology* (2nd ed.; trans. Frank Chance). Robert M. DeWitt, New York.

158. Visakorpi, R. 1972. Effect of irradiation of established delayed hypersensitivity. Supression of skin reactions, recovery and the effect of cell transfer. *Acta Path. Microbiol. Scand.* B 80: 788–794.

159. Visakorpi, R. 1974. The effect of irradiation on macrophage migration inhibition. *Immunol.* 27: 145–149.

160. Vorbrodt, A., Hliniak, A., and Krzyzowska-Gruca, S. T. 1972. Ultrastructural studies on the behavior of macrophages in the course of X-ray therapy on human skin cancer. *Acta Histochem.* 43: 270–280.

161. Vorbrodt, A., Hliniak, A., and Niepolomska. 1971. Histochemical studies on cellular response of human skin cancer in the course of X-ray therapy. *Rad. Biol. Ther.* 12: 15–24.

162. Vorbrodt, A., Hliniak, A., and Niepolomska. 1971a. Further histochemical studies on cellular response of human skin cancer in the course of fractionated X-ray therapy. *Rad. Biol. Ther.* 12: 547–558.

163. Walls, R. S., Basten, A., Leuchars, E., *et al.* 1971. Mechanisms for eosinophilic and neutrophilic leucocytosis. *Brit. J. Med.* 3: 157–159.

164. Wara, W. M., Phillips, T. L., Wara, S. W., Ammann, A. J., and Smith, V. 1975. Immunosuppression following radiation therapy for carcinoma of the nasopharynx. *Amer. J. Roent.* 123: 482–485.

165. Wasserman, J., Glas, U., and Blomgren, H. 1975. Auto antibodies in patients with carcinoma of the breast. *Clin. Exp. Immunol.* 19: 417–422.

166. Wohl, H., and Ghossein, N. A. 1971. Complement levels before and after radiotherapy in cancer patients. *Oncology* 25: 344–346.

167. Yantorno, C., Soarnes, W. A., Gonder, M. J., *et al.* 1967. Studies in cryoimmunology. 1. The production of antibodies to urogenital tissue in consequence of freezing treatment. *Immunology* 12: 395–410.

168. Yoffey, J. M., and Courtice, F. C. 1956. *Lymphatics, Lymph and Lymphoid Tissue* (2nd ed.). Edward Arnold, London.

169. Yoshida, T., Benacerraf, B., McClusky, R., Vasselli, P. 1969. The effects of intravenous antigen on circulating monocytes in animals with delayed hypersensitivity. *J. Immunol.* 102: 804–811.

170. Young, R. C., Corder, M. D., Berard, C. W., and DeVita, V. T. 1973. Immune alterations in Hodgkin's disease. *Arch. Int. Med.* 131: 446–454.

171. Zeidman, I., and Buss, J. M. 1954. Experimental studies on the spread of cancer in the lymphatic system: I. Effectiveness of the lymph nodes as a barrier to the passage of embolic tumor cells. *Cancer Res.* 114: 403–405.

172. Zeromski, J. O., Gorny, M. K., and Jarczewska, K. 1972. Malignancy associated with antinuclear antibodies. *Lancet* 2: 1035–1036.

CHAPTER 7

EVALUATION OF SPECIFIC IMMUNE REACTIVITY IN HUMAN PATIENTS WITH SOLID CANCERS

Jean C. Hager
and G. H. Heppner

Department of Medicine
Roger Williams General Hospital
Division of Biology and Medicine
Brown University
Providence, Rhode Island 02912

A number of techniques have been described for detecting and measuring specific immune reactivity to antigens of solid cancers in human patients. These techniques include those to detect humoral antibody (precipitation, immunofluorescence, complement fixation, immune adherence, and cytotoxicity), and cell-mediated immunity (colony inhibition, cytotoxicity, leucocyte indicator assays, and blastogenesis). Modifications of cell-mediated immune assays have been developed to measure CMI-humoral interaction. Assays to measure CMI in vivo are also available. For a variety of technical and philosophical reasons, none of the assays so far described are satisfactory for the purposes of either detecting or monitoring immune reactivity in cancer patients.

I. INTRODUCTION

An area of great hope in clinical tumor immunology is the development of techniques to detect and quantitate immune reactivity to tumor associated antigens in patients with cancer. Should such methodology exist it would be possible to use it both in early detection and diagnosis of cancer and in assessment of prognosis and response to therapy. What follows is a description of some of the techniques which have been developed for use in patients with solid cancers. Because of the unrealistically high claims which have been repeatedly made for these approaches, we are here emphasizing the difficulties encountered in attempting to actually apply them in the clinic.

II. METHODS USED TO DETECT SPECIFIC DEFENSES IN HUMAN PATIENTS

A. In Vivo Methods

It is generally believed that testing patients directly *in vivo* for evidence of immune reactivity to their own or related tumors will give a more accurate picture of the tumor-host relationship than will testing patients' sera or cells *in vitro* where only a narrow, preselected aspect of the problem is investigated. In fact, it is also difficult to design methods of testing *in vivo* in which the test antigens are either valid or presented to the patients' immune system in a way appropriate to natural disease events. There are generally two approaches which have been tried: measurement of transplantation resistance, and skin testing with tumor cells or extracts.

1. TRANSPLANTATION RESISTANCE. The concept that immune mechanisms might operate in a tumor-bearing individual so as to result in immunological rejection of the tumor load left medical lore and entered the experimental laboratory when Foley (22), and then Prehn and Main (89), showed that animals could be sensitized by a primary tumor growth so that, following tumor removal, they could reject the growth of a second tumor challenge. These experiments gave birth to the field of tumor immunology, and to the naive hope that after considerable study enough would be known about the underlying immune mechanisms to establish programs to eliminate cancer, analogous to vaccination programs in infectious diseases.

Although studies of transplantation resistance in animals are laborious and costly, they are at least feasible and have provided valuable insights into the relationship of the animal and his tumor. In humans, however, these experiments generally cannot be repeated, for obvious reasons.

a. Skin Testing with Extracts.   The general rationale behind skin testing is that an *in vivo* assessment of delayed hypersensitivity might be a close reflection of the state of systemic cellular immunity. Most of the skin tests have been performed with soluble membrane extracts of tumor cells, and for control, of normal tissues (43, 47, 71, 93, 99, 110). Patients are tested concurrently with the membrane preparations and a battery of standard recall antigens to determine if their general cellular reactivity is intact, although the ability to react to such antigens is not necessarily related to the ability to respond to tumor-associated antigens. Most investigators have defined a positive reaction to be 5 mm or more of induration at 48 hours after inoculation. This definition is derived from experience with tuberculin testing and may not always represent the peak timing of the reaction to membrane extracts (43).

On a technical level skin testing is claimed to be relatively simple, not requiring specialized equipment or extensive training of personnel (43). The major advantage of the technique lies in the use of tumor tissues taken directly from the patients. This eliminates the difficulties in obtaining cultured cells both from the solid tumors, and, more especially, from the normal tissues which are exquisitely difficult to culture. This method also avoids problems of microbial contamination or *in vitro* acquired antigenic changes, although the extraction procedures used to solubilize the antigens may result in their alteration (46).

There are some serious problems encountered with the skin testing technique. In several studies, particularly in breast cancer (48), melanoma (14), and lung cancer (49), it has been found that a high frequency of reactions occur in patients tested with the designated "normal" tissue preparations. Thus, it is necessary to differentiate reactivity to tissue-associated antigens from that elicited by tumor-associated antigens. In some studies further purification of the antigen has been successful in separating the specific antigens (14).

Another serious problem with the control preparations is the selection of relevant "normal" tissue. Also there may be quite a low yield of soluble antigen from both normal and cancer tissues. Further, the procedures are tedious and must be done individually for each tumor, and for each patient. The preparations are limited in numbers and it is difficult to standardize them. These procedures are also limited because considerable time and cooperation is required from the patients.

Patients are tested with doses quantified by ranges of protein/ml solution (not per original starting material) extracted from the appropriate tissues. The elicited reactions do not follow a dose response curve (43). Quantitation of the induration observed is difficult. Induration is only measured conveniently in two dimensions, whereas the reaction occurs in three dimensions. A positive test depends on the presence of adequate numbers of mononuclear cells to accumulate at the reaction sites. The final result evaluated is, therefore, several steps removed from the initiating event. The clinical evaluation of the test is properly validated by the correlation of histological studies of skin punch biopsy, i.e., a positive reaction should consist of lymphocytic and histiocytic perivascular infiltrates in the upper dermis (43).

Perhaps one of the most serious difficulties in the skin testing procedures is the ethical prohibition of testing healthy normal individuals with extracts of cancer tissues to obtain baseline values. Generally, controls consist of patients tested with extracts of patients with other types of cancers or with designated "normal" tissue surgically removed from cancer patients. The choice of "normal" tissue may be inappropriate or, even if truly normal in character, may be inadequate, since the amounts of represented cell types may vary from those in the tumor tissue.

b. Skin Testing with Cryostat Sections. The skin window test provides an alternative in vivo test to the intradermal injection of soluble tissue extracts. This procedure, a modification of the Rebuck test, was pioneered in tumor immunology by Black and Leis (5, 6, 7). It has been extensively used by these investigators and associates for breast cancer studies. An ether-alcohol fixed cryostat section of autologous tissue, mounted on a coverslip, is applied to an abraded area of the patients' skin for a period of 30 hours to allow "infiltration," or collection, of exudate cells on the coverslip. The test measures the delayed hypersensitivity reaction of the patient to his own tumor tissues which have been altered only by fixation and freezing.

The technique itself is exquisitely simple and is closer than most immunological assays to the biological composition of the tumor-host relationship. However, this procedure requires great cooperation on the part of the patients. The success of the assay also depends on the involvement of an experienced pathologist for evaluation and choice of the areas of tissues used as antigens, both the representative tumor sections and the control, non-involved or benign disease tissues. The pathologist must also assist in correlations of the test reactions with lymphoreticular activity in the patient. Reading the exudates on the skin windows also requires certain skill in characterization of the inflammatory response (5, 6, 7).

One of the major disadvantages of this technique is the inability to quantitate the amount of antigen presented to the patient. Further, the patients' immune response is evaluated in qualitative terms. The response itself is dependent upon a similar series of events as is the intradermal skin testing, i.e., presensitized lymphocytes which can be antigenically stimulated to release soluble factors and then sufficient numbers of reactive cells to produce the basophil-associated mononuclear cell response. Another problem is that only autologous tissues can serve as a source of antigen due to ethical considerations. Therefore, controls for the technique are less than optimal.

B. In Vitro Methods

1. HUMORAL IMMUNITY.   Immunoglobulins have been demonstrated on solid human tumors *in vivo* (51, 53, 54, 57, 68, 108, 111). This finding suggests that the tumor-associated antigens stimulate a humoral immune response which results in localization of antibody on the tumor surface. The resultant immune complex may even bind complement (51, 53). Whatever the role of these antibodies *in vivo*, they may be useful in defining and localizing either cell surface or intracellular antigens of potential use of immunological testing.

a. Precipitation.   Immunologists have traditionally taken advantage of the formation of a precipitate by antigen and antibody to get a handle on these constituents in unknown mixtures. Some tumor immunologists have tried to follow this classic approach to detect antibody in patients' sera (12, 50, 65, 68) or in tumor extracts (91). The main approach is use of an Ouchterlony double diffusion system or the related immunoelectrophoretic analysis. These methods require an antigen preparation which is capable of combining specifically with antibody to form a precipitate when optimal ratios of antigen and antibody concentrations are reacted. Antigens have been prepared as tumor extracts, i.e., by freeze-thaw and homogenization. The use of these methods has met with little success in tumor studies since many sera positive by other tests have either failed to precipitate with the provided extract antigen (50), or have reacted with normal tissue extracts and other tumor extracts as well as specific tumor extracts (12, 68). Further, so few tumor-bearer sera may react with the antigen that the test is useless (50). The problem may be the lack of the appropriate concentrations of antigen and antibody to form a precipitate, or it may be lack of specificity in the reagents. In studies using specific sera eluted off an immunoabsorbant column (65) it was possible to separate the specific antibodies and form precipitates. However, a significant difficulty in this assay is that when positive reactions are encountered, they may be unique events with patients followed serially (12) with no standard time postoperatively at which antibody can be detected.

A promising departure from these techniques (25) uses tumor antigens from body fluids entrapped in polyacrylamide gels to absorb specific antibodies from pooled cancer-bearer sera. These antibodies are then radioiodinated and used in a radioimmunoassay to detect antibodies in individual patient sera. The specificity of this assay needs further refinement before it will be useful.

b. Immunofluorescence.

Immunofluorescence assays are modifications of precipitation detection assays. Antigen and antibody are allowed to react to form microprecipitates which are visualized by the addition of a fluorochrome label, commonly fluorescein isothiocyanate, to either the antibody (direct test) or an anti-antibody (indirect test). The reaction is observed microscopically when the fluorochrome is excited by UV or blue light. It is a highly sensitive technique which can be used to detect either antibodies against known antigen, or tissue antigens with specific reagent antisera. Such assays are quantitated by either titration of serum or enumeration of the positive cells. Immunofluorescence assays are simple to perform but, because many artifacts can occur, do require some skill in interpretation.

The major difficulties lie in the realm of specificity. Test sera, and even reagent sera, contain substances which can nonspecifically bind to cellular constituents. Sera may contain antibodies which cross-react with cellular antigens, i.e., heterophile reactions (29), or they may contain antibodies to normal cellular, tissue, or species antigens, i.e., to blood group antigens (Hager, unpublished data). These contaminating antibodies result in positive reactions which are misleading. There are also problems in variability between laboratories which probably stem from lack of technical standardization (for review, see Ref. 63). It is especially important in performing immunofluorescence tests to include stringent controls for specificity, and for technique, i.e., blocking reactions, testing buffer in place of serum, properly matching controls.

Certain spurious reactions can be eliminated by absorption of sera with various tissue powders, cells, or by purification of the immunoglobulin fractions. Generally the investigator does not have the luxury of sufficient amounts of sera to perform these preparatory steps and is left to interpretation by comparison with controls. A good positive control is valuable but it is difficult to find such a control for screening patient sera. Negative controls are essential and easier to obtain.

If the cells or tissues are fixed prior to the fluorescent antibody reaction, intracellular antigens are revealed and membrane antigens are destroyed. In our experience the choice of fixative can have a profound effect on the reaction observed and certain fixatives destroy antigenicity. We recommend trying a battery of fixatives before establishing an assay procedure. Buffer controls are essential in the test since we have found fixation makes cells markedly autofluorescent. In fact, the specific fluorescence is difficult to evaluate against the brilliant fluorescent background of fixed cells.

When mixed cell preparations are used, cytological controls are important to determine which cells are involved in the reaction, particularly since leukocytes can nonspecifically react. Cytology is also valuable because the most popular fixatives, acetone and methanol, markedly disrupt cellular architecture.

The fixed-cell assay has been widely used since the early demonstrations of its applicability to a variety of cancers (64, 78, 90). Despite its wide usage, the nature of the intracellular tumor-associated antigens is uncertain.

A viable cell membrane immunofluorescence test was devised by Möller (77) to demonstrate cell surface isoantigens. The Kleins (59) adapted the technique to study tumor cell surface antigens, presumably transplantation antigens, and to detect antibodies in patients' sera to these antigens. This sensitive assay reveals surface immunological reactions because live cell membranes will exclude the antibody and conjugate (60). Caution is urged in interpretation of data since tumor antigens are only one type of cell membrane antigen and appropriate controls are demanded.

The membrane immunofluorescence assay can be done with cultured tumor cells or with freshly dissociated tumor materials. The problems in culturing tumor cells restrict the available antigenic material. Also it must be remembered that cultured cells may acquire antigens *in vitro* (52) or possibly might lose antigens with successive passages. When cultured cells are used, appropriate control cells are generally not available and cells cultured from other types of tumors, or normal fibroblasts must serve as controls. On the other hand, if freshly dissociated tumor material is used, and the appropriate normal tissue control, it is impossible to determine which cells are reacting with the antibody since all cells look alike in suspension.

c. Complement Fixation.   The detection of antibody in a patient's serum by complement fixation is a familiar technique that has found wide and practical application in virology. In tumor immunology it has been used in a most limited way (21, 50, 91). Primarily, the tumors to which this technique has been applied are representatives of those in which a viral etiology is actively sought, i.e., breast cancer, melanoma, and sarcoma. The complement-fixing antigen is an intracellular one prepared in these studies by extraction, including freezing and thawing of either fresh tumor material (50) or cultured tumor cells (21). An alternative preparation involves homogenization and fluorocarbon extraction of tumor cells (91). In one study (92) the KCl-extracted antigen used in skin testing failed to fix complement, but rather inhibited the "standard" complement fixation test (21) which suggests preparation of antigen is a limiting factor in this technique.

Complement fixation assays can be made quantitative by inhibition assays. However, this assay as applied to tumors is of unknown specificity at this time since the antigens are not characterized. In fact, there may be multiple antigens present in extracts (50). Further, the antigens from one tumor may cross-react with antigens extracted from other cancers (50). The assay is also troubled by finding that certain sera are anticomplementary (50). This procedure does offer an advantage over serum cytotoxicity assays in that the antibody is detected by an indicator system of proven sensitivity. Serum cytotoxicity assays are affected by variabilities in tumor cell sensitivity to complement-mediated lysis.

d. Immune Adherence.   The immune adherence (IA) reaction, first described by Nelson in 1953 (80), was introduced to tumor immunology in 1969 (30, 81), and rapidly developed into a micromethod (101). Despite its long period of availability, the technique has had little application in human solid tumor immunology, finding use primarily in melanoma studies (i.e., 18, 50, 79, 94).

IA is a highly sensitive technique for detection of antigen, antibody and complement on cell membranes. Indicator cells, either primate erythrocytes or non-primate platelets, attach by means of the C3 receptor for antigen-antibody complexes. The observations are made microscopically or by reading the hemagluttination patterns. IA can be used to detect antibody or surface antigens. Since it is an excellent means of detecting histocompatibility antigens, sera must be absorbed for studies of other surface antigens, such as the tumor-associated antigens. The IA technique is more sensitive than several other assays, and has greater sensitivity for detection of IgM than IgG: *130 times more sensitive than complement fixation and 1000 times more than agglutination in detecting IgG* when tested with antibodies to bacteria (18). Tumor immunologists also acclaim its high sensitivity compared to other techniques (18).

The assay may be applied to biopsy material (51) or cultured tumor cells (18, 79, 94). Apparently there is some difficulty in keeping target cells in good shape throughout the assay. Most investigators allow an incubation period for regeneration of surface antigens after dispersion by enzyme digestion, although the enzymes purportedly do not affect antigenicity (97). Reproducibility in the test is a major problem (18, 79, 94). Patient sera react differently over a period of time and differences do not correlate with the course of the disease (18, 94). There is also a flux in the antigenic expression of cultured cells (18, 79). The antigens of cultured tumor cells are reported to be stabilized by mild formalin fixation (79). It may be possible to detect spurious antibodies (57), so necrotic tissues must be carefully cleaned away when using biopsy material, and all cells must be free of microbial contaminants. The specificity of the reaction must be confirmed by inhibition using antibody to C3 (51). Initially, the test system must be evaluated with complement from various species since this may be a source of variability (80, 101).

The IA assay has the advantages of high sensitivity and detection of the antigen, antibody and complement complex without requiring participation of the entire series of complement components or actual tumor cell lysis. Its major difficulties are the familiar problems of lack of a standard source of antigen, all the complications of the use of cultured cells or restrictions of biopsy material. The methods of observation are a further limitation and more quantitative methods would be desirable.

e. Serum Cytotoxicity.   The serum cytotoxicity test is a technique for evaluating the ability of antibody directed against tumor surfaces antigen to bind complement and cause immune lysis of the tumor cells. Lewis reported in 1967 (62) that the sera of patients with melanoma would cause their own cultured tumor cells to round up and come off the walls of the culture vessel suggesting that the sera were cytotoxic. The colony inhibition assay, and various similar microdetection assays, were subsequently applied for evaluation of this phenomenon in human solid cancers (13, 23, 33, 112). Essentially, tumor cells are plated in known amounts, serum and complement are added, the cells are incubated, and then the remaining numbers of cells are scored microscopically or with the aid of a radioactive label (24).

The difficulties involved with the source of antigen, plating of cells and scoring techniques will be discussed with the assays of cell-mediated immunity (CMI). The major difficulties in the special adaptation of these techniques to studies of humoral immunity, rather than the effects of humoral factors on CMI, are the variable sensitivity of tumor cells to complement-mediated lysis and the variability of individual patient reactivity over a period of time as has been seen in the previously discussed assays of humoral immunity.

2. CELL-MEDIATED IMMUNITY.   One of the dogmas of cancer immunology is that cell-mediated immune reactions are of prime importance to host defense against solid tumors. Although this dogma is certainly an oversimplification—if not an outright error—there is a great deal of interest in methods capable of accurately measuring specific CMI in patients to their own, or related, tumor cells. The assays which have been developed fall broadly into three categories: cytotoxicity, blastogenesis, and leukocyte indicator tests.

a. Cytotoxicity and Colony Inhibition Assays.

One of the major thrusts to the study of CMI in humans was the development by the Hellströms of the colony inhibition (CI) assay (31, 32). In this test CMI is measured by the ability of lymphocytes to interfere with the development of colonies of tumor cells. The colonies are allowed to develop in a cell culture system following exposure to lymphocytes from patients with various types of tumors, or from normal donors, and then are counted under magnification (19, 32). CMI is indicated by a difference in the number of colonies following treatment with specific patient lymphocytes versus that in the control groups. Although the endpoint of the CI test is colony formation, in actuality, this test measures three events: cytostasis, cytotoxicity, and inhibition of colony development.

CI assays have a major drawback which has limited their use, the difficulty encountered in the cell culture phase of the test in getting tumor cells, particularly human solid cancers in short term cultures, to reproducibly and frequently produce colonies. Therefore, tests with less demanding cell culture requirements were devised, namely, the microcytotoxicity (MC) assays of Tagasugi and Klein (102) and of the Hellströms (34). These tests, and other modifications, principally differ in well size of the microcytotoxicity plates, a factor which to these reviewers has more to do with convenience than with substance.

In the MC assays the endpoint is the number of individual tumor cells present following treatment with various types of lymphocytes and also following a several day culture period. Thus, these assays also measure cytostasis and cytotoxicity.

A further modification of the MC and CI tests has been the introduction of radioactively labeled tumor cells for use as target cells in order to eliminate the tedious, time-consuming, and subjective visual counting methods. A variety of labels have been used, including 3H-thymidine (55), 51Cr (45, 97), 3H-proline (4, 82), and 125I-IUdR (16, 84). A further advantage is seen with those labels which are suitable to labeling target tumor cells prior to addition of lymphocytes, as opposed to a postlabeling procedure, in that cytotoxicity, rather than cytostasis, is more clearly measured (4). In our opinion, aside from convenience, the radioactive label assays have not solved any of the real problems of CI and MC testing, and have added further problems associated with the use of radioactivity (spontaneous release, reutilization of label, etc.).

What then are the problems of CI and MC testing? Most simply they can be divided into those due to the target cells and those due to the effector cells (lymphocytes?). In the first case cultivation of human solid tumors is an art, and one which unfortunately is quite rare. Although there are some differences between different tumor types and different investigators, generally speaking less than 20% of tumor samples can be cultivated at all, and of these few grow well enough to be used in a meaningful number of assays. This hard fact has had two consequences: the vast majority of assays have been performed with allogeneic combinations of tumor cells and lymphocytes, and many investigators have turned to long-term cell lines rather than fresh cultures, as a source of target cells. The allogeneic problem will be discussed below. The use of long-term cells has been, with the exception of some bladder cancer lines (4, 84, 104), fraught with frustration in that rarely have they been suitable for the detection of specific, tumor-type-related, killing by appropriate patient lymphocytes (105). Indeed, with some lines lymphocytes from controls have been observed to be more cytotoxic than were patient lymphocytes (104). Further, in experiments in which we used the same tumor cell lines over periods of time ranging from initiation to either loss or establishment of continuous growth, we found marked variations with passage number in regards to sensitivity to appropriate patient lymphocyte killing, as well as to killing by lymphocytes from other, unrelated patients or from normal donors. The sensitivity to these three lymphocyte populations varied independently, as did the pattern of killing exhibited by different lines, over the course of passage (40). Accordingly, we have concluded that the use of passaged lines for MC assays is not a viable alternative to short-term cultures.

Another target cell problem encountered in CI and MC assays is the general inability to identify definitively which cells growing out of a tumor sample are in reality cancer cells and which are normal contaminants. With the exception of neuroblastoma and some melanoma cultures, most tumor cells are non-distinctive when grown in monolayer, the usual mode for these assays. Thus, in the case of visual counting, it is a matter of judgment which cells are counted, and in the radioactive label assays, no distinction is made at all. We have described a modification of the CI assay in which the colony formation is carried out in dilute agar—a procedure which is selective for cancer, as opposed to normal, cells (19). In any event, it should be appreciated that the only tumor cells capable of acting as targets in MC or CI tests are those capable of survival and growth in the cell culture system employed—and it is by no means certain that such cells are the most clinically appropriate.

One final but very important problem with target cells is the selection of control cells. Normal cell counterparts to solid cancer cells are even harder to culture than are the cancer cells. Because of this it is impossible to compare lymphocyte reactivity on, say breast cancer cells to normal mammary gland parenchyma, leaving aside the problem of which cell type would be appropriate to which cancer. One is left with two alternatives: comparison to tumor cells of another histological type and comparison to easily grown normal cells, generally fibroblasts. The first alternative results in selection of the results since the only possible toxicity which could be detected would have to be specific for histological type. The second is invalid since fibroblasts may differ in sensitivity to killing irrespective of the tumor status of the lymphocyte donor (40).

The problems associated with the effector cells in the MC and CI assays are, if anything, more severe than those due to target cells. Above we have referred to these effector cells as lymphocytes, by which we mean whatever peripheral white cells are left after a wide variety of "purification" procedures used by the various workers in this field (3). Although it is probably true that different lymphoid cell subpopulations will prove to be important in relation to tumor type (100), stage of disease, non-selective killing (58), and so forth, there is clearly no method of preparation of effector cells which yields uniform, expected results, even though the various methods vary enormously in the final makeup of lymphoid subpopulations (3, 86).

Probably the greatest problem in MC assays has been the repeated observation of toxicity of tumor cells of lymphocytes from normal donors (40, 44, 104)—not infrequently, as mentioned above, of a greater magnitude than that seen with patient lymphocytes (11, 40). Although there may be good reasons for normal cytotoxicity, including sensitization to ubiquitous tumor virus or other environmentally-associated antigens (36, 103), in vitro sensitization of lymphocytes to antigens during the culture period, or "immune stimulation" of tumor cell survival by patient, but not control lymphocytes (41), it is nevertheless a detriment in a test which is supposed to measure immunological effects of tumor-bearing. The problem is further compounded by the ability of control lymphocytes to be selectively toxic for different target cells and for fluctuations in control reactivity to be observed in serial evaluations, much the same as can be seen with patient lymphocytes (40, 44). There have been a variety of solutions to this problem, including selection of the control lymphocytes on the basis of least toxicity, use of a frozen, standard, low toxicity control lymphocyte preparations, and elimination of a lymphocyte control in favor of a "media" control, but none of these seem satisfactory from a scientific aspect. Nor has matching of lymphocyte donors to target cells on the basis of blood group specificity proven, in our hands, to alleviate the problem (42), despite another report to the contrary (67).

The problem of normal cytotoxicity is also related to the other major problem of CI and MC testing, namely assessment of specificity to the observed reactions. Basically, since the baseline of control reactivity is high, and since this reactivity will be, in the vast majority of tests, directed against allogeneic target cells, it is difficult to determine how much cytotoxicity of patient lymphocytes for allogeneic tumor cells of the same histological type as their own can be attributed to true immunological cross-reactivity and how much is a function of the same reactivity seen with normal allogeneic lymphocytes. The fact that occasionally "criss-cross" experiments, in which lymphocytes from cancer patients with two different types of cancer are cytotoxic only for the appropriate type, are successful (34, 97) suggests that some tumor-associated, cross-reactive reactivity does exist, but this reactivity may be only the tip of a vast iceberg of nontumor-associated reactivity, and hence of limited significance. Surely, this is our conclusion from analysis of a large number of experiments which in total suggest tumor-type-associated specificity, even though most of the individual experiments fail to clearly demonstrate this (40). A further difficulty in deciding whether or not cross-reactivity according to histological type is a general phenomenon is the relatively few experiments done with autochthonous combinations (3), so that data on degree and amount of toxicity for allogeneic cells cannot readily be compared to autochthonous data, and hence cannot really be evaluated. In our opinion the widespread belief that cell-mediated immunity to human tumor cells cross-reacts on the basis of histological type is a delusion based upon an initial assumption that this is so and subsequent experimental designs which reinforced that assumption (82). It should be noted that these assumptions are not peculiar to CI and MC assays, but also underlie the other tests for CMI described below.

b. Leukocyte Indicator Assays.   A variety of assays for CMI exist in which the endpoint is some effect on monocyte function as a consequence of the elaboration of soluble factors by sensitized lymphocytes exposed to appropriate antigen. The most used method is the leukocyte migration inhibition (LMI) test in which peripheral white cells are incubated in the presence or absence of tumor cell antigen and the relative degree of migration of leukocytes out of a capillary pipette or well into liquid or agarose medium is measured (1, 28, 93, 115). The test may either be done in a one-stage procedure, in which the lymphocytes and migrating indicator cells are incubated together with antigen, or as a two-stage test, in which supernatents from antigen-lymphocyte cultures are added to indicator cells which may be of human or guinea pig origin (28). This latter procedure may be preferable from the point of view of test standardization or when the lymphocyte suspensions do not contain sufficient numbers of functional migrating cells as with lymph node suspensions (28) or previously frozen peripheral blood leukocytes.

Generally, the antigens used in LMI tests are soluble extracts of cultured or fresh tumor cells (11, 75, 76) or, in the case of breast cancer, soluble viral glycoproteins (9). Black and co-workers have also described an assay in which cryostat sections of tumors are used, rather than extracted antigens (8, 9).

The data are described in terms of a migration index (M.I.) in which the average area of migration for cells exposed to lymphocytes and antigen is divided by the average area for lymphocytes and saline. The highest M.I. giving the best separation between patients and controls and between patients tested against the same versus another tumor or normal antigen preparation is usually used as the limit for a positive response. This value, which may be set retrospectively, assures that normal reactivity and lack of specificity are not problems with this test. Whether this is scientifically justified, or another manifestation of designing experiments to fit initial assumptions, is not clear. Again, relatively little has been done with autochthonous tumor antigens, but where done there is reason to question the assumption of complete cross-reactivity between tumors of same histological type. Modifications have been described for using test tubes (26) and capillary tubes (106). This latter assay can be performed very quickly (3 hours), a decided advantage over other CMI tests. It is likely that other modifications, perhaps involving radioisotope labeling of the monocytes (85), may further reduce the cumbersome technical aspects of the test. As with the LMI tests uncertainties are present in the area of antigen quantitation. So far most investigators claim detection of remarkable specificity for tumor type, as well as cross-reactivity related to histological type of cancer (26, 69, 88), although this has not been universally found (2).

The basis for the LAI test is not fully established at this writing. Although Maluish and Halliday (69) seem to favor a mechanism involving production of a monocyte-reactive lymphokine by lymphocytes, Marti, Grosser, and Thomson (27, 70), have presented strong evidence for the presence of anti-tumor cytophilic antibody on the surface of the monocytes, which, upon reacting with soluble tumor antigen, results in changes in the adherent properties of the cells.

A new test seemingly related to the LAI has recently been described in which soluble antigens are used to inhibit "spreading" or monocytes from tumor patients (74). This test also needs further evaluation in regard to specificity, etc.

c. Blastogenesis Assays.

The third method which has been used to detect CMI in humans with solid tumors is induction of blastogenesis, as measured by uptake of 3H-thymidine, in autologous lymphocytes following incubation with antigen. The tumor antigens used are either whole cells, treated with mitomycin C (98, 107) or irradiation (this latter is reported to be preferable (73)), or tumor extracts (72) or soluble antigens from other sources (20, 56).

The use of soluble extracts as antigens in LMI tests has both advantages and disadvantages. The advantages are that the need for extensive cell culture as in CI and MC tests may be circumvented and that the same antigens tested in vitro can often be used for in vivo skin testing. The disadvantages relate to the preparation of active antigens which must be done empirically and to a certain extent in the dark. The amount of testing necessary to see whether an active preparation has been obtained may also use up most of the material. Further the preparation of control antigens is a problem. Since one does not know what a given antigen in fact is, it is difficult to select an appropriate control source. In the case of adenocarcinomas, the difference in degree of cellularity between a tumor and a normal sample may be quite large, and in addition there may be quite a different mix of cells. Expression of extracted antigen in terms of milligrams of protein does not eliminate the problem since one has no way of knowing whether the "antigen" is proportional to total protein, or whether the proportion of cells responsible for the antigen is the same in cancer versus normal tissue samples. Dose response curves for the various tissue extracts would be helpful, but they have not been routinely performed for LMI testing. Once again the concentrations chosen for testing are those which give the expected results.

Another leukocyte indicator assay which is currently being evaluated is the leukocyte adherence inhibition (LAI) test. This test measures the ability of soluble antigens to prevent adherence of blood monocytes. The original procedure of Maluish and Halliday (69) involved incubation of leukocytes and antigen, placing the cells in hemocytometers, and then counting them before and after washing away non-adherent cells. An advantage to this method is that general lymphocyte reactivity can simultaneously be measured with mitogens such as PHA and Con A. A disadvantage is that when the antigen is whole cells the assay cannot be used to investigate the question of cross-reactivity between tumors of same histological type, or normal reactivity, since allogeneic lymphocytes will respond positively because of histo-incompatibility differences and irrespective of tumor status. Further the level of response is usually quite low, as compared to that achieved with nonspecific mitogens. Finally, appropriate control stimulator cells are seldom available for solid tumors and the common use of autologous lymphocytes for such controls is not completely satisfactory.

3. HUMORAL-CELLULAR IMMUNE INTERACTIONS. The methods used to detect CMI in patients with solid cancer have also been used to study the presence of factors in serum capable of modifying CMI in both a positive and negative direction. Clearly these studies of serum factors are subject to the same procedural difficulties as have been described for the CMI assays. Further, it is abundantly clear that there are numerous factors in patient, and control, sera which can non-specifically modify in vitro measurements of CMI. These are seldom controlled for in studies designed to detect tumor specific serum factors. Further, investigations of the specificity of the serum factors, the extent to which cross-reactivity is seen between them, and their molecular nature are, in truth, meager—a situation which in large part is due to the technical problems of the CMI assays.

The most often discussed specific serum factor able to modulate CMI in vitro is the serum blocking factor (SBF) described by the Hellströms and associates with CI and MC assays (38). These factors are measured by their ability to block expression of CMI by cytotoxic lymphocytes. Similar observations have been reported by many other workers using both cytotoxicity and other CMI assays (17, 27, 42, 76, 96). Several immune factors, including soluble antigen, antibody, and antigen-antibody complexes, have been shown to be capable of blocking under experimental conditions (39), but which is responsible in any given individual test with human sera is seldom known.

A related serum effect is that of "unblocking" activity. In this phenomenon serum from a second individual is able to prevent blocking of CMI by serum otherwise positive for SBF (35, 69). The nature of unblocking has not been elucidated.

Finally, numerous reports exist on the detection of serum factors able to either increase lymphocyte killing of reactive cells or to arm normal lymphocytes and turn them into killers (37, 42, 61, 87, 109). This activity is no doubt related to antibody-dependent cellular cytotoxicity as described in human allogeneic and experimental systems (61). Its evaluation in regard to human specific tumor immunity is only beginning, although it seems to be a fairly infrequent finding (42, 61, 87).

III. CONCLUSION

A variety of methods have been described to measure immunity to solid tumor antigens. For reasons described above, none of these methods have so far yielded the type of results needed for useful, clinical testing. Clearly many technological improvements are needed, including standardization of antigen preparation and evaluation procedures. However, the greatest need in immunological testing is an honest, objective approach which does not prejudge, and hence preselect, for the type of reactions which are detected.

ACKNOWLEDGMENT

This work was supported in part by Grant Number CA 13943 awarded by the National Cancer Institute.

REFERENCES

1. Anderson, V., Bjerrum, O., Bendixen, G., Schildt, T., and Dissing, I. 1970. Effect of autologous mammary tumor extracts on human leucocyte migration *in vitro*. *Int. J. Cancer* 5: 357–363.

2. Armitstead, P. R., and Gowland, G. The leukocyte adherence inhibition test in cancer of the large bowel. *Brit. J. Cancer* 32: 568–573.

3. Bean, M. A., Bloom, B. R., Herberman, R. B., Old, L. J., Oettgen, H. F., Klein, G., and Terry, W. D. 1975. Cell-mediated cytotoxicity for bladder carcinoma: Evaluation of a workshop. *Cancer Res.* 35: 2902–2913.

4. Bean, M. A., Pees, H., Fogh, J. E., Grabstald, H., and Oettgen, H. F. 1974. Cytotoxicity of lymphocytes from patients with cancer of the urinary bladder: Detection by a 3H-proline microcytotoxicity test. *Int. J. Cancer* 14: 186–197.

5. Black, M. M., and Leis, H. P., Jr. 1970. Human breast carcinoma. Part III. Cellular responses to autologous breast cancer: Skin-window procedure. *N.Y. State J. Med.* 70: 2583–2589.

6. Black, M. M., and Leis, H. P., Jr. 1971. Cellular responses to autologous breast cancer tissue: Correlation with stage and lymphoreticuloendothelial reactive. *Cancer* 28: 263–273.

7. Black, M. M., and Leis, H. P., Jr. 1973. Cellular responses to autologous breast cancer tissue: Sequential observations. *Cancer* 32: 384–389.

8. Black, M. M., Leis, H. P., Shore, B., and Zachrau, R. E. 1974. Cellular hypersensitivity to breast cancer. Assessment by a leukocyte migration procedure. *Cancer* 33: 952–958.

9. Black, M. M., Moore, D. H., Shore, B., Zachrau, R. E., and Leis, H. P. 1974. Effect of murine milk samples and human breast tissues on human leukocyte migration indices. *Cancer Res.* 34: 1054–1060.

10. Boddie, A. W., Holmes, E. C., Roth, J. A., and Morton, D. L. 1975. Inhibition of human leukocyte migration in agarose by KCl extracts of carcinoma of the lung. *Int. J. Cancer* 15: 823–829.

11. Boddie, A. W., Urist, M. M., Chee, D. O., Holmes, F. C., and Morton, D. L. 1975. Inhibition of leukocyte migration in agarose by KCl extracts of a human melanoma cell line grown in serum-free medium. *Int. J. Cancer* 16: 1035–1041.

12. Boehm, O. R., Boehm, B. J., and Humphrey, L. J. 1974. The natural history of the antibody response to breast antigens. *Clin. Exp. Immunol.* 16: 31–40.

13. Bubeník, J., Perlmann, P., Helmstein, K., and Moberger, G. 1970. Cellular and humoral immune responses to human urinary bladder carcinomas. *Int. J. Cancer* 5: 310–319.

14. Char, D. H., Hollinshead, A. C., Cogan, D. G., Ballintine, E. J., Hogan, M. J., and Herberman, R. B. 1974. Cutaneous delayed hypersensitivity reactions to soluble melanoma antigen in patients with ocular malignant melanoma. *N. Engl. J. Med.* 291: 274–277.

15. Cochran, A. J., Mackie, R. M., Thomas, C. E., Grant, R. M., Cameron-Mowat, D. E., and Spilg, W. G. S. 1973. Cellular immunity to breast carcinoma and malignant melanoma. *Brit. J. Cancer* 28: Suppl. I 77–82.

16. Cohen, A. M. 1973. Host immunity to growing sarcomas. *Cancer* 31: 81–89.

17. Cohen, A. M., Ketcham, A. S., and Morton, D. L. 1972. Cellular immunity to a common human sarcoma antigen and its specific inhibition by sera from patients with growing sarcomas. *Surgery* 72: 560–567.

18. Cornain, S., deVries, J. E., Collard, J., Vennegoor, C., van Wingerden, I., and Rumke, P. 1975. Antibodies and antigen expression in human melanoma detected by the immune adherence test. *Int. J. Cancer* 16: 981–997.

19. Cummings, F. J., Heppner, G. H., Stolbach, L., and Calabresi, P. 1973. Demonstration of cell-mediated and blocking immune responses to tumor antigens in cancer patients with the colony-inhibition-in-gel test. *Israel J. Med. Sci.* 9: 308–316.

20. Cunningham-Rundles, S., Feller, W. F., Cunningham-Rundles, C., Dupont, B., Wanebo, H., O'Reilly, R., and Good, R. A. 1976. Lymphocyte transformation *in vitro* to RIII mouse milk antigen among women with breast disease. *Cell. Immunol.* 25: 322–327.

21. Eilber, F. R., and Morton, D. L. 1970. Sarcoma-specific antigens: detection by complement fixation with serum from sarcoma patient. *J. Natl. Cancer Inst.* 44: 651–657.

22. Foley, E. J. 1953. Antigenic properties of methylcholanthrene-induced tumors in mice of the strain of origin. *Cancer Res.* 13: 835–837.

23. Fossati, G., Colnaghi, M. I., Della Porta, G., Cascinelli, N., and Veronese, U. 1971. Cellular and humoral immunity against human malignant melanoma. *Int. J. Cancer* 8, 344–350.

24. Goodman, W. S. 1961. A general method for quantitation of immune cytolysis. *Nature* 190: 269–270.

25. Gorsky, Y., Vanky, F., and Sulitzeanu, D. 1976. Isolation from patients with breast cancer of antibodies specific for antigens associated with breast cancer and other malignant diseases. *Proc. Natl. Acad. Sci. USA* 73: 2101–2105.

26. Grosser, N., and Thomson, D. M. P. 1975. Cell-mediated antitumor immunity in breast cancer patients evaluated by antigen-induced leukocyte adherence inhibition in test tubes. Cancer Res. 35: 2571–2579.

27. Grosser, N., and Thomson, D. M. P. 1976. Tube leukocyte (monocyte) adherence inhibition assay for the detection of anti-tumour immunity. III. "Blockade" of monocyte reactivity by excess free antigen and immune complexes in advanced cancer patients. Int. J. Cancer 18: 58–66.

28. Cuillou, P. J., Brennan, T. G., and Giles, G. R. 1975. A study of lymph nodes draining colorectal cancer using a two-stage inhibition of leukocyte migration technique. Gut 16: 290–297.

29. Hager, J. C., and Tompkins, W. A. F. 1976. Antibodies in normal rabbit serum that react with tissue-specific antigens on the plasma membranes of human adenocarcinoma cells. J. Natl. Cancer Inst. 56: 339–344.

30. Harris, H., Miller, O. J., Klein, G., Worst, R., and Tachibana, T. 1969. Suppression of malignancy by cell fusion. Nature 233: 363–368.

31. Hellström, I. 1967. A Colony Inhibition (CI) technique for demonstration of tumor cell destruction by lymphoid cells in vitro. Int. J. Cancer 2: 65–68.

32. Hellström, I., Hellström, K. E., Bill, A. H., Pierce, G. E., and Yang, J. P. S. Studies on cellular immunity to human neuroblastoma cells. Int. J. Cancer 6: 172–188.

33. Hellström, I. E., Hellström, K. E., Pierce, G. E., and Bill, A. H. 1968. Demonstration of cell-bound and humoral immunity against neuroblastoma cells. Proc. Natl. Acad. Sci. USA 60: 1231–1238.

34. Hellström, I., Hellström, K. E., Sjögren, H. O., and Warner, G. H. 1971. Demonstration of cell-mediated immunity to human neoplasms of various histological types. Int. J. Cancer 7: 1–16.

35. Hellström, I., Hellström, K. E., Sjögren, H. O., and Warner, G. A. 1971. Serum factors in tumor-free patients cancelling the blocking of cell-mediated tumor immunity. Int. J. Cancer 8: 185–191.

36. Hellström, I., Hellström, K. E., Sjögren, H. O., and Warner, G. A. 1973. Destruction of cultivated melanoma cells by lymphocytes from healthy black donors (North American Negro) Int. J. Cancer 11: 116–122.

37. Hellström, I., Hellström, K. E., and Warner, G. A. 1973. Increase of lymphocyte-mediated tumor cell destruction by certain patient sera. Int. J. Cancer 12: 348–353.

38. Hellström, I., Sjögren, H. O., Warner, G., and Hellström, K. E. 1971. Blocking of cell-mediated tumor immunity by sera from patients with growing neoplasms. Int. J. Cancer 7: 226–237.

39. Heppner, G. H. 1972. Blocking antibodies and enhancement. Ser. Haemat. 4: 41–66.

40. Heppner, G., Henry, E., Stolbach, L., Cummings, F., McDonough, E., and Calabresi, P. 1975. Problems in the clinical use of the microcytotoxicity assay for measuring cell-mediated immunity to tumor cells. Cancer Res. 35: 1931–1937.

41. Heppner, G., Kopp, J. S., Medina, D. 1976. Microcytotoxicity assay of immune responses to non-mammary tumor virus-induced, pre-neoplastic, and neoplastic mammary lesions in Balb/c mice. Cancer Res. 36: 753–758.

42. Heppner, G. H., Stolback, L., Byrne, M., Cummings, F. J., McDonough, E.,

and Calabresi, P. 1973. Cell-mediated and serum blocking reactivity to tumor antigens in patients with malignant melanoma. *Int. J. Cancer* 11: 245–260.

43. Herberman, R. B. 1974. Delayed hypersensitivity response toward autochthonous tumor extracts, *in* G. Mathé and R. Weiner (ed.), *Recent Results in Cancer Research: Investigation and Stimulation of Immunity in Cancer Patients*, pp. 140–146. Springer-Verlag, New York.

44. Herberman, R. B., and Oldham, R. K. 1975. Problems associated with study of cell-mediated immunity to human tumors by microcytotoxicity assays. *J. Natl. Cancer Inst.* 55: 749–753.

45. Hersey, P., Edwards, A., Adams, E., Kearney, R., and Milton, G. W. 1975. Comparison of ^{51}Cr release and microcytotoxicity assays against human melanoma cells. *Int. J. Cancer* 16: 164–172.

46. Hollingshead, A. 1972. Discussion: Skin tests. *Natl. Cancer Inst. Monogr.* 37: 206–212.

47. Hollingshead, A., Glew, D., Bunnag, B., Gold, P., and Herberman, R. 1970. Skin-reactive soluble antigen from intestinal cancer-cell-membrane and relationship to cancinoembryonic antigens. *Lancet* 1: 1191–1195.

48. Hollingshead, A. C., Jaffurs, W. T., Alpert, L. K., Harris, J. E., and Herberman, R. B. 1974. Isolation and identification of soluble skin-reactive membrane antigens of malignant and normal human breast cells. *Cancer Res.* 34: 2961–2968.

49. Hollinshead, A. C., Stewart, T. H. M., and Herberman, R. B. 1974. Delayed-hypersensitivity reactions to soluble membrance antigens of human malignant lung cells. *J. Natl. Cancer Inst.* 52: 327–338.

50. Humphrey, L. J., Estes, N. C., Morse, P. A., Jewel, W. R., Boudet, R. A., and Hudson, M. J. K. 1974. Serum antibody in patients with mammary disease. *Cancer* 34: 1516–1520.

51. Irie, K., Irie, R. F., and Morton, D. L. 1974. Evidence for *in vivo* reactions of antibody and complement to surface antigens of human cancer cells. *Science* 186: 454–456.

52. Irie, R. F., Irie, K., and Morton, D. L. 1974. Natural antibody in human serum to a neoantigen in human cultured cells grown in fetal bovine serum. *J. Natl. Cancer Inst.* 52: 1051–1058.

53. Irie, K., Irie, R. F., and Morton, K. L. 1975. Detection of antibody and complement complexed *in vivo* on membranes of human cancer cells by mixed hemadsorption techniques. *Cancer Res.* 35: 1244–1248.

54. Izsak, F. C., Brenner, H. J., Landes, E., Ran, M., and Witz, I. P. 1974. Correlation between clinico-pathological features of malignant tumors and cell surface immunoglobulins. *Israel J. Med. Sci.* 10: 642–646.

55. Jagarlamoody, S. M., Aust, J. C., Tew, R. H., and McKhann, C. F. 1971. *In vitro* detection of cytotoxic cellular immunity against tumor-specific antigens by a radioisotopic techniques. *Proc. Nat. Acad. Sci.* 68: 1346–1350.

56. Jehn, U. W., Nathanson, L., Schwartz, R. S., and Skinner, M. 1970. *In vitro* lymphocyte stimulation by a soluble antigen from malignant melanoma. *N. Engl. J. Med.* 283: 329–333.

57. Johansson, B., and Ljungqvist, A. 1974. Localization of immunoglobulins in urinary bladder tumours. *Acta Pathol. Microbiol. Scand. A.* 82: 559–563.

58. Kiuchi, M., and Takasugi, M. 1976. The nonselective cytotoxic cell (N cell). *J. Natl. Cancer Inst.* 56: 575–582.

59. Klein, E., and Klein, G. 1964. Antigenic properties of lymphomas induced by the Moloney agent. *J. Natl. Cancer Inst.* 32: 547–568.

60. Klein, G., Clifford, P., Klein, E., Smith, R. T., Minowada, J., Kourilsky, F. M., and Burchenal, J. H. 1967. Membrane immunofluorescence reactions of Burkitt lymphoma cells from biopsy specimens and tissue cultures. *J. Natl. Cancer Inst.* 39: 1027–1044.

61. Kodera, Y., and Bean, M. A. 1975. Antibody dependent cell-mediated cytotoxicity for human monolayer target cells bearing blood group and transplantation antigens and for melanoma cells. *Int. J. Cancer* 16: 579–592.

62. Lewis, M. G. 1967. Possible immunological factors in human malignant melanoma in Uganda. *Lancet* 3: 921–922.

63. Lewis, M. G. 1974. Technical and interpretative problems with immunofluorescence, *in* G. Mathé and R. Weiner (ed.), *Recent Results in Cancer Research: Investigation and Stimulation of Immunity in Cancer Patients,* pp. 58–66. Springer-Verlag, New York.

64. Lewis, M. G., Ikonopisov, R. L., Nairn, R. C., Phillips, T. M., Fairley, G. H., Bodenham, D. C., and Alexander, P. 1969. Tumour-specific antibodies in human malignant melanoma and their relationship to the extent of the disease. *Brit. Med. J.* 3: 543–547.

65. Lewis, M. G., and Phillips, T. M. 1973. Separation of two distinct tumor-associated antibodies in the serum of melanoma patients. *J. Natl. Cancer Inst.* 49: 915–917.

66. Lewis, M. G., Proctor, J. W., Thomson, D. M. P., Rowden, G., and Phillips, T. M. 1976. Cellular localization of immunoglobulin within human malignant melanomata. *Brit. J. Cancer* 33: 260–266.

67. Levy, N. L. 1973. Use of an *in vitro* microcytotoxicity test to assess human tumor specific cell mediated immunity and its serum-mediated abrogation. *Natl. Cancer Inst. Monogr.* 37: 85–92.

68. Mahoney, J. C., Boehm, O. R., Boehm, B. J., and Humphrey, L. J. 1972. Studies of serum from patients with breast cancer. *Surg. Forum* 23: 87–88.

69. Maluish, A., and Halliday, W. J. 1974. Cell-mediated immunity and specific serum factors in human cancer: the leukocyte adherence inhibition test. *J. Natl. Cancer Inst.* 52: 1415–1420.

70. Marti, J. H., Grosser, N., and Thomson, D. M. P. 1976. Tube leukocyte adherence inhibition assay for the detection of anti-tumor immunity. II. Monocyte reacts with tumor antigen via cytophilic anti-tumor antibody. *Int. J. Cancer* 18: 48–57.

71. Mavligit, G., Gutterman, J. H., McBride, C. M., and Herish, E. M. 1972. Multifaceted evaluation of human tumor immunity using a salt extracted colon carcinoma antigen. *Proc. Soc. Exp. Biol. Med.* 140: 1240–1245.

72. Mavligit, G. M., Gutterman, J. U., McBride, C. M., and Hersh, E. M. 1974. Cell-mediated immunity to human solid tumors *in vitro* detection by lymphocyte blastogenic responses to cell-associated and solubilized tumor antigens. *Recent Results Cancer Res.* 47: 84–86.

73. Mavligit, G. M., Hersh, E. M., and McBride, C. M. 1973. Lymphocyte blastogenic responses to autochthonous viable and nonviable human tumor cells. *J. Natl. Cancer Inst.* 51: 337–343.

74. Mazuran, R., Mujagic, H., Malenica, B., and Silobrevic, V. 1976. *In vitro* detection of cellular immunity to melanoma antigens in man by the monocyte spreading inhibition test. *Int. J. Cancer* 17: 14–20.

75. McCoy, J. L., Jerome, L. F., Dean, J. H., Cannon, G. B., Alford, T. C., Doering, T., and Herberman, T. B. 1974. Inhibition of leukocyte migration by tumor-associated antigens in soluble extracts of human breast carcinoma. *J. Natl. Cancer Inst.* 53: 11–17.

76. McCoy, J. L., Jerome, L. F., Dean, J. H., Perlin, E., Oldham, R. K., Char, D. H., Cohen, M. H., Felix, E. L., and Herberman, R. B. 1975. Inhibition of leukocyte migration by tumor-associated antigens in soluble extracts of human malignant melanoma. *J. Natl. Cancer Inst.* 55: 19–23.

77. Möller, G. 1961. Demonstration of mouse isoantigens at the cellular level by the fluorescent antibody technique. *J. Exp. Med.* 114: 415–434.

78. Morton, D. L., and Malmgren, R. A. 1968. Human osteosarcomas: Immunologic evidence suggesting an associated infectious agent. *Science* 162: 1279–1281.

79. Müller, D., and Sorg, C. 1975. Use of formalin-fixed melanoma cells for the detection of antibodies against surface antigens by a micro-immune adherence technique. *Eur. J. Immunol.* 5: 175–178.

80. Nelson, R. A., Jr. 1953. The immune-adherence phenomenon. *Science* 118: 733–737.

81. Nishioka, K., Irie, R. F., Kawana, T., and Takeuchi, S. 1969. Immunological studies on mouse mammary tumors. III. Surface antigens reacting with tumor-specific antibodies in immune adherence. *Int. J. Cancer* 4: 139–149.

82. Oldham, R. K., Djeu, J. Y., Cannon, G. B., Siwarski, D., and Herberman, R. B. 1975. Cellular microcytotoxicity in human tumor systems analysis of results. *J. Natl. Cancer Inst.* 55: 1305–1318.

83. Oldham, R. K., and Herberman, R. B. 1973. Evaluation of cell-mediated cytotoxic reactivity against tumor associated antigens with ^{125}I-iododeoxyuridine labelled target cells. *J. Immunol.* 111: 1862–1871.

84. O'Tolle, C. 1973. Standardization of micrototoxicity assay for cell-mediated immunity. *Natl. Cancer Inst. Monogr.* 37: 19–24.

85. Pierce, G. E., and DeVald, B. L. 1974. Leukocyte adherence inhibition as measured by a radioisotopic technique for detection of cell-mediated tumor immunity. *Int. J. Cancer* 14: 833–839.

86. Pierce, G. E., and DeVald, B. L. 1975. Effects of human lymphocytes on cultured normal and malignant cells. *Cancer Res.* 35: 1830–1839.

87. Pierce, G. E., and DeVald, B. L. 1975. Effects of human sera on reactivity of lymphocytes in microcytotoxicity assays. *Cancer Res.* 35: 2729–2737.

88. Powell, A. E., Sloss, A. M., Smith, R. N., Makley, J. T., and Hubay, C. A. 1975. Specific responsiveness of leukocytes to soluble extracts of human tumors. *Int. J. Cancer* 16: 905–913.

89. Prehn, R. T., and Main, J. M. 1957. Immunity to methylcholanthrene-mediated sarcomas. *J. Natl. Cancer Inst.* 18: 769–778.

90. Priori, E. S., Seman, G., Dmochowski, L., Gallager, H. S., and Anderson, D. E. 1971. Immunofluorescence studies on sera of patients with breast carcinoma. Cancer 28: 1462–1471.

91. Romsdahl, M. M., and Cox, J. S. 1973. Immunological studies on malignant melanomas of man. Yale J. Biol. Med. 46: 693–701.

92. Roth, J. A., Holmes, E. C., Reisfeld, R. A., Slocum, H. K., and Morton, D. L. 1976. Isolation of a soluble tumor-associated antigen from human melanoma. Cancer 37: 104–110.

93. Segall, A., Weiler, O., Genin, J., Lacour, J., and Lacour, F. 1972. In vitro study of cellular immunity against autochthonous human cancer. Int. J. Cancer 9: 417–425.

94. Shiku, H., Takahashi, T., Oettgen, H. F., and Old, L. J. 1976. Cell surface antigens of human malignant melanoma. II. Serological typing with immune adherence assays and definition of two new surface antigens. J. Exp. Med. 144: 873–881.

95. Sinkovics, J. G., Ahmed, N., Hrgovicic, M. J., Cabiness, J. R., and Wilber, J. R. 1972. Cytotoxic lymphocytes II. Antagonism and synergism between serum factors and lymphocytes of patients with sarcomas as tested against cultured tumor cells. Texas Reps. Biol. Med. 30: 347: 360.

96. Sjögren, H. O., Hellström, I., Bansal, S. C., Warner, G. A., and Hellström, K. E. 1972. Elution of "blocking factors" from human tumors, capable of abrogating tumor-cell destruction by specifically immune lymphocytes. Int. J. Cancer 9: 274–283.

97. Steele, G., Sjögren, H. O., and Stadenberg, I. 1976. In vitro cell-mediated immune reactions of melanoma and colorectal carcinoma patients demonstrated by long term ⁵¹chromium assays. Int. J. Cancer 17: 27–39.

98. Stjernswärd, J., Vánky, F., and Klein, E. 1973. Lymphocyte stimulation by autochthonous human solid tumours. Brit. J. Cancer 28: Suppl. I, 72–76.

99. Stewart, T. H. M. 1969. The presence of delayed hypersensitivity reactions in patients toward cellular extracts of their malignant tumors. The role of tissue antigen nonspecific reactions of nuclear material and bacterial antigen as a cause for this phenomenon. Cancer 23: 1368–1379.

100. Stevenson, G. T., and Laurence, D. J. R. 1975. Report of a workshop on the immune response to solid tumors in man. Int. J. Cancer 16: 887–896.

101. Tachibana, T., and Klein, E. 1970. Detection of cell surface antigens on monolayer cells. I. The application of immune adherence on a micro scale. Immunol. 19: 771–782.

102. Tagasugi, M., and Klein, E. 1970. A micro-assay for cell-mediated immunity. Transplantation 9: 219–227.

103. Takasugi, M., and Mickey, M. R. 1976. Interaction analysis of selective and nonselective cell-mediated cytotoxicity. J. Natl. Cancer Inst. 47: 255–261.

104. Takasugi, M., Mickey, M. R., and Terasaki, P. I. 1973. Reactivity of lymphocytes from normal persons on cultured tumor cells. Cancer Res. 33: 2898–2902.

105. Takasugi, M., Mickey, M. R., and Terasaki, P. I. 1974. Studies on specificity of cell-mediated immunity to human tumors. J. Natl. Cancer Inst. 53: 1527–1538.

106. Urist, M. M., Boddie, A. W., Holmes, E. C., and Morton, D. L. 1976. Capillary tube leukocyte adherence inhibition: an assay for cell-mediated immunity in cancer patients. *Int. J. Cancer* 17: 338–341.

107. Vánky, F., Stjernswärd, J., and Nilsonne, U. 1971. Cellular immunity to human sarcoma. *J. Natl. Cancer Inst.* 46: 1145–1151.

108. Vánky, F., Trempe, G., Klein, E., and Stjernswärd, J. 1975. Human tumor-lymphocyte interaction *in vitro*: Blastogenesis correlated to detectable immunoglobulin in the biopsy. *Int. J. Cancer* 16: 113–124.

109. Vanwijck, R., Bouillenne, C., and Malek-Mansour, S. 1975. Potentiation and arming of lymphocyte mediated immunity by sera from melanoma patients. *Eur. J. Cancer* 11: 267–276.

110. Wells, S. A., Burdick, J. R., Christiansen, C., Ketcham, A. S., and Adkins, P. C. 1973. Demonstration of tumor-associated delayed cutaneous hypersensitivity reactions in patients with lung cancer and in patients with carcinoma of the cervix. *Natl. Cancer Inst. Monogr.* 37: 197–203.

111. Witz, I. P. 1973. The biological significance of tumor-bound immunoglobulins, *in* W. Arger, R. Haas, W. Henle, P. H. Jofschneider, N. K. Jerne, P. Koldovsky, H. Koprowski, O. Maaloe, R. Rott, H. G. Schweiger, M. Sela, L. Syrucek, P. K. Vogt, and E. Wecker (eds.), *Current Topics in Microbiology and Immunology*, vol. 61, pp. 151–171. Springer-Verlag, New York.

112. Wood, W. C., and Morton, D. L. 1970. Microcytotoxicity test: Detection in sarcoma patients of antibody cytotoxic to human sarcoma cells. *Science* 170: 1318–1320.

CHAPTER 8

CELLULAR AND HUMORAL IMMUNITY IN PATIENTS WITH SOLID TUMORS

F. J. Cummings
and G. H. Heppner

Department of Medicine
Roger Williams General Hospital
Division of Biology and Medicine
Brown University
Providence, Rhode Island 02912

The colony inhibition technique and microcytotoxicity assays have demonstrated cell-mediated reactivity of peripheral blood lymphocytes and serum blocking activity in groups of patients with various histological types of tumors, including carcinoma of the bladder, breast, colon, and lung and malignant melanoma. Frequent toxicity or reactivity of control lymphocytes from normal individuals makes it extremely difficult to interpret sequential assay results in any given patient. This information may be of biological importance to a group of patients with a particular type or stage of tumor, but these trends may not be evident in each case. Thus, currently these assays have little clinical relevance to the individual cancer patient.

Introduction

Following the introduction of the colony inhibition (CI) technique for demonstration of tumor cell destruction by lymphoid cells *in vitro* (22), many investigators hoped to apply such methods to study antitumor immune responses in cancer patients as an adjunct to the clinical management of their disease. The work of Hellström and Hellström, performed in neuroblastoma patients and their close relatives (23, 24), preceded numerous studies in humans with a variety of other histological types of cancer (26). Simplification of the CI technique was achieved with the microcytotoxicity (MC) assays of Takasugi and Klein (52) and of the Hellströms (25), and the widespread acceptance of these and their modifications (13, 29, 35) has resulted in countless reports of cell-mediated immunity to human tumors and blocking of this effect by soluble serum factors, as well as other reports concerning more complex interactions of lymphoid cells and tumor cells and/or serum, i.e., unblocking factor, antibody-dependent cell-mediated cytotoxicity or "arming" (4, 50).

The aims of these investigations, and the hopes of their investigators, was to determine if such techniques would be able to provide some correlation with the presence or absence of disease, or its activity, or with response to therapeutic manipulations. If achieved, such correlations would add more sophisticated diagnostic and prognostic parameters to the clinical evaluation both of groups of cancer patients of similar histological types and of individual cancer patients during the course of disease.

There has now been eight years experience with the application of these procedures to the study of human cancer. The initial years were primarily devoted to accumulating information related to the presence or absence of immunity to different types of cancer in groups of patients or in individual patients. Recent years have been more concerned with a critical evaluation of the utility, practicality, and specificity of the MC assay and its application to the study of human malignancy in general and to the individual patient in particular. Do the results that are obtained really mean anything? Is the assay really worth the effort it takes to get results? These questions are appropriate at this point in time, in order to provide direction to future investigations of human tumor immunity.

This chapter will describe selected reports involving the application of the CI technique and the MC assay to the study of cell-mediated and blocking immune responses seen in cancer patients. We will particularly emphasize studies in which sequential measurements, made in relation to changing disease or therapy were attempted since only these will reveal the *clinical* usefulness of the tests.

After outlining the work that has been accomplished, we shall discuss what we feel are some of the major limitations with the assays that are presently available. This will be done in the context of a review of our own experiences with the CI technique and the MC assay in the assessment of tumor immunity in patients with malignant melanoma and with breast carcinoma. A more comprehensive discussion of the *technical* difficulties encountered with these assays is given in this volume (see preceding chapter). We will conclude with a discussion of the requirements for a useful test. What can we expect with the present assays? What magnitude of difference of results between a patient and a normal individual is important, and what magnitude can we now achieve? The answers to these questions can only be speculative, until we have developed more discriminating assays and they have withstood the challenges of time and clinical experience and have proved their usefulness.

Studies in Melanoma Patients

Melanoma patients are an obvious choice for immune evaluation because of evidence for antitumor antibody (21, 38), reputed occasional spontaneous regression, and the variable clinical course noted in many patients. Thus, not only may immune responses play a role in modifying the melanoma process, the variability and oftentimes unfortunately short duration of this disease provides a useful system in which to do studies aimed at correlating clinical change with *in vitro* immune measurement.

Many authors have reported CI and MC assay results in melanoma patients (see review by Stevenson (51)). Initially groups of patients were compared to controls, but subsequently individual patients were studied with respect to time or to treatment. The Hellström group described syngeneic cell-mediated immunity in 23 of 23 patients and on 41/41 occasions with allogeneic lymphocyte-tumor cell combinations (26). These results were confirmed by several authors, although the frequency of positive responses was not so high. Fossatti *et al.* found cell-mediated immunity in 21 of 31 (68%) tests in 16 patients (18, 54), whereas DeVries and associates observed lymphocyte cytotoxicity in 35 of 61 (57%) patients using the MC assay (16). We published our experience with CI and MC tests in 33 melanoma patients, observing reactivity on 65/82 (79%) occasions (30). On the other hand, Mukherji and co-workers reported cell-mediated responses 3/14 (21%) times, although with significantly higher levels in patients free of disease or with disease regressing after therapy (39), and Currie *et al.* found cell-mediated immunity in only 3/22 (14%) patients (15). The disparity between these results and those of other investigators may be due to the techniques used, however.

The Hellströms were the first to introduce the term "blocking factor" to describe the abrogation by serum of lymphocyte-mediated cytotoxicity to tumor cells. In their original reports on melanoma patients, they observed this in 67 of 81 (83%) patients with growing neoplasms and in only 3 of 19 (16%) patients who were symptom-free after therapy (27). We found serum blocking activity on 24/52 (46%) occasions using normal serum-immune lymphocyte controls (30). Mukherji and co-workers reported serum blocking in 5/12 (42%) tests (39).

Most workers found that cell-mediated responses with appropriate allogeneic lymphocytes were similar to those using lymphocytes from autochthonous sources. Most felt there was no correlation between the degree of reactivity and age, sex or the extent of disease. Serum blocking activity, however, tended to be more frequently observed in patients whose disease had spread beyond the local area or was clinically active, although this was not universally the case (12).

Sequential determinations of cell-mediated reactivity and serum blocking activity in individual melanoma patients initially looked promising. The Hellström group followed 10 patients with at least 8 determinations on each patient (28). They observed 3 patterns of reactivity. In patients who had their primary melanoma removed and had had no recurrence during the testing period, they found cell-mediated reactivity but no blocking activity. In patients with progressing metastatic melanoma, they noted both cell-mediated and serum blocking reactivity, although the latter fluctuated at different times. In patients who were clinically tumor-free but who had blocking serum activity, they saw a recurrence of melanoma within months of testing and, with successful treatment, their sera even potentiated the cytotoxic effects of their immune lymphocytes. Byrne working in our laboratory reported sequential data on 13 patients, and found that cell-mediated immunity was present fairly constantly in those patients whose disease was relatively stable, but it was lost with rapidly-spreading disease or if the test were performed within one week of death (12). He noted, however, that serum blocking factor, while generally associated with a poor prognosis, might also be found in patients without active disease.

The influence of therapy upon in vitro reactivity measured sequentially has been evaluated by several authors. We studied 12 patients who were treated using chemotherapy with imidazole carboxamide derivatives (14). Eight of the twelve patients had no change in cell-mediated reactivity and five had no change in serum blocking factor. Three patients demonstrated a fall in both parameters and an additional 3 patients showed a fall in serum blocking factor only. It was concluded that there was no significant depression of cell-mediated reactivity by chemotherapy, but results on serum blocking factor were less conclusive, since depression to undetectable levels may be due to a change in disease status rather than to coincident drug use. However, no clear pattern of changing reactivity, either of cell-mediated or blocking activity, could be associated with changes in clinical status. Indeed, lymphocytes from normal donors were found to fluctuate in ability to show cytotoxicity on melanoma cells to as great an extent as did patient lymphocytes (32).

The sequential reactivity of patients who received immunotherapy with irradiated melanoma tumor cells and BCG was measured by Berkelhammer and associates using frozen stored lymphocytes for effector cells (7). They noted significant increases in reactivity following immunotherapy. This increase was not specific for melanoma antigens, since they observed a similar pattern of reactivity against a specificity control, bladder carcinoma cells. In general, lymphocyte reactivity *in vitro* did not correlate with the clinical course of disease. Levy previously had reported the appearance of serum blocking factor in association with accelerated clinical deterioration 3 weeks following an injection of BCG into a small tumor nodule, but this was on a single patient (37). The influence of tumor burden and therapy was studied by Unsgaard and O'Toole (53). They noted tumor specific reactivity mainly during a 3–4 week interval after surgery. This was in marked contrast to other investigators who found tumor specific immunity from 6 months to 2 years after surgery in a similar group of patients (28). The majority of tumor-free patients given preoperative radiotherapy did not show tumor-specific immunity when tested after surgery.

Studies in Patients with Bladder Carcinoma

Aside from melanoma patients, patients with bladder carcinoma have been investigated most thoroughly and comprehensively. In 1970, Bubenik's group reported that 17 of 19 (89%) bladder carcinoma patients had lymphocytes that were cytotoxic to both autochthonous and allogeneic bladder carcinoma cells *in vitro* (11). All 11 cell lines tested were susceptible to this cytotoxic effect. In contrast, no cytotoxicity was seen with lymphoid cells from patients with other tumors or when normal bladder epithelium was used as target cells. Both peripheral blood leukocytes and purified lymphocytes were cytotixic. Bean has suggested that this cytotoxicity is both specific and nonspecific for the bladder cell line used, as determined by measuring the loss of ^{3}H-proline from prelabelled monolayer target cells (5).

It was also noted that 8 of 13 (62%) bladder carcinoma patients had complement-dependent antibody in their serum which was cytotoxic to cultured bladder carcinoma cells. This was not a consistent finding, however, since when patients were observed sequentially it was present on some occasions but not on others. In addition, 4 of 9 (44%) patients had serum blocking factor and 1 of 9 (19%) patients had serum that was not cytotoxic without lekuocytes but became cytotoxic when normal leukocytes were added. This latter effect was thought to be the result of opsinizing antibody; it was complement-dependent and probably IgM (11).

In 1972, O'Toole, Perlmann, and co-workers reported that the incidence of cytotoxicity varied with clinical staging. Fourteen of 16 (88%) patients with localized (TNM Stages T-1 and T-2) disease and 7 of 17 (41%) patients with Stages T-3 and T-4 had lymphocytes that were cytotoxic to cultured antochthonous and allogeneic bladder carcinoma cells (42). Studies suggested that the effector cells were non-thymus-derived lymphoid cells (44).

These authors also published studies concerned with the influence of radiation therapy upon MC assay results (46). Local radiation therapy in doses ranging from 3500–8400r destroyed or diminished existing cytotoxicity when it was administered continuously, but it returned promptly in 3–7 days following completion of therapy in some patients. After radiation, all Stage T-2 patients redeveloped a response usually within 7 days, whereas 80% of Stage T-3 and 50% of Stage T-4 patients did so. Those patients whose lymphocytes were not cytotoxic after radiotherapy were those who had large residual tumor or who had distant metastases detected within 3 months of testing. The same was true if they had only weak cytotoxicity and were followed for up to 9 months. Those who were clinically free of tumor when tested anywhere from 1–10 years after radiation therapy usually had no cytotoxic lymphocytes. Thus, it was assumed that the requirement for cytotoxicity was the presence of viable tumor or tumor-derived material.

Extending their investigations to the influence of surgery upon microcytotoxicity assay results, O'Toole, Perlmann and their colleagues evaluated a group of bladder carcinoma patients who were treated with either local resection or total cystectomy (43). Surgery resulted in a loss of cell-mediated immunity to bladder carcinoma cells, but recurrence led to a reappearance of cell-mediated immunity. Thus, their results again suggest that maintenance of a cellular response to a bladder carcinoma is dependent upon the presence of tumor material in the body, either from a localized primary tumor or from the systemic release of necrotic tumor material. Cell-mediated immunity before treatment was influenced by the tumor burden and changes in the former were a result of treatments that altered the amount of tumor in the body (45). On the other hand, Elhilali and associates found that bladder carcinoma patients who had positive lymphocyte or serum cytotoxicity were without tumor recurrence up to 3 years following therapy (17).

Other investigators have studied additional patients with bladder carcinoma and have correlated cell-mediated reactivity with their clinical course (10). Hakala *et al.* noted an increase in immunity following tumor removal or during the administration of Bacillus Calmette-Guerin (BCG) (20). A progressive decrease in cytotoxicity was observed by O'Boyle and co-workers in patients with progressive disease, although the general range of cytotoxicity was small and variability was too great to allow direct comparisons between different patients and to assess the effects of therapy (41).

Studies in Breast Carcinoma Patients

Although there is little direct evidence that immune responses can influence the balance between breast cancer and the tumor host, there is suggestive evidence that such is the case both in mouse mammary tumors and in humans (31). Considerable evidence is available to suggest the presence of immune responses to human breast cancer from results obtained by using many different procedures. Histologic evidence, such as sinus histiocytosis or lymphocytic predominance of regional nodes, correlates with increased survival in breast cancer patients (6, 8). *In vivo* antitumor cell-mediated immunity, as measured by Black's group with the Rebuck skin window technique using cryostat sections of autologous breast cancer as antigen, is frequently more positive in patients with noninvasive *in situ* or invasive breast carcinoma with negative nodes than in patients with invasive tumor and positive lymph nodes (9). The presence of antitumor antibody has also been described, but its specificity has been questioned because of positivity noted in some controls, other tumor patients and in some patients with benign breast conditions (34). Leukocyte migration inhibition and leukocyte adherence inhibition have revealed more reactivity both to autologous and homologous breast tumor material than to benign breast tissue or controls (2, 19).

Only a few studies have been reported using the CI technique and the MC assay. Hellströms' group reported cell-mediated reactivity in 7 of 8 (88%) patients using autochthonous lymphocytes and on 13/15 (86%) occasions using allogeneic cells (26). We reported 6 of 9 (67%) patients having reactivity with autochthonous cells and 9 of 12 (75%) tests demonstrating cross-reactive inhibition (31).

Anderson and co-workers found significantly greater killing of allogeneic target cells by lymphocytes obtained from breast cancer patients who had undergone mastectomy, postoperative radiation therapy and had received an autograft or irradiated tumor cells from 40–66 months before testing, when compared to age-matched control groups of breast cancer patients not receiving an irradiated autograft and of noncancer-bearing women (1). These data are questionable, however, because the overall mean percentage tumor cell kill by both normal women and nonauto-grafted breast cancer patients was greater than that observed with auto-grafted patients, although paired comparisons of tumor cell kill demon-strated autografted patients exceeded nonautografted patients and the latter exceeded normal women.

Serum blocking activity has been demonstrated in breast cancer pa-tients. Hellström reported this in 3 of 5 (60%) patients using autochtho-nous cells and on 10/17 (59%) occasions with allogeneic cells (26), and we noted this in 5 of 7 (71%) patients using autochthonous cells and in 3 of 6 (50%) patients with allogeneic cells (31).

The significance of the above results in relation to *in vivo* tumor progression has been questioned by Jeejeebhoy, who found that lympho-cytes from normal disease-free women, those with cystic disease, and those with breast carcinoma were equally capable of inactivating breast tumor cells *in vitro* (36). He also observed that humoral factors from both normal and breast cancer patients could block, potentiate, or leave unaf-fected lymphocyte-mediated tumor cell inhibition. We have also observed significant breast cancer cell killing by lymphocytes from normal donors, although overall with some breast cancer target cells, the amount of inhi-bition by patient lymphocytes is greater than that with normal effector cells. The extent of the normal cell killing is so great and of such variable intensity, however, that interpretation of an individual test in a sequential series is impossible.

Studies in Patients with Other Tumors

Patients with several other histologic types of carcinoma have been investigated for cell-mediated reactivity and serum factors as-sociated with their tumor. Among these have been patients with car-cinoma of the colon or lung. Pierce and associates used the CI assay to study lymphocytes from 15 patients with carcinoma of the colon and 50 controls. When tested against 8 different adenocarcinomas of the colon, strong inhibition of tumor growth was observed with both autochthonous and allogeneic lymphocytes (47). Serum blocking factor was also noted in 6 experiments. Nairn and his group studied 60 cases of colonic carcinoma for antitumor immunoreactivity, as determined by lymphocyte cytotoxic-ity, complement-dependent serum cytotoxicity, and immunofluorescence staining (40). They found that 19 of the 60 cases showed at least one type of reactivity. Lymphocytoxicity against cultured colonic carcinoma cells was seen in 8 of 24 (33%) patients in this series, and later this was confirmed in 34% of 263 cases using a microassay. Pihl and co-workers reported on the clinicopathological correlation with immunoreactivity in 132 patients with colonic carcinoma. Of these patients, 43 out of 132 (33%) were found to have cytotoxic lymphocytes. Only 9 of 53 (17%) patients with cytotoxic lymphocytes had regional lymph node (Duke's stage C) metastases, whereas 34 of 79 (43%) patients had this reactivity if their colon carcinoma was limited to the bowel wall (Duke's stages A, B1, or B2). Lymphocyte reactivity was also more common in patients with well-differentiated (64%) as opposed to less-differentiated tumors (25%) (49).

Patients with bronchogenic carcinoma have been studied by Pierce and DeVald (48). Cytotoxicity was seen on 39/76 (51%) occasions in lung cancer patients, but also on 16/44 (36%) occasions using target cells of tumors other than lung cancer. The frequency of reactivity correlated with clinical status, in that it was observed on 30/40 (75%) occasions in patients without evidence of disease postresection for lung cancer, but only on 9/36 (25%) occasions in patients preoperative, inoperable, or with clinically evident disease postresection. Vose and associates reported that 73% of patients with lung carcinoma demonstrated cytotoxicity in a MC assay when they were studied postoperatively or while receiving radiation therapy (55).

Discussion

The preceding pages represent an attempt to outline the pertinent publications that have appeared concerning the clinical application of the CI technique and the MC assay to the study of human tumor immunity. The outline is not all-inclusive but does reflect the general trend of studies that have been done with these procedures. It is now appropriate to assess critically what information we have gained from this experience. This will prove helpful not only in telling us just how useful these tests are, but also in determining the requirements for future assays. Obviously, our own experience with these methods in patients with melanoma or with breast cancer is the major basis for this discussion.

The main concept that must be understood in interpreting MC assay or CI results is that, even though they may reveal trends in a group of patients with a particular type or stage, say, of tumor, the trends may not be so evident in each individual patient within that group. Thus, the results may indicate important trends for the group of patients as a whole, but they may not be predictive for the individual patient. The reasons for this are unclear. It may be that each group of patients has not been stratified sufficiently well enough with regard to all prognostic variables.

Important prognostic variables for malignant melanoma include sex, stage of disease, depth or level of invasion into dermis of primary melanomas and location of primary lesions. Most published studies have only considered the first two parameters in classifying patients. The investigations on bladder carcinoma patients, on the other hand, have always considered clinical stage in classifying patients and since this correlates well with grade of differentiation of the tumor, it has been rather easy to define subsets of patients. It is certainly true that the most consistently predictive results have been obtained in patients with bladder cancer. With breast carcinoma patients, the situation is extremely complex. Not only are age, menopausal status, histology of the tumor, and size of the primary and clinical stage important prognostic variables, but also in patients with recurrent or metastatic disease one must consider disease-free-interval, dominant metastatic sites (organ involvement is dominant to bone and bone involvement is dominant to soft tissue), previous therapy and the presence or absence of estrogen receptors in predicting survival or response to therapy with surgery, hormones, or chemotherapy. Little attention has been given to these variables in the reported studies on breast cancer patients.

In addition to these clinical short-comings in studies of human tumor immunity, there are major technical difficulties in CI and MC methodology. Perhaps the most disturbing factor is the frequent toxicity or reactivity of lymphocytes obtained from normal individuals who serve as controls in these studies (32, 48). Control lymphocytes inhibit the growth of target cells with high frequency, particularly in our experience, with cell line, as opposed to short-term, cultures. This inhibition is not found for all target cells tested at a given time with a single preparation of lymphocytes, that is, it is "specific." Our sequential studies over a 2-year period with lymphocytes from the same control donors show major fluctuations in inhibition against the same target cells. Target cells also change with serial passage in their susceptibility to destruction by control lymphocytes. Whatever the reasons for this degree of control lymphocyte reactivity, it is extremely difficult to interpret the assay results of any given test in any given patient. Whether or not one detects inhibition of target cell survival by a cancer patient's lymphocytes on a particular day depends on the toxicity of the control lymphocytes. Whether specificity of inhibition by patients' lymphocytes for appropriate tumor cells can be demonstrated depends upon a lack of specificity by control lymphocytes. Selection of control lymphocytes (or elimination of them from the protocol) selects the results. Thus, although we found that lymphocytes from melanoma patients showed greater reactivity on melanoma target cells in 238/300 (79%) tests and lymphocytes from breast cancer patients showed greater reactivity on breast cancer cells in 49/76 (64%) tests, and both showed more than that seen with control lymphocytes (32), we also found that sequential testing gave no data *consistently* correlating with clinical status or therapy, leaving those selected sequential studies anecdotal at best. In the last analysis this lack of consistent correlation between microcytotoxicity results and any clinical or therapeutic parameter, not the technical problem or control cytotoxicity, is the real reason why we feel the methodology is not clinically useful. Simply stated, it does not tell us what we need to know in regards to selection of therapy or assessment of prognosis.

Well then, what requirements are necessary for a meaningful test of antitumor immune reactivity in cancer patients? Obviously, any improvements in methodology that would eliminate control variability and allow selection of the most appropriate controls and target cells for study would be essential to providing reliable technical data. However interesting the observations of control cytotoxicity may be, it cannot be forgotten that the aim of the testing is to detect meaningful *differences* between controls and patients and between patients of different clinical status. Further reliable technical data may not be enough to insure that this information is a true reflection of a patient's immunity to his tumor. Even with the crude methods available, the majority of patients tested do have cell-mediated reactivity. Thus, there may be no reason to believe that measurement of this parameter alone will really matter, although quantitative differences may exist. What may matter, however, is a true measurement of circulating factors that are capable of moderating cell-mediated responses. With the present methodologies, it is impossible to determine this independently of measuring cell-mediated immunity. If procedures are developed that will allow detection of blocking factors independent of determining cell-mediated reactivity, this may provide a more reliable clinically useful assay of human tumor immunity.

Another factor to consider is what magnitude of difference from normal can we detect with the present assays or improvements in them. An important question will be what magnitude of difference is going to be significant, in terms of correlating with prognostic variables, survival or response to therapies. Until now, it has been extremely difficult to determine just how much change in reactivity is necessary to allow a correlation, because of the problems with control variability, target cell susceptibility, etc. Also, the prognostic factors chosen for attempted correlation to immune reactivity must be independently meaningful to the particular disease being studied.

In conclusion, one can say that experience with CI and MC testing has provided a conceptual stimulus to understanding the basic elements of human tumor immunity, even though the actual data obtained must be interpreted with caution. This information is of biological importance to cancer patients as a group, but presently these assays have little clinical relevance to the individual cancer patient. Hopefully with refinements in methodology and better stratification of cancer patients, a true reflection of an individual patient's tumor immunity will be possible.

REFERENCES

1. Anderson, J. M., Kelly, F., Wood, E., Roger, K. D., and Freshney, R. I. 1973. Evaluation of leukocyte functions six years after tumour antograft in human mammary cancer. Brit. J. Cancer 28: 83–96.
2. Anderson, V., Bjerrum, O., Bendixen, G., Schiødt, T., and Dissing, I. 1970. Effect of autologous mammary tumor extracts on human leukocyte migration in vitro. Int. J. Cancer 5: 357–363.
3. Baldwin, R. W., Price, M. R., and Robbins, R. A. 1972. Blocking of lymphocyte-mediated cytotoxicity for rat hepatoma cells by tumor-specific antigen-antibody complexes. Nature New Biology 238: 185–187.
4. Bansal, S. C., and Sjögren, H. O. 1971. "Unblocking" serum activity in vitro in the polyoma system may correlate with antitumour effects of antiserum in vitro. Nature New Biology 233: 76–78.
5. Bean, M. A., Pees, H., Fogh, J. E., Grabstald, H., and Oettgen, F. 1974. Cytotoxicity of lymphocytes from patients with cancer of the urinary bladder: Detection by a ³H-proline microcytotoxicity test. Int. J. Cancer 14: 186–197.
6. Berg, J. W. 1959. Inflammation and prognosis in breast cancer. A search for host resistance. Cancer 12: 714–720.
7. Berkelhammer, M. J., Mastrangelo, J., Laucius, J. F., Bodurtha, A. J., and Prehn, R. T. 1975. Sequential in vitro reactivity of lymphocytes from melanoma patients receiving immunotherapy compared with the reactivity of lymphocytes from healthy donors. Int. J. Cancer 16: 571–578.
8. Black, M. M. 1970. Lymphoreticuloendothelial reactivity as a component of the tumor-host relationship, in L. Severi (ed.), Immunity and Tolerance in Oncogenesis, pp. 863–876. Division of Career Research, Perugia University, Perugia, Italy.
9. Black, M. M., and Leis, H. P. 1970. Cellular responses to autologous and breast cancer tissue. Sequential observations. Cancer 32: 384–389.
10. Bloom, E. T., Ossorio, C., and Brosman, S. A. 1974. Cell-mediated cytotoxicity against human bladder cancer. Int. J. Cancer 14: 326–334.
11. Bubenik, J., Perlmann, P., Helmstein, K., and Moberger, G. 1970. Cellular and humoral immune responses to human urinary bladder carcinomas. Int. J. Cancer 5: 310–319.
12. Byrne, M., Heppner, G., Stolbach, L., Cummings, F., McDonnough, E., and Calabresi, P. 1973. Tumor immunity in melanoma patients as assessed by colony inhibition and microcytotoxicity methods: A preliminary report. Natl. Cancer Inst. Monogr. 37: 3–8.
13. Cummings, F. J., Heppner, G. H., Stolbach, L., and Calabresi, P. 1973. Demonstration of cell-mediated and blocking immune responses to tumor anti-

gens in cancer patients with the colony-inhibition-in-gel test. *Israel J. Med. Sci.* 9: 308–316.

14. Cummings, F. J., Heppner, G. H., and Calabresi, P. 1975. Evaluation of cell-mediated reactivity and serum blocking factors in melanoma patients on chemotherapy. *Med. Pediat. Oncol.* 1: 195–206.

15. Currie, G. A., Lejeune, F., and Fairley, G. H. 1971. Immunization with irradiated tumour cells and specific lymphocyte cytotoxicity in malignant melanoma. *Brit. Med. J.* 2: 305–310.

16. De Vries, J. E., and Rumke, P. 1976. Tumour-associated lymphocyte cytotoxicity superimposed on "spontaneous" cytotoxicity in melanoma patients. *Int. J. Cancer* 17: 182–190.

17. Elhilali, M. M., and Nayak, S. K. 1975. Immunologic evaluation of human bladder cancer: in vitro studies. *Cancer* 35: 419–431.

18. Fossati, G., Colnaghi, M. I., Della Porta, G., Cascinelli, N., and Veronesi, U. 1971. Cellular and humoral immunity against human malignant melanoma. *Int. J. Cancer* 18: 344–350.

19. Grosser, N., and Thomson, D. M. P. 1975. Cell-mediated antitumor immunity in breast cancer patients evaluated by antigen-induced leukocyte adherence inhibition in test tubes. *Cancer Res.* 35: 2571–2579.

20. Hakala, T. R., Lange, P. H., Elliott, A. Y., and Elwin E. Fraley. 1976. Changes in cell-mediated cytotoxicity during the clinical course of patients with bladder carcinoma. *J. Urology* 115: 268–273.

21. Fairley, G. H., Lewis, M. G., Ikonopisov, R. L., Nairn, R. C., and Alexander, P. 1971. Detection of tumor specific immune reactions in human melanoma. *Ann. N.Y. Acad. Sci.* 177: 286–289.

22. Hellström, I., Hellström, K. E., Pierce, G. E., and Yang, J. P. S. 1968. Cellular and humoral immunity to different types of human neoplasms. *Nature* 220: 1352–1354.

23. Hellström, I., Hellström, K. E., Pierce, G. E., and Bill, A. H. 1968. Demonstration of cell-bound and humoral immunity against neuroblastoma cells. *Proc. Natl. Acad. Sci.* 60: 1231–1238.

24. Hellström, I., Hellström, K. E., Bill, A. H., Pierce, G. E., and Young, J. P. S. 1970. Studies on cellular immunity to human neuroblastoma cells. *Int. J. Cancer* 6: 172–188.

25. Hellström, I., and Hellström, K. E. 1971. Colony inhibition and cytotoxicity assays, *in* Bloom, B. R. and Glade, P. R. (eds.), *In vitro Methods in Cell Mediated Immunity 1971.* Pp. 409–414. Academic Press, New York.

26. Hellström, I., Hellström, K. E., Sjögren, H. O., and Warner, G. A. 1971. Demonstration of cell-mediated immunity to human neoplasms of various histological types. *Int. J. Cancer* 7: 1–16.

27. Hellström, I., Sjögren, H. O., Warner, G., and Hellström, K. E. 1971. Blocking of cell-mediated tumor immunity by sera from patients with growing neoplasms. *Int. J. Cancer* 7: 226–237.

28. Hellström, I., Warner, G. A., Hellström, K. E., and Sjögren, H. O. 1973. Sequential studies on cell-mediated tumor immunity and blocking serum activity in ten patients with malignant melanoma. *Int. J. Cancer* 11: 280–292.

29. Heppner, G. H., and Kopp, J. S. 1971. A dilute agar colony inhibition (CI) test for studying cell-mediated immune responses against tumor cells. *Int. J. Cancer* 7: 26–33.

30. Heppner, G. H., Stolbach, L., Byrne, M., Cummings, F. J., McDonnough, E., and Calabresi, P. 1973. Cell-mediated and serum blocking reactivity to tumor antigens in patients with malignant melanoma. *Int. J. Cancer* 11: 245–260.

31. Heppner, G. H. 1973. Is there evidence that immunity influences tumor-host balance in breast cancer? *Recent Results Cancer Res.* 42: 63–72.

32. Heppner, G., Henry, E., Stolbach, L., Cummings, F., McDonough, E., and Calabresi, P. 1975. Problems in the clinical use of the microcytotoxicity assay for measuring cell-mediated immunity to tumor cells. *Cancer Res.* 35: 1931–1937.

33. Heppner, G. H. 1977. Immunology: Breast cancer. *Recent Results in Cancer Research* 57: chap. 9. Springer-Verlag, Heidelberg.

34. Humphrey, L. J., Estes, N. C., Morse, P. A., Jewell, W. R., Boudet, R. A., Hudson, M. J. K. 1974. Serum antibody in patients with mammary disease. *Cancer* 34: 1516–1520.

35. Jagarlamoody, S. M., Aust, H. C., Tew, R. H., and McKhann, C. F. 1971. In vitro detection of cytotoxic cellular immunity against tumor-specific antigens by a radio-isotopic technique. *Proc. Nat. Acad. Sci. (Wash.)* 68: 1346–1350.

36. Jeejeebhoy, H. F. 1975. Immunological studies of women with primary breast carcinoma. *Int. J. Cancer* 15: 867–878.

37. Levy, N. L., Mahaley, M. S. Jr., and Day, E. D. 1972. Serum-mediated blocking of cell-mediated anti-tumor immunity in a melanoma patient association with BCG immunotherapy and clinical deterioration. *Int. J. Cancer* 10: 244–248.

38. Lewis, M. G., Ikonopisov, R. L., Narin, R. C., Phillips, T. M., Fairley, G. H., Bodenham, D. C., and Alexander, P. 1969. Tumor-specific antibodies in human malignant melanoma and their relationship of the extent of the disease. *Brit. Med. J.* 3: 547–553.

39. Mukherji, B., Nathanson, L., and Clark, D. A. 1973. Studies of humoral and cell-mediated immunity in human melanoma. *Yale J. Biol. Med.* 46: 681–692.

40. Nairn, R. C., Nind, A. P. P., Guli, E. P. G., Davies, D. J., Rolland, J. M., McGiven, A. R., and Hughes, E. S. R. 1971. Immunological reactivity in patients with carcinoma of colon. *Brit. Med. J.* 4: 706–709.

41. O'Boyle, P. J., Cooper, E. H., and Williams, R. E. 1974. Evaluation of immunological reactivity in bladder cancer. *Brit. J. Urol.* 46: 303–308.

42. O'Toole, C., Perlmann, P., Unsgaard, B., Moberger, G., and Edsmyer, F. 1972. Cellular immunity to human urinary bladder carcinoma. I. Correlation to clinical stage and radiotherapy. *Int. J. Cancer* 10: 77–91.

43. O'Toole, C., Perlmann, P., Unsgaard, B., Almgard, L. E., Johansson, B., Moberger, G., and Edsmyr. 1972. Cellular immunity to human urinary bladder carcinoma. II. Effect of surgery and preoperative irradiation. *Int. J. Cancer* 10: 92–98.

44. O'Toole, C., and Perlmann, P. 1973. Lymphocyte cytotoxicity in bladder cancer: No requirement for thymus-derived effector cells? *Lancet* 1: 1085–1088.

45. O'Toole, C., Unsgaard, B., Almgard, L. E., and Johansson, B. 1973. The cellular immune response to carcinoma of the urinary bladder: Correlation to clinical stage and treatment. *Brit. J. Cancer* 28: 266–275.

46. O'Toole, C. 1973. Effect of therapy and tumor stage on cellular immunity to bladder carcinoma. *Adv. Exp. Med. Biol.* 29: 477–482.

47. Pierce, G. E., Hellström, I. E., Hellström, K. E., and Yang, J. P. 1969. Demonstration of cellular immunity against human tumors. *Surg. Forum* 20: 112–113.

48. Pierce, G. E., and DeVald, B. 1975. Microcytotoxicity assays of tumor immunity in patients with bronchogenic carcinoma correlated with clinical status. *Cancer Res.* 35: 3577–3584.

49. Pihl, E., Hughes, E. S. R., Nind, A. P. P., and Narin, R. C. 1975. Colonic carcinoma: Clinicopathological correlation with immunoreactivity. *Brit. Med. J.* 3: 742–743.

50. Pollack, S., Heppner, G., Brown, R. M., and Nelson, K. 1972. Specific killing of tumor cells *in vitro* in the presence of normal lymphoid cells in sera from hosts immune to the tumor antigens. *Int. J. Cancer* 9: 316–323.

51. Stevenson, G. T., and Laurence, D. J. R. 1975. Report of a workshop on the immune response to solid tumors in man. *Int. J. Cancer* 16: 816–887.

52. Takasugi, M., and Klein, E. 1970. A microassay for cell-mediated immunity. *Transplantation* 9: 219–227.

53. Unsgaard, B., and O'Toole, C. 1975. The influence of tumour burden and therapy on cellular cytotoxicity responses in patients with ocular and skin melanoma. *Brit. J. Cancer* 31: 301–316.

54. Veronesi, U., Cascinelli, N., Fossati, G., Canevari, S., and Balzarini, G. 1973. Lymphocyte toxicity test in clinical melanoma. *Eur. J. Cancer* 9: 843–846.

55. Vose, B. M., Moore, M., and Jack, G. D. 1975. Cell-mediated cytotoxicity to human pulmonary neoplasms. *Int. J. Cancer* 15: 308–320.

CHAPTER 9

REVIEW OF TUMOR ENHANCEMENT

Vilas V. Likhite

Harvard Medical School
Boston, Massachusetts 02115

The presence of enhancing factors is becoming more completely delineated in the animal host. It appears that antigen excess and the subsequent antibody effecting immune complexes (and their subsequent properties in the zone of equivalence) may be the major culprit in the human host. The effects of immune complexes in man appear to be similar to those observed in animal models and have been documented by the increased presence of antigen-antibody complexes and their manifestations (i.e., their deposition on the glomerular membrane). However, there needs to be a better correlation of these deleterious effects as observed in the *in vitro* system which could be employed for predetermining *in vivo* outcome. The availability of these parameters may allow for a more efficient surveillance of the cancer patient.

Introduction

Immunological enhancement has been most often defined as the inhibition or delay by antibodies or cells of an immune response to specific antigens. Unexpected accelerated growth of tumors in immunized animals led to the finding that the immunological specificity of the phenomenon was mediated by a serum factor (37). These observations were reproduced in connection with normal alloantigens and tumor antigens, and the subsequent correlation of in vitro results in vivo generated new concepts of the blocking of lymphocyte-mediated cytotoxicity (54, 117, 128). The participation of this process in host-tumor relationships reflected an undesirable occurrence of essential, normal immunologic functions. It was suggested that forbidden clones of self-reactive lymphoid cells were not completely eliminated, as evidenced by the finding that circulating self-reactive lymphocytes of healthy rodents were observed in cytotoxicity assays. The serum factors blocking these reactions were thought to play a major role in the prevention of autoimmune disease (47, 199). In addition, maternal lymphocytes were also observed to react with fetal antigens expressed by normal embryonic cells and the reaction could be abrogated using autologous sera (32, 166). These serum-blocking factors of lymphocyte-mediated cytotoxicity were also found to be effective in the tolerance to certain grafts, bone marrow transplants, and parabiosis, and in tetraparental or allophenic mice (95–97, 227). Graft-vs.-host disease could also be ameliorated using the sera which blocked the cytotoxic effect on target cells of the recipient, and the phenomenon of enhancement facilitation was thus recognized (221). These effects, known as serum-mediated enhancement of tumor growth, were subsequently recognized in host-tumor systems. Solubilized or shed cell surface antigens, antibodies, and antigen-antibody complexes with antigen excess were found to be commonly responsible for the phenomenon, which could act not only on the target cell, but also on the effector lymphocyte (28, 35, 73, 149, 218). In order to provide an adequate background in the subject of tumor enhancement and in order to better display the range of modern views of the factors controlling this entity, many views which are considered untenable by the author will be presented individually.

Antibody

Several studies have revealed that antibodies that mediate tumor enhancement belong to the IgG class with other immunoglobulin classes being presently excluded (119, 211, 212, 234, 235). Of the subclasses of IgG, the most exacting work has implicated IgG_2 in both spontaneous and transplanted tumors (31, 119, 190, 191, 211, 233, 234), although a few investigators have observed enhancing factors to be present in the IgG_1 subclass (43, 220) (the problems may lie in the method of separation). Recent studies have suggested the presence of IgG_3 in addition to IgG_1, as the enhancing factor in man (123). IgG immunoglobulins evidencing enhancing behavior have also been associated with hemagglutinating and cytotoxic activities, although the reverse is not true (65).

The effective mechanism may lie in the finding that IgM antibodies have extremely potent cytotoxic abilities; IgM is a pentamer of IgG, with five pairs of Fc chains, any one of which can fix complement (49) and only one molecule of which is sufficient for sensitizing one red cell for immune lysis (26). A minimum of two molecules of IgG is required on the surface of a red cell for C_1 binding and lysis (26). Thus, one can assume that whenever two or more molecules are needed, the distribution of H-2 antigens on tumor cell surfaces (which may be at sites far from each other) becomes relevant. If they are at sites too distant for effective binding of complement, the cell may become more resistant to cytotoxicity. Blocking antibodies exhibit a paradoxical effect which is more likely related to their ability to fix and activate the complement cascade. Both in vivo and in vitro, small doses of antibody have been observed to promote tumor growth or protect tumor cells from injury, whereas larger amounts of the same antibody either inhibit tumor progression or destroy target tumor cells (84, 116). The opposing effects may thus depend upon the antigenic density over the cell surface, the ratio of antibody molecules to antigenic sites, and the ability of antibody to activate complement.

It seems as though slow-moving IgG (IgG_2) may be the most suitable factor responsible for mediating tumor enhancement. It has good avidity to antigen (allowing for poor disassociation from the cell surface) and has a half-life of 5 to 15 days, thereby allowing sufficient time for grafts to take (50). It may inhibit the production of IgM (217). It will not cause passive cutaneous anaphylaxis, i.e, it is not bound, as is IgG_1, to tissue mast cells. Most of all, it does not activate complement unless two or more chains in close proximity are available on the surface of a membrane (26, 49). If this is one requirement for an immunoglobulin to participate in tumor enhancement (and since complement is fixed on the Fc fragment of the immunoglobulin molecule), then the Fab fragment of any molecule should be effective in exhibiting tumor enhancement, as it binds antigen without activating complement. This theory is supported by the finding that light chains of IgG₁ did indeed exhibit tumor enhancement (31, 43).

Cell-Mediated Immunity

Whereas antibodies are efficient in the rejection of certain cell types only, the cell-mediated immune responses are effective against neoplastic cells or cells transplanted between genetically dissimilar individuals. This is evidenced by the ability of immune lymphoid cells to transfer transplantation immunity passively to unsensitized hosts in situations where humoral isoantibodies were inefficient (21, 163). In addition, Mitchison (164) demonstrated that immunity to tumor allografts containing foreign H-2 antigens could be adoptively transferred with lymphoid cells but not serum. This was followed by evidence which showed similar results using heavily irradiated syngeneic sarcoma cells (transfer of cytotoxicity with lymphoid cells but not serum), an effect which was negated if the lymphoid effector cells were killed by freezing and thawing (134).

The involvement of cell-mediated immunity towards syngeneic tumor cells was first demonstrated by Yoshida and Southam (192, 229) and subsequently confirmed by investigators using various techniques including the colony-inhibition assay developed by Hellström and Hellström (91, 92), which allowed for better quantification of the effects. This finding was significant as it indicated that the host possessed the immunological ability to react against its own neoplasm, although this ability might not be sufficient for effecting tumor rejection.

Cell-mediated immunity can commonly be detected at least as early as 5 to 7 days after transplantation of syngeneic tumor cell grafts (100, 229). Processes that depress this type of reaction can precipitate an aligned tumor development in both animals and man (154, 179). Specific cell-mediated responses to human tumors have been detected through reduction in growth of autologous tumor transplants (63, 64, 115, 177) and in vitro studies (76, 114, 197) involving colony inhibition studies which correlate with quantitative demonstration of cell-mediated immunity (57, 99). Three most important facts have emerged from these studies: (1) in the absence of autologous serum, specific cell-mediated in vitro inhibition of tumor cells occurs regardless of the clinical state of the patient, in contrast to most carcinogen-induced animal tumors; (2) specific cellular recognition and colony inhibition are cross-reactive among human tumors of similar origin and similar histological type; and (3) in some situations, in vitro and in vivo manifestations of cell-mediated immunity sometimes may correlate with clinical disease (11, 33, 34, 63, 64, 102).

Antigen

A number of experiments have revealed that histocompatibility (H) antigens, particularly of the H-2 locus, were involved in the induction of enhancing antisera (167–169, 205, 206). These antigens are also involved in the induction of transplantation immunity (206). It is unknown whether all or only some of the H antigens will induce blocking antibody, although non-H-2 antigens have been observed to do so (39). In one instance, a single H antigen difference between donor and recipient permitted the expression of immunological enhancement (228). Tumor-specific antigens, also located on the cell surface, are also capable of effecting enhancing antibody, whether the tumor cells were obtained from spontaneous, virally or chemically induced tumors (129, 166).

The manner of presentation of antigen to the living host may also determine if the enhancing factor will be induced. It seems that viable tissue may be more effective than nonviable tissue, and the route of administration of antigen, whether with or without adjuvant, may be crucial in effecting the outcome of production of enhancement (126, 206). Of additional importance in affording or not affording complement fixation are the density and spatial distribution of cell surface antigens present on the cell surface membrane (148), the lack of which is essential for enhancement (137).

Host

The host provides an ingredient integral to the process of immunological enhancement, the nature of which is partially obscure. The role of immunosuppression in facilitating the growth of antigenic tumor cells has been well studied. Neonates and thymectomized or immunosuppressed hosts receiving grafts exhibit prolongation of graft survival beyond the usual time of rejection in experimental animals (228, 234) and in immunodefiency syndromes in man (78). A relative decrease of various immune reactions has been well-documented in old age (38), and also following virus infection (23, 113). The genetic composition of the host may influence the development of enhancement. Whether or not an animal responds to an antigen depends on its histocompatibility genes and, therefore, the genetic composition of the host is additionally important. Although some investigations have revealed that the genetic determination of the immune response may lie in the same process as that of the synthesis of immunoglobulins (22), others propose that genes may be more important in antigenic recognition (150). Animals of the same H-2 type exhibit the same pattern of immune response and marked antigen-specific polymorphism with respect to their patterns of response between strains of different H-2 types (151).

Mechanisms of Tumor Enhancement

The effect of enhancement in relation to both tumor growth and peripheral lymphocyte levels can be interpreted three ways: (a) enhancement in the face of increased numbers of immune lymphocytes should mean that antibody may be protecting target cells from the effects of immunity and afferent enhancement; (b) failure to achieve enhancement and inhibition of lymphocytosis after sensitization imply afferent enhancement, since these effects are accomplished before sensitization; and (c) successful enhancement coupled to inhibition of lymphocytosis after sensitization would indicate that blocking factors turn off the central machinery of the immune response. Thus, the afferent arc is the part of the response that begins with the presentation of immunogenic host and includes recognition, preparation, and meeting of the antigen with immunocompetent cells. The afferent arc reflects the events that occur in the already-immunized host and describes the phenomena associated with antigen-antibody reactions, antigen-cell interactions, activation of the complement system, and evolution of injury.

The rationale for afferent enhancement is based on the postulation that antiserum is in some way able to block the development of cellular immunity in the nodes and other lymphoid organs draining the graft (21, 206). Since the destruction of the graft is usually dependent on cellular immunity, a blockage of this sort would permit the graft to grow and is thus referred to as afferent inhibition of transplantation immunity, or walling off the graft by circulating antibody. The concept of afferent blockade rests on two findings: (i) in vitro: when immersed in blocking antibodies, target tumor cells or tissue grafts will bind to antibody and will be enhanced when grafted into allogeneic recipients (116, 120, 125, 235); and (ii) in vivo: specific uptake of labeled antibodies of enhancing antibodies of enhancing antiserum may be detected in the grafts (121).

Evidence against the afferent inhibition theory of enhancement postulates that all available antigenic sites of tumor cells are covered by blocking antibodies (182) and the inhibited state would depend on the continued unavailability of the antigenic site (4). Also, both enhancement and second-set rejection of homologous tumor grafts can be demonstrated in the same animal, that is, a first (sensitizing) tumor graft inoculated concomitantly with an excess of antibody is enhanced, whereas a second tumor graft one week later suffers accelerated rejection (no afferent inhibition). The graft destined for enhancement provides the necessary immune stimulus (no afferent inhibition) for homograft rejection reaction. Another observation casting doubt on the afferent inhibition theory of enhancement is that alloantiserum injected into mice 6 or 7 days after sensitizing tumor inoculum (at a time when the homograft intensity should be at peak level) enhances the tumor (65, 125). Afferent inhibition has been invoked to explain this on the assumption that continued antigenic stimulation is required to maintain the cellular response. Afferent inhibition is untenable, however, if an analogy between delayed hypersensitivity and tumor graft rejection is valid (164), for passive antibody will not diminish the delayed hypersensitivity reaction once sensitization has occurred (10). Kaliss (125) and Chantler (41) have emphasized that both enhancement and resistance may exist in animals prepared for active enhancement of a neoplasm and that enhancement cannot occur in the absence of an immune response. In tumor systems, resistance to neoplastic can be detected prior to the appearance of enhancement (42).

If peripheral inhibition (both afferent and efferent) were the principal cause of enhancement, then IgM and IgG_1 antibodies would also be expected to inhibit the development of immunity by reacting with and covering the antigens. Even if IgM were discounted on the basis of its rapid metabolic decay and its chemical configuration (43), the inability of IgG_1, with the same hemagglutinating property as IgG_2, to enhance tumor growth casts considerable doubt on the efficacy of peripheral inhibition (211, 212). However, the unique ability of IgG_2 to suppress immunity implicates a central effect. In order to test the hypothesis that removal of antigen blocks the continuation of the immune response, tumor cells were inoculated in the tail of experimental mice (212). The tail with the tumor was amputated 6 days later. Lymphocytosis continued at the same rate as that in tumor-bearing mice during the subsequent two-week observation period. Mice receiving antiserum 6 days after grafting exhibited curtailed lymphocytosis, which may be evidence against afferent inhibition. The final argument involves the differential effect of antibody on the humoral versus the rejection response. H-2 antigens are apparently fully represented on all nucleated cells of the body and are controlled by a single though complex gene locus (207, 212). If one can assume that the same antigens are responsible for both antibody formation and allograft rejection, afferent inhibition is untenable if one considers the strong antibody response observed in mice exhibiting tumor enhancement. The discovery that allograft rejection may be suppressed while serum antibody production continues suggests the presence of at least two separate lines of lymphoid cells responsible for these functions. Thus, if one line of lymphoid cells is inhibited, but the other is stimulated, afferent blocks against the same antigen can be excluded.

Efferent inhibition (see Fig. 1) postulates that effector elements (either

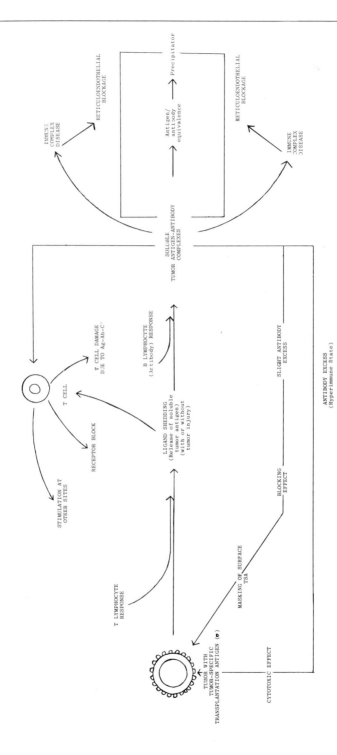

Fig. 1. Schematic representation of events associated with enhancement.

sensitized cells, antibodies, or both) are prevented from reaching and reacting with the antigens. The block is presumed to be in two places: at the periphery of the graft where blocking antibodies cover the antigens and thereby prevent effector elements from seeing their targets or centrally, in reticuloendothelial and lymphoid organs, where blocking complexes depress or inhibit cellular immunity (i.e., they bind to effector cells and prevent them from interacting with target antigens). In order to evaluate efferent enhancement, recipient animals were immunized with tissues from donors. Tumor cells from donors were then incubated with blocking antibodies or normal serum and washed, to remove excess serum. Subsequently the treated tumor cells were incubated with sensitized lymph node cells of the recipient, and the extent of destruction compared between experimental (tumor plus blocking serum) and control (tumor plus control serum) target cells. Alternately, the treated tumor cells may be injected into sensitized recipients (166–169).

Lymph node cells from mice, exhibiting rejection of Moloney sarcomas, have been shown to inhibit colony formation (93). A similar inhibition using lymph node cells from mice with progressively growing tumors resulted in their deaths. This finding may be explained by the demonstration that progressor serum contains immunoglobulins which can specifically block the colony-inhibiting effect of immune lymph node cells by protecting the target cells (98). The antagonistic effect of humoral antibodies on cytotoxicity caused by cell-mediated immunological reactions may explain the observation by Möller (168) that lymph node cells are more efficient in killing target cells in tissue culture than spleen cells from the same animal. It has also been demonstrated that hyperimmunization usually abolishes the cytotoxic effect of spleen cells, whereas it does not affect the efficiency of lymph node cells (166). Since spleen cells are known to be a main source of humoral antibody synthesis and it seems conceivable that spleen cells from the hyperimmune hosts contained a mixed population of humoral antibody-producing cells and cellular antibody, there is the suggestion that the humoral antibodies produced in tissue culture may have combined with the target cells and protected them from destruction by the cell-mediated immune factors. In subsequent studies involved with efferent enhancement (or prolonged survival), it was demonstrated that perfusion of rabbit donors' ear skin with antidonor alloantiserum, followed by transplantation, resulted in prolonged survival (86, 210). In addition, enhanced proliferation of allogeneic ascites tumor cells has been found to parallel a marked histiocytosis within the host receiving passive antibody (17). These studies also revealed a lack of adherence of these histiocytes to tumor cells, as well as a lack of the usual mutual necrobiosis. Chantler (41) also found an elevated histiocytosis in mice, with enhanced growth of ascites tumors following pretreatment with irradiated tumor cells. The histiocytes from these animals, when washed free of ascites fluid, could adoptively immunize other animals against the tumor. The enhancement could be reproduced if normally sensitized histiocytes (no enhanced tumor) were mixed with ascites fluid containing alloantibody, thereby preventing the transfer of adoptive immunity.

A major argument against efferent enhancement is that blocking antisera given repeatedly to recipients with enhanced neoplastic or normal tissue grafts do not prolong survival of grafts indefinitely (228). If blocking factors operate by covering antigenic sites of target grafts or by inhibiting effector lymphocytes, then multiple doses of these antibodies (administered over an extended period of time) should be capable of covering antigenic sites that have been uncovered by dissociation of antibodies or that have been recently synthesized. Otherwise such doses should be capable of reacting with effector lymphocytes that are being formed continuously. To date, these procedures have not extended the period of enhancement. Evidence against afferent enhancement is provided in experiments where varying amounts of blocking antibody and constant amounts of tumor antigen are employed. Relatively large quantities of cytotoxic antisera (0.5–1.0 ml), in the presence of complement, destroy target cells, whereas minute quantities of the same antibodies (0.1–0.5 ml) tend to enhance tumor growth or protect them in vitro from destruction (4, 112, 116). The enhancement of small quantities of passive antibody may argue against peripheral inhibition, but whether the amount of antibody was sufficient to cover all antigenic sites on the allograft remains speculative. It is significant that depression of the primary five-day hemolysin response of mice to sheep erythrocytes has been observed with the use of passive hyperimmune anti-erythrocyte antibody administered in a quantity sufficient to cover no more than about 1% of the antigenic sites of the cells (112).

As total destruction often results when antibodies react with a target cell in the presence of complement, one might expect that efferent inhibition could be mediated by nontoxic antibodies. However, there is evidence that a cytotoxic mouse antibody (eluted early from DEAE cellulose columns) suppressed growth of tumor cells in mice, whereas a slower eluting antibody produced enhancement (43). In addition, several investigators have shown that enzymatic digestion, which removes the Fc portion of complement-fixing IgG antibodies, converts them from cytotoxic to enhancing antibodies (31, 43, 119, 212). It has been well established that complement-dependent cytotoxic reactions are strongly influenced by cell surface antigen density (148). There is also evidence indicating that immunological enhancement of the efferent inhibition type is affected by antibody class; concentration, affinity and cell surface density of antigen; the presence of sensitized lymphoid cells; and the ability of the antibodies to fix complement (148, 203). Thus, it may be proposed that when target cells are introduced into the host having specific antibody of the IgG class, this antibody coats a variable portion of the antigenic determinants on the cell surface. Perhaps due to a number of factors, including a limitation in the amount of antibody, a low density of antigenic determinants on the cell surface, inability of the IgG subclass to fix complement, or to a combination of these factors, few or no complement-fixing doublets of IgG will be produced. Consequently, the reaction of the target cell with enhancing antibody fails to trigger complement-dependent reactions (such as adherence to macrophages, chemotaxis, enhanced phagocytosis, immune adherence, and immune cytobiosis), and there is continued presence and duplication of the target tumor cell. If the proper amount of enhancing antibody still persists at the time the host begins to produce sensitized lymphoid cells, tumor cell cytolysis by the lymphoid cells will be blocked. A flaw in this theory is that cytotoxic and enhancing antibodies appear to be distinct from each other.

The theory of central blockade states that blocking antibodies regulate or inhibit either the production of antibodies that contribute to graft rejection or the number, motility, and efficacy of sensitized lymphocytes that may react specifically to target cell antigens and effect their destruction (45, 104, 127, 153, 211, 212, 217). The block is presumed to be at the level of the effector cell, most likely within the confines of the lymphoid centers, such as the lymph nodes and the spleen. A central effect of antiserum is indicated in experiments where BP_8 tumor cells syngeneic to C_3H mice were incubated with anti-BP_8 serum produced in $C_{57}B1$ mice (the excess serum washed) and then incubated with $C_{57}B1$ lymphoid cells from mice sensitized against BP_8 tumor. Enhancement of tumor growth was observed when these lymphoid cells were admixed with BP_8 cells and injected into $C_{57}B1$ mice (4). Incubation of BP_8 cells with serum from normal $C_{57}B1$ mice in the above experiment resulted in a lack of enhancement. In another study (suggesting either afferent or central inhibition), two groups of mice were sensitized to a tumor allograft and the second group, in addition, received enhancing serum at tumor inoculation (a third group was untreated). Grafts of mixtures of tumor cells with lymphocytes from the first group (into unsensitized syngeneic mice) were inhibited in growth, whereas grafts of tumor cells mixed with lymphocytes from the serum-treated second group grew at rates equalling those of grafts derived from mixtures of lymphocytes derived from normal animals (212).

Brief exposure to mixtures of antigen and antibody tend to produce a significant reduction in the capacity of mouse spleen cells to respond to antigenic challenge (69). The kinetics of such immune suppression *in vitro* to polymerized flagellin of *Salmonella adelaide* follows an exponential time course and closely parallels the kinetics of immune tolerance induced *in vitro* (58). A significant reduction of immune capacity was found to occur within 15 minutes of exposure of cells to antigen and antibody, while marked suppression required treatment for 4 to 6 hours, thereby suggesting that the immune suppression is due to a specific process of interaction of antigen and antibody (with the relevant cells) rather than a mere physical carry-over of antibody which could neutralize subsequently added antigen. In addition, further direct proof of the existence of the central effect was obtained by testing the splenic content of immunocompetent cells of mice injected with antigen and antibody, which then exhibited a significant reduction in the number of immunocompetent cells reactive to the polymerized flagellin.

The most cogent argument for central blockade may come from investigations that have demonstrated that IgG_2 in mice effects immunological enhancement of tumor inocula, a property that is lacking in IgG_1 and IgM (20, 21). In addition, passive transfer of IgG_2 (into mice receiving tumor cell grafts) inhibited the lymphocytosis in the circulation that usually accompanies the immune response to the tumor. Neither IgM nor IgG_1 was capable of abolishing the lymphocytosis in inoculated recipients. This suggests that IgG_2 inhibited these cells from synthesized IgG_2, thereby permitting tumor enhancement, although direct data demonstrating IgG_2 feedback inhibition of production of IgG_2 were provided in these experiments. However, this proposal is attractive and supported by evidence of feedback regulation of production of antibody purported to operate in the immunological centers of immunized animals (153, 182, 211, 212, 217). The production of IgG antibodies can result in the suppression of IgM synthesis in previously uncommitted cells either by direct competition, perhaps through a higher affinity for the receptor or perhaps by induction of tolerance.

In another study, Halliday (87, 88) employed the inhibition of macrophage migration assay to study sarcoma induced in mice with either methylcholanthrene or Moloney sarcoma virus. Sera and peritoneal cells were obtained from mice bearing primary or transplanted tumors (progressor mice) and from mice in which these tumors had spontaneously regressed or had been surgically removed (regressor mice). Peritoneal cells from the two types of tumor-treated animals were distinguishable, as cells from regressor mice exhibited inhibition of migration from sarcoma-soluble antigen, whereas those from the progressor mice did not and mixtures of peritoneal cells from both types of mice were not inhibited in the presence of antigen. In addition, sera from progressor mice blocked the migration inhibition found in the peritoneal cells from the regressor mice. Serum from regressor mice lacked this property and was also unable to unblock peritoneal cells from progressor mice so that the mixture of the latter cells with this serum was inhibited by tumor antigen. Here it appeared likely that a soluble factor was responsible for the suppression observed, since the culture medium from peritoneal cells harvested from tumor-bearing mice could suppress the migration inhibition seen with cells from immune mice while the culture medium from tumor-free or from untreated control mice could not. Furthermore, it was demonstrated that the addition of sera from mice with Moloney sarcomas that had regressed could bestow a specific reactivity upon nonreactive peritoneal cell populations from progressor mice. This might also suggest that sensitized lymphocytes were also present in the tumor-bearing animals, but were prevented from reacting, thereby blocking factors released from other cells within the same population, i.e., the action of the blocking sera was abolished by an "unblocking" effect of regressor sera.

Evidence against the central theory of enhancement is provided in studies showing that serum from progressor mice with Maloney sarcomas was found to abrogate the inhibitory effect on lymph node cells from regressor mice in the presence of tumor cells (93, 98). The serum appeared to affect the target cells rather than the lymph node cells, since incubation with tumor cells with serum abrogated the destruction by immune lymph node cells while incubation with lymph node cells did not. Washing the target cells following inoculation with serum removed part of the protective effect (201, 202).

However, all the above studies seem to give support to the notion that blocking factors may also be immune complexes, already demonstrated to be capable of acting directly on lymphocytes, as the blocking effect on lymphocytes is often transient and quickly lost in the absence of blocking factor (201). This is supported by the finding that in addition to the antibody component, blocking factors also contain antigen (202). The blocking effect is apparently reversible, since it has been shown in autochthonous systems that peripheral lymphocytes from patients, when washed, can exhibit cytotoxicity to target tumor cells in vitro (204). This blocking factor can be absorbed specifically from serum by tumor cells, indicating that a free antibody site is present in the complex. The factor appears to direct its specificity at the lymphoid cell rather than the target cell in the system, indicating probable free antigen ligand in the complex. Kantiainen and Mitchison (130) have demonstrated that activated thymus cells can take up detectable amounts of antigen and antigen-antibody complexes. Complexes obtained by immunization using antigen admixed with adjuvant can be activated by trypsinizing spleen cells. These studies also reveal that trypsinization of T and B cell populations results in detectable amounts of complexes on T cells and attention is focused on the ligand as a source of free antigen in the complex and a possible source of specificity in blocking. Also focused on are mechanisms whereby specific lymphocyte recognition can be "defused," masked, deviated, or otherwise prevented from being triggered toward cytotoxic activity.

Evidence supporting the idea of immune complexes as blocking factors is also provided by Sjögren and co-workers (201, 202). It was shown that sera from mice with either methylcholanthrene or Moloney-virus-induced sarcomas can be separated into two components by ultrafiltration at pH 3.1, one with a molecular weight greater than 100,000 and another with a molecular weight between 10,000 and 100,000. Neither component alone can exhibit the blocking effect, which can be demonstrated when the two components are mixed. The smaller component can block by itself only when it is added to the lymphocytes rather than target cells, whereas the larger component (which contains antibodies) cannot effect blocking when added to either target cells or lymphocytes. This evidence argues against seeing the blocking in these experiments as being caused by a simple blindfolding mechanism under conditions where the amounts of antibody are right for efficient covering of the target cell antigens.

Findings analogous to those obtained with tumor-specific immunity have been reported from investigations dealing with enhancements of tumor allografts. Incubation of target cells with antibodies to their H-2 antigens was found to release a factor that could make lymphocytes non-reactive when added to them. This factor, called "immunosuppressive substance" by Amos (4), may have been a complex of enhancing antibodies and released or shed H-2 antigens or some other molecule with an immunosuppressive effect formed by the tumor cells, the lymphocytes, or both. Free antibodies, when added to lymphoid cells which were then washed and added to the tumor cells, did not give enhanced tumor growth—again, casting doubt on the afferent theory of enhancement.

In another study by Cohen and co-workers (48), a fraction was isolated from a mixture of alloantiserum and ascitic fluid that was capable of blocking cell-mediated cytotoxicity and of enhancing sarcoma I tumor allografts in $B_{10}D_2$ mice. Initially, this fraction had little precipitable IgG and no detectable H-2 antigen, but on further purification, the fraction disassociated into an IgG component and a smaller molecule analogous to an H-2 fragment of the Class I type, thereby suggesting that the purified material was an H-2-IgG immune complex, which accounted for its effects. When effector lymphocytes were pretreated with this fraction, their cytotoxic capacity was considerably diminished.

Still other evidence that antigen-antibody complexes are blocking factors was provided by Baldwin (12), who showed that when a tumor antigen and its specific antibody are mixed, the mixture alone (and not antigen or antibody alone) exhibits blocking activity, although the antigen can in some cases effect blocking of lymphocyte-mediated cytotoxicity. However, there is additional evidence that although the blocking effect can sometimes be mediated by free antigen, the effect may not have immunological specificity. Studies have shown that three out of four bursectomized progressor quails had blocking activity (89). The blocking effect of sera from these progressors could not be removed with Rous sarcoma cells and was detectable only when the sera was allowed to interact with effector cells. The fact that bursectomized animals cannot express antibody production suggests that antigen-ligand was shed *in vivo*, thereby resulting in deviation of the effective response and/or in reticuloendothelial blockage, although their T cell function remains unaffected. This system may be analogous to that studied by Diener and Feldman (69) and Jose and Seshadri (122), who worked with a system in which B cells were made nonreactive to salmonella antigen, and addition of antibodies increased the immunosuppressive effect of free antigen.

Thus, one can postulate that the action of blocking factors is perpetrated on lymphocytes, by blocking their receptor sites with antigen, and that the antibody part of the antigen-antibody complex acts by carrying the antigen to the lymphocyte as well as by cross-linking it to the lymphocyte receptor site. This antibody may be needed particularly when the amount of free antigen is relatively small. A simple explanation of unblocking would then be that it is mediated by antibody that binds to the antigenic sites of blocking complexes, as well as to antigen molecules, in such a way that there is no longer any free antigen to interact with the lymphocytes and block their cytotoxic activity. Yet, under certain conditions, an efferent blockage may be made possible by the unblocking serum, and one can envision that unblocking serum could also blindfold target antigens. If the assumption that blocking factors are antigen-antibody complexes is correct, it follows that the release or shedding of the antigen-containing ligand from a growing tumor could be of fundamental importance in that it has escaped immunologic surveillance. It may be hypothesized that one way in which tumors can become independent of immune surveillance may be by the appearance of all varients with great abilities to shed antigen ligands (105). Such antigen could then stimulate immunologically competent cells to form antibody component, which, in the presence of continued release of antigen ligand during tumor cell growth, could form immune-blocking complexes. Furthermore, the antigen might be capable of abrogating lymphocyte cytotoxicity even in the absence of antibody, if the amount of free antigen is sufficient. The role of immune complexes in enhancement is further suggested by the presence of these aggregates on glomerular membranes of tumor-bearing animals and man.

Blocking Factors

Even when an antibody acts alone to mediate blocking, it is probable that shedding of membrane antigens from the cell surface occurs and rapid formation of immune complexes takes place on the tumor cell surface or in close proximity to the target cell itself (see Fig. 1). This is evidenced by the finding that tumor cells exposed to autologous sera have a tendency to shed antigens, which, in the presence of excess antibody, formed complexes. The significance of blocking serum factors is substantiated by the demonstration of accelerated tumor growth in recipients of globulins eluted from target tumor cells (13). Splenectomy and/or surgical excision of large tumors have been known to reduce the of blocking factors, which have been similarly affected by immunosuppression, plasmaphoresis, or thoracic duct drainage (72, 108, 109). However, larger doses of antimetabolites employed in immunosuppression have been known to depress cell-mediated immune reactions (109). "Autoenhancement" has been employed to cover the initial survival of allografts in a recipient, a process facilitated by injection of blocking serum until the established allograft immunizes the recipient into production of blocking factors (65). In addition, tumor cells themselves are capable of producing globulin-like substances that may conceal surface antigens (44). Furthermore, tumor cells may produce lysozomal enzymes that may degrade the reactive cytotoxic antibodies and render them incapable of activating complement, but may remain complexed with antigens which can negate lymphocyte-mediated cytotoxicity (55). Figure 1 provides a hypothetical scheme of events with regard to enhancement.

Miscellaneous Mechanisms of Tumor Enhancement

Several hypotheses have advocated either a physiological, antigenic, or metabolic alteration in the character of the primary neoplasm, to the extent that the host does not respond in the same fashion that it would to an unaltered tumor. Kaliss (125) initially interpreted enhancement as being due to some physiological alteration in the tumor, induced by its contact with antiserum, which insures its survival despite the hostile response of the host. This interpretation was based on the demonstration that originally the strain-specific tumors acquired the ability to grow in untreated, incompatible hosts after one passage in an antiserum-treated foreign host. Kaliss explained his theory in terms of experiments in which the first graft is accepted and the second is rejected in an accelerated fashion. He postulated that the first graft had time to undergo "pre-enhancement" change before the rejection reaction of the host had reached full potency, and that the second inoculum was rapidly destroyed by the already-heightened resistance of the host, before the graft had time to go through the initial phase of enhancement. These studies have been confirmed by several investigations (166, 167), but the changes were expressed long after enhancement had already been observed. Gorer (83) has suggested that antiserum may actually result in stimulation of tumor cell mitosis. There have been isolated examples of growth stimulation by antibody (6), but most data do not confirm this hypothesis.

Several reports establish that antigenic composition of cell surfaces may fluctuate (139, 189). This is particularly true for mouse lymphocytes, in which cell-membrane antigens such as TL, Ly, and even H-2 may increase or decrease under certain environmental conditions or may be modulated by antibody. Antigenic modulation (the loss of TL antigens from TL+ cells exposed to TL antibody in the absence of lytic complement) has been demonstrated in vitro. H-2 and TL isoantigens of the mouse are specified by the closely linked genetic loci H-2 and TLa. The phenotypic expression of TL antigens was found to reduce the demonstrable amount of certain H-2 antigens to as little as 34% of the quantity demonstrated on TL thymocytes (29, 175). An antigenic modulation (change of TL phenotype from TL+ to TL− produced by TL antibody) is known to entail a compensatory increase in H-2 (D) antigen.

A mutative metabolic change in enhanced tumor grafts has been suggested by Hutchin et al. (116) and Amos et al. (5). Changes in cytoplasmic organelles of the mouse ascites sarcoma BP_8 (C_3H tumor) were studied histochemically during enhanced growth in $C_{57}B1$ mice. Increased amounts of oxidative enzymes (succinic dehydrogenase and glucose-6-phosphate dehydrogenase) and decreased amounts of lysozymal acid phosphatase were demonstrated regularly in tumor cells in the enhanced $C_{57}B1$ mice. But these investigators did not demonstrate any relationship between the metabolic disturbances and immunological enhancement, nor did they rule out the possibility that the enzymatic alterations within tumor cells reacting with antibody might have occurred from injury with nonimmunological agents. However, as a group, the hypotheses suggesting that antiserum acts by changing tumor cell characteristics are rendered unlikely by several findings. Of particular relevance in this respect is the demonstration that enhancement depends upon the specificity of the antiserum employed. Strong enhancement is observed only when all H-2 antigens on the tumor cells (which are foreign to the recipients) are coated with antibodies and the degree of enhancement increases with the number of uncoated H-2 isoantigens (167). Thus, one particular antiserum directed against the genotype of one tumor may completely fail to induce enhancement in one particular host because it does not react against all tumor antigens foreign to the recipients, but the same antiserum may be fully active in another host. Since the same antibodies react with the same tumor cells in both cases, but can induce enhancement only in one particular host, it is unlikely that antibodies act by changing the tumor cell properties.

One escape mechanism from immunological control is apparent from the evidence that certain molecules, such as sialomucin, often bound to the surfaces of tumor cells, are able to block the tumor antigens from being fully exposed in vivo, and are able to repel sensitized lymphocytes (196, 225). Tumor cells have been reported to have a lower mutual adhesiveness than normal cells and often an increased negative charge (51). Although less adhesive to other cells, tumor cells are said to show more nonspecific stickiness, with a tendency to cling to foreign substances (52). Neuraminidase enzyme extracted from Vilirio cholera removes sialic acid groups from the cancer cell membrane—a procedure which may more readily expose the antigens and thereby facilitate immune recognition. It is not known how significant this masking of tumor antigens is in vivo, for the tumors usually escape immunological control. The fact that host reactivity to tumor antigen in vitro correlates well with tumor growth in vivo, and that an immunotherapeutic event can be seen in at least some systems, indicates that masking cannot be absolute.

Potentiating and Arming Effect of Sera

There has been ample evidence that in vitro killing of neoplastic target cells can occur in the presence of nonsensitized lymphoid cells and heat complement inactivated sera either from mice which bear the respective tumors or from mice in which the tumors have been removed (186). This phenomenon has been observed in both autochthonous and transplanted tumors. In these studies, target cell death was dependent on the simultaneous presence of both nonsensitized lymphoid cells and heat-inactivated sera, as neither nonsensitized lymphocyte cells nor sera alone could mediate such an effect. This finding seems to be analogous to that of Moller (166), who observed that cytotoxicity to a murine sarcoma line was observed in the presence of normal allogeneic or semi-syngeneic lymph node cells and rabbit antimouse serum. It has also been observed that human polyploid Chang liver cells undergo cytolysis in the presence of anti-Chang antiserum and nonsensitized allogeneic or xenogeneic lymphoid cells (101, 155, 180). In addition, sera from certain tumor-bearing patients can increase the cytotoxic effect of reactive lymphocytes or antitumor cells in vitro. This potentiating effect was found to be specific, i.e., sera from one patient with sarcoma potentiated the cytotoxic effect of lymphocytes from another patient with sarcoma or sarcoma cells, but did not influence the cytotoxic effects of lymphocytes from melanoma patients with melanoma target cells.

Pollak (185) has reported a more frequent detection of arming with a smaller dose of serum per mouse, suggesting that there may have been enough blocking factors (immune complexes) in the larger dose to inhibit the passively armed lymphoid cell reactions, and that blocking and arming factors may be present in different concentrations in the sera (94). The arming factor could be an antigen-antibody complex (in antibody excess situations) which may link the antigen-sensitive lymphocyte to tumor-specific antigens at the target cell. The arming factor could also be antibody, which would bind to the Fc receptor on the lymphocytes (93, 98), while the Fab end of the molecule would bind to the target cell antigen. Either mechanism could initiate cytotoxic activity, but there is evidence that antigen-antibody complexes, in different ratios than those of blocking complexes, and not antibodies alone, are required to induce cytotoxic activity in human lymphocytes (178).

An arming activity has also been observed with sera from bursectomized quails, indicating that it was not bursa-dependent (89). Some of the arming sera studied could potentiate the cytotoxic effect of regressor spleen cells (observed with both bursectomized and nonbursectomized quail), and could have been due either to bursa-nondependent IgM antibodies, or bursa independence at low antibody concentration. It is alternately possible that bursectomy may have only depressed and not totally inhibited antibody levels (141). It is worth noting that in most of these experiments, the lymphoid population used contained other cells besides lymphocytes—namely, macrophages. Although small lymphocytes have been implicated as the effector cells (20), it has also been reported that the synergistic cytotosic reaction proceeds more rapidly in the presence of mixed lymphoid cell populations (180). Among the possible types of interactions between the immune sera and different types of nonsensitized lymphoid cells which could cause target cell death are arming of macrophages by cytophilic antibody (181), opsonizing of target cells (34), arming of lymphocytes (59, 61), and destruction of target cells by cytolytic antibodies in the presence of complement produced by lymphoid cells (214).

In conclusion, the molecules responsible for this potentiating effect remain to be delineated, as do the cells associated with the reaction. The potentiating molecules may be antigen-antibody complexes present during antibody excess; perhaps they are just antibodies and the cells upon which they act are non-T lymphocytes, but the evidence is unclear. One possibility is that the potentiating serum factors are "unblocking factors," which may decrease the blocking effect of tumor antigen-antibody complexes and/or antigen which may be present with the lymphocyte suspensions tested, which then may free from restraint the cytotoxic potential of the patient's lymphocytes. It is also possible that the factors may act by arming reactive lymphoid cell populations in a way similar to that seen when nonimmune lymphocytes are studied. The combination of such an arming effect and the cytotoxic activity of immune lymphocytes (detected in the absence of serum) may, in a synergistic way, produce a high cytotoxicity even when the arming activity by itself is low.

Unblocking Antibodies

Circulating lymphocytes of rats carrying progressively growing polyoma tumors are especially cytotoxic to polyoma cells in vitro (98, 102). The sera from these rats have been observed to block this lymphocyte cytotoxicity, an effect mediated most likely by tumor-specific antigen-antibody complexes (104, 201). Inoculation of blocking sera into rats has previously been shown to facilitate tumor growth (13), but an unblocking effect can be produced following immunization with tumor cells in those rats that had been previously inoculated with live BCG (14, 15). These antibodies can counteract the effect of specific blocking sera and tumor eluate in vitro. An unblocking effect has also been demonstrated in the sera from mice with Moloney sarcomas that have regressed. They not only lack blocking activity, but also cancel the blocking effect of sera from syngeneic mice with the same growing Moloney sarcoma tumors (94). This serum effect has been demonstrated as unblocking (or deblocking), and the factors associated with the effect have the same specificity as the blocking activity and cell-mediated immunity. The phenomenon has also been observed in a few patients who were cured of neoplastic disease (103).

The mechanisms associated with the therapeutic unblocking effect remain to be clarified. It could be that the inhibitory effect on tumor growth was due to complement-dependent antibodies, as "unblocking sera" have been demonstrated to be cytotoxic in the presence of rat complement (14). However, such a mechanism is difficult to reconcile with the fact that the tumors in these animals grew as rapidly as in the controls and exhibited only slight inhibition for two weeks, after which they started regressing rapidly (15). A more likely mechanism is that the inoculated antiserum had an unblocking effect in vivo (either by means of neutralizing the activity of blocking antibodies, or of antigen-antibody complexes), when they were produced, or perhaps the antibody prevented their formation by masking the antigenic determinants on the tumor cells, or caused feedback inhibition (217). The result of this "deblocking" would be that the tumor commences regressing as soon as the host begins to confer an effective cell-mediated immune response. The effect could also be due to a competition between the unblocking and blocking antibodies on the surface of the target tumor cells. However, in view of the finding that blocking activity is mediated by antigen-antibody complexes, one might anticipate that an interaction between the antibodies and the antigen part of the blocking complex could take place, which may result in the abolishment of blocking activity if a reaction between the antigen part of the complex and the immune lymphocyte is essential to the blocking phenomenon. Other possible mechanisms may lie within the macrophage effect, where arming by cytophilic antibodies could account for this type of effect (172), or it may be opsonizing antibodies that render the target cell easily ingestible (51). This effect may be also an arming-type effect on previously unsensitized lymphocytes by some immunoglobulin molecules (Igx) (60), or by perhaps other repressors of tumor growth, such as interferon.

Unblocking and Potentiating Serum Factors

Thus, the complexity of tumor cell destruction by serum factors and effector cells (macrophages and lymphocytes) has been well defined. Allografts of this mouse plasmacytoma in rats resulted in immune reactions against these tumors in mice: (a) direct killing of tumor cells by immune lymphocytes; (b) killing of tumor cells by either normal or immune lymphocytes mediated by either IgG or IgM immune globulins; (c) phagocytosis of tumor cells augmented by either IgG or IgM immune globulins; and (d) tumor cell lysis by IgM antibodies and complement.

The mechanism of action of this tumor-specific lymph node cell-arming serum factor has not been determined, although the factor could be cytophilic antibody and macrophage or the Fc receptor-bearing lymphoid cell. The arming factor could thus attach to antigens on the tumor cell surface by its Fab fragments and to the lymphocyte by its activated Fc fragment. The arming factor could also be a cytophilic antibody with the lymphocyte providing complement to mediated cytolysis.

T Cells in Enhancement

In some systems, antigen-specific T lymphocytes have been termed true regulators of the immune response (132), as they have the ability to augment or to suppress the induction and expression of immunity (30, 79, 132). The function of T cells in the mediation of immunity can often be replaced by their humoral products (67, 79, 173), suggesting that the suppressor T cells (or suppressive effects of T cells) may be mediated by humoral products or by factors from other cells that were stimulated by the T cells (200). The immunotherapeutic approach to the cancer problem has been seriously challenged by the observation that tumor allografts may grow better in animals which have been actively or passively immunized against these tumors (127). Although tumor enhancement has been generally accepted as a phenomenon dependent on the serum (4), it has also been obtained by adoptive transfer of lymphoid cells both under syngeneic (188) and allogeneic conditions (117). It has been shown that lymph node cells sensitized against allogeneic tumors could either antagonize or promote tumor growth, depending on the time interval between sensitization and lymphocyte transfer. These studies have revealed that there is a difference between the behavior of early and late lymphocytes removed from the immunized host. The terms early and late refer to the time elapsed between the inoculation of tumor and removal of the lymph node cells, and this varies from days to weeks, depending on the tumor system employed. Generally speaking, lymphocytes removed (and tested) within days following tumor inoculation destroy target tumor cells and inhibit progressive tumor growth in vivo (25, 118), whereas lymphocytes removed much later seem to help promote tumor growth, or are inactive. The ratio between tumor and lymphoid cells also appears to be critical—while a high lymphoid cells/tumor cells ratio led to protection, a low ratio resulted in enhancement (188). Thus, there remains increasing evidence for the direct involvement of T cells in the suppression of cell-mediated immune responses (79, 85). Lymphoid cells from the thymus or bone marrow, when adoptively transferred and administered in a mixture with tumor cells to previously unsensitized syngeneic hosts, revealed that the enhancing phenomenon was present only in the cells of the thymic origin (218). This conclusion is also supported by the finding that neonatally thymectomized mice often have a higher resistance to induction of tumor by murine mammary virus than their control siblings (107), and this procedure can also lead to decreased rates of tumor growth (157). Furthermore, the inoculation of syngeneic thymocytes depressed the graft-vs.-host reaction of parental thymocyte in irradiated F_1 recipients, as well as the ability of primed T cells to kill tumors in irradiated hosts. The characterization of T cell populations endowed with enhancing properties requires additional investigation.

Tolerance

The classic concepts of transplantation immunity are based on the development of immunological homeostasis in fetal and neonatal life, which assures the distinction between self and nonself. If an antigen or infectious agent enters the fetus, it may be accepted as self which then becomes tolerant or poorly responsive to such substances as oncogeneic viruses and which may thus reflect the properties of the substance (194, 222), perhaps in the presence of immune complexes occurring as a result of antibody responses. Tolerant mice are capable of allowing for replication and shedding of lymphocytic choriomeningitis virus during their entire life span without exhibiting clinical illness, which can be present in nontolerant mice—an effect that can be abrogated with thymectomy (142). These findings have been reproduced, with a reasonable facsimile, in oncogenic virus systems, where immune complexes were also observed (176) (although the tolerance was modified and may have reflected an immunological tardiness and lack of coordination of the immune faculties). Several investigations furnish support for these views, as well as for the weaknesses in the hypotheses, and even for the concept of split tolerance, i.e., inhibition of cell-mediated, but not humoral, immunity. Tolerance differs from immune deficiency or immune suppression by its antigen specificity. Tolerance of the B lymphocyte induced by a hapten on a nonimmunogenic carrier often consists of the elimination of the antigen-reactive B cell clone, whereas tolerance mediated by T cells involves an active proliferation of a clone of cells that can transfer the state of tolerance to normal recipients. These cells die on exposure to radioactively labeled antigen, a phenomenon referred to as antigen suicide.

Macrophages in Tumor Rejection

There is increasing evidence concerning the role of macrophages as effector cells of tumor immunity, based on the presence of macrophages at the site of tumor rejection (80), as well as in vitro killing of syngeneic tumor cells by macrophages (62, 231). Macrophages from lymphoma-immune mice have been demonstrated to prevent in vitro replication of lymphoma cells; incubation of normal macrophages with product released from immune lymphocytes conferred the ability to kill lymphoma cells to macrophages. The decreased ability of immune spleen cells to neutralize tumor cells in newborn mice or in preirradiated adult recipients supports the contention that there is cell cooperation at the effector level of tumor immunity (231). Transplantation of normal bone marrow in irradiated animals restored the function needed for elicitation of tumor cell neutralization by immune lymphocytes, which confirms the studies showing the need for marrow-derived cells for the manifestation of delayed hypersensitivity reactions (216). It has also been confirmed that the macrophage is a bone marrow-derived cell necessary for the manifestation of the delayed-type response elicited by immune lymphocytes and antigen in irradiated hosts (223).

The macrophage may have the same function in tumor immunity, as in the manifestation of the delayed hypersensitivity response. It has been shown that the lymphocytes from peritoneal exudates from immune animals are more effective than macrophages in the specific initiation of tumor rejection (233), but the final steps can be nonspecific, as unrelated tumor cells were killed at the site of rejection of sensitizing tumor cell grafts in the recipients (232). Evidence for the role of macrophages in this system (the final tumor cell killing) is supported by the finding that it was possible to prevent the development of tumors by local inoculation of a preparation containing Migration Inhibition Factor activity (19). Normal macrophages can be converted to killer cells by prior incubation with immune lymphocytes or with soluble products released from immune lymphocytes. In addition, tumor cell neutralization by immune lymphoid cells can be negated in mice following their treatment with silica which tied up and destroyed macrophages (62, 231).

Thymic Deficiency

Artificial neonatal thymectomy in experimental animals results in immune deficiency disease, with an increased incidence of spontaneous neoplasia and decreased resistance to transplanted, virus-induced and chemically induced tumors (143, 152, 160). An exception is in the incidence of thymus-dependent AKR lymphoma, which is reduced following this procedure (226), although the B lymphocyte responses are unaffected. Restoration of immune competence in these mice (with thymic tissue, cells, or extracts) prevents the polyoma virus-induced oncogenesis. Thymosin, a humoral thymic factor, has been shown to restore immunologic competence. The effects of thymectomy in adult animals have not been fully assessed (7). The short-lived lymphocyte population in the healthy host appears to be highly dependent on the intact thymic function, and thus, the precursor lymphocytes that develop into cytotoxic cells become depleted, whereas those lymphocytes that react with proliferator in the mixed lymphocyte culture are spared.

Antithymocyte Serum

Rabbit antimouse thymocyte serum administered to mice simulates surgical thymectomy, although the rates of oncogenesis have varied depending on the tumor system employed (2, 111, 124, 140). The results—using antilymphocyte serum, which blocks both humoral and cell-mediated immune responses—are conclusive only in promoting increased replication of oncornaviruses (110). The unexpected effect of thymectomy on the depression of virally induced mammary tumors has been well-established (208). Treatment of these virally infected mice with antilymphocyte also inhibited mammary carcinogenesis and these animals established antiviral antibodies. In these instances, the mammary tumor virus-carrier mice may be tolerant to the virus-associated cell surface antigens, but not to mature virions; the former may elicit only cell-mediated immune reactions, whereas the virion antigens evoke antibody responses. The virus is incorporated into the host cells and the surface antigens of the virus genome-carrier cells may be accepted as self, and immunosuppression with antilymphocyte serum may subsequently result in virus activation.

Although neonatal thymectomy is effective in the augmentation of growth of most virally, but not chemically, induced tumors, treatment with antilymphocyte serum effected accelerated growth of chemically induced tumors (3, 40) and increased metastasis was observed.

Suppressor Cells

The cooperation (synergism and antagonism) between immunocompetent cells is extremely complicated. Generally speaking, in responses against thymus-dependent antigen, helper activity of T lymphocytes is essential for antibody production by B cells. A response to these antigens in the absence of T cells is ineffective. Thus, binding of the antigen by its carrier determinant to a T cell and by its inducing determinant to a B cell may provide a bridge whereby these cells can be brought in close proximity (165). Recent evidence also indicates that helper T cells proliferating in response to antigen release soluble mediators that render B cells responsive to antigen (68, 198). Also, T cell receptor and antigen complexes may be presented to macrophages, which would then determine whether to augment or suppress the antibody response to these antigens by B cells (66). In addition to this helper function, B cell unresponsiveness has been found to be T cell-dependent (224). Suppressor effects of T cell subpopulations have been repeatedly demonstrated in antigenic competition, tolerance, graft-vs.-host disease, skin sensitivity, and reactions to thymus-independent antigens (85, 211, 212), and these effects can be transferred from tolerant mice to normal mice in order to induce tolerance (9, 161). These suppressor cells appear to be short-lived, rapidly proliferating T cells which can be affected preferentially by cyclophosphamide (184, 187) or splenectomy (138).

The suppression of immune T cell activity by B lymphocytes or their products has been well-authenticated and the cells have been found to be of intermediate size, between T cells and B cells (82). These suppressor cells carry immunoglobulin moeities on their cell surfaces, and the suppressive effects are not immunologically specific, that is, suppressor effects against one sensitized antigen can be concomitant with effects against other antigens without requiring previous sensitization towards the latter antigens. These effects can be abrogated by splenectomy, BCG vaccination, and administration of cyclophosphamide (138).

T cells can exist in several subclasses, with two types being identified in mice (24). T_1 cells are abundantly present, sessile, and relatively insensitive to antilymphocyte serum; whereas T_2 cells form a minority of thymocytes, abound in lymph nodes, but circulate and are very sensitive to antilymphocyte serum. T_1 cells decrease shortly and substantially following thymectomy, and T-dependent areas become depleted in the spleen but not in the lymph nodes. The cortical thymic cells are also sensitive to corticosteroids, whereas the minority medullary B cells are not. Paradoxically, large doses of medullary cells are responsible for graft-vs.-host disease in suitable recipients, whereas in smaller doses there is inhibition of graft-vs.-host disease, brought about by parental lymph node cell grafts in F_1 hybrids. The cortical cells cannot by themselves cause graft-vs.-host disease, and serve as good examples of cell populations involved in synergium acd antagonism occurring in the T cell compartments (24).

Suppressor T lymphocytes separated from thymuses of tumor-bearing mice have been known to enhance tumor growth in recently inoculated mice with tumor cells of the same type (218). Enhancement was evidenced by a higher number of takes, early appearance of tumors, and increased metastasis. Bone marrow-derived cells, when administered to these animals, had an antitumor effect, whereas adult thymectomy, followed by tumor transplantation, resulted in delayed tumor growth and reduced metastasis. This suggested that depletion of the short-lived thymocyte population coincided with the recovery of antitumor immune reactions in the host.

Tumor rejection mechanisms and tumor-directed reactions by previously sensitized recipients of tumor cells coated with antibody can be switched off, and the sensitized lymphocytes have been observed to function as the suppressor cells (4). Large doses of sensitized T cells have been observed to suppress tumor growth, whereas smaller doses of the same cells administered with small amounts of antitumor antibody against methylcholanthrene-induced tumors resulted in enhanced tumor growth (133). Hyperimmune antibody, when administered prior to inoculation of L 1210 leukemia cells in DBA/2 mice have been observed to inhibit the development of leukemia-specific, cell-mediated immunity (162). Peritoneal cells from this system were unable to accept cytophilic antibodies and may have been due to loss of specific surface receptors on the macrophages therein. There is also evidence that oncogenic viruses may (directly or indirectly, by means of virion-antibody complexes) activate suppressor cell proliferation (131). Suppressor function of immune responsiveness has been attributed to a special subclass of T lymphocytes that maintain homeostasis by preventing autoimmune reactions. This may be accomplished either by suppressing helper and amplifier T cells, or by suppressing specifically the activity of non-T cells, such as antibody-producing B cells. Therefore, removal of the suppressor effect by the induction of graft-vs.-host disease or chimerism or by adult thymectomy may result in the improvement of host defense against various tumors (193, 215).

Suppressor T cells may mechanize their effect on the tumor-bearing host by the secretion of molecular mediators (77). The targets of regulatory activity of suppressor T cells can be both the T and B lymphocyte cells through specific mediators with well-balanced interaction involving a balance between T-cell-dependent helper and amplifier function, with opposite T-cell-directed suppressor function, whether specifically or nonspecifically.

Coinfection with Viruses

Virus infections in the tumor-bearing host can inhibit the neoplastic process by being directly cytotoxic, as in oncolytic viruses, or by evoking lymphocyte unresponsiveness or suppressor cells. On the other hand, they can facilitate incidence and tumor growth in the presence of extremely subthreshold levels of chemical carcinogens and may act by being a carrier of the chemical to the genetic apparatus of the cell (156). They may also enhance leukenogenesis by providing helper function (209).

Sialic Acid Coat of Tumor Cells

The cell surface sialic acid reflects internal changes within the cell (36), which vary during the G_4 phase and mitosis (increased levels). Transformed cells have been known to produce higher levels of glycopeptides (than do resting cells), thereby accounting for the higher levels of surface sialic acid, which may thus mask antigens and prevent their recognition (75). The increased presence of these factors may also determine the ability of these cells to metastasize (27).

Immune Deficiency

The most important genes controlling viral leukenogenesis in mice are the dominant Fr-2 gene controlling splenic transformation by the Friend virus complex, and the Fr-1 gene, which determines the susceptibility to the Friend helper virus—genes which most likely interact within the H-2 region and which determine the surface virion antigens (146, 147). The Rgv-1 gene of the resistance-Gross virus within the Ir-1 genes regulates the immune response to most oncornaviruses (171). Correlation has been found between the susceptibility to methyl-cholanthrene-induced fibrosarcomas and the hepatic inducibility of aryl-hydrocarbon hydroxylase, in that animals inducible for the enzyme were more susceptible to oncogenesis (136). The autosomal dominant gene has no correlation with viral oncogenesis. Thus, gene products can influence antigenic strength and the immune response to neoplastic cells. Hereditary immunodeficiency, such as thymic aplasia in nude mice, results in an increased susceptibility to oncogenesis (56).

Immunosuppression by Oncogenic Viruses

The presence of immune defects in mice infected with leukemia viruses has been most profound (183). For example, infection with Gross virus in mice resulted in a compromised humoral and cell-mediated immune response to bacteriophage antigens or to skin grafts across weak histocompatibility barriers (53); otherwise, the viruses may depress either the cell-mediated or humoral immune responses (81, 195). Antigenic competition between oncornaviruses and tumor cells (virions) has resulted in augmentation of tumor growth in the hosts which failed to exhibit immune responses towards the virions. In these studies, IgG antibody production was depressed more than IgM, and antigen-reactive cells were affected more than the antibody-producing cells, and there was an increased susceptibility to virus infection (18). However, the mechanism of immunosuppression is not clear, as it has not been resolved whether immunosuppression is essential for oncogenesis (90).

Immunoselection

The quantitative expression of antigen on the tumor cell has been shown to be a major determinant of the host's immune response. Chemically induced tumors (which are highly antigenic) have been found to express an inverse relationship between the amount of tumor associated and histocompatibility antigens (213), whereas decreased amounts of H-2 and increased amounts of tumor antigen were demonstrated on tumor cell surfaces of virally induced tumors (70, 71, 72). Antigenic loss has been observed in passage of tumors and chemical treatment with actinomycin D has been observed to increase expression of H-2 and tumor antigens (46, 174). It appears that low antigenicity of the tumor cell also results in increased ability to metastasize. Another documented escape mechanism has been demonstrated by the ability of tumor cells to excessively produce and release tumor cell ligand-antigens, which can induce immune tolerance in neonatally inoculated mice, and tumor-specific immunity in tumor-bearing mice (8). Spleen cells, but not sera, from mice bearing these tumors were useful in adoptive immunotherapy, an effect that was negated by ascites fluid from these mice.

Failure of Recognition and Response

The production of antitumor antibodies may, through feedback inhibition, prevent the further production of the same antibody. In addition, the tumor cell may decrease the expression or production of target antigen during the policed environment, or else a massive release of antigen may cause immune paralysis in the host or activate suppressor T and B cells. However, a small colony of tumor cells, within the total tumor cell mass, may actually be unable to elicit immune responses in the host or may adapt to the effective primitive surveillance mechanism in the host (16, 74, 135).

Mediators Released by Tumors

Tumor cells have been known to produce biologically active molecular mediators and poorly defined toxic substances. For example, the tumor angiogenesis factor (m.w. 100,000), which is sensitive to protease and ribonuclease, containing protein, carbohydrate, and RNA, has been found in the placenta, but not in normal regenerating tissue (144). Poly IC, a synthetic nucleic acid homopolymer-pair polyriboinosinic acid, may inhibit the RNA component of the angiogenesis factor and effect massive necrosis of tumors (145, 170). Tumor cells may also produce immunosuppressive substances, some of which may be directly toxic to the lymphoid system (158, 170).

REFERENCES

1. Abercrombie, M., and Ambrose, E. J. 1969. The surface properties of cancer cells. A review. *Cancer Res.* 22: 525.
2. Allison, A. C., and Law, L. W. 1968. Effects of antilymphocyte serum on virus oncogenesis. *Proc. Soc. Exp. Biol. Med.* 127: 207.
3. Allison, A. C., and Taylor, R. B. 1967. Observations on thymectomy and carcinogenesis. *Cancer Res.* 27: 703.
4. Amos, D. B., Cohen, I., and Klein, W. J., Jr. 1970. Mechanisms of immunological enhancement. *Transplant. Proc.* 2: 68.
5. Amos, D. B., Prioleau, W. H., and Hutchin, P. 1968. Histochemical changes during growth of C3H ascites tumor BP8 in C57B1 mice. *J. Surg. Res.* 8: 122.
6. Amos, D. B., and Wakefield, J. D. 1959. Growth of mouse ascites tumor cells in diffusion chambers. II. Lysis and growth inhibition by diffusible antibody. *J. Natl. Cancer Inst.* 22: 1077.
7. Anderson, L. C., Hayry, P., and Boch, M. A., et al. 1974. Differences in the effects of adult thymectomy on T cell-mediated responses *in vitro*. *Nature* 252: 252.
8. Andrews, E. J. 1974. Failure of immunosurveillance against chemically induced *in situ* tumors in mice. *J. Natl. Cancer Inst.* 52: 729.
9. Asherson, G. L., Zembala, M., and Barnes, R. M. R. 1971. The mechanism of immunological unresponsiveness to picryl chloride and the possible role of antibody-mediated depression. *Clin. Exp. Immunol.* 9: 109.
10. Axelrod, M. A. 1968. Suppression of delayed hypersensitivity by antigen and antibody. Is a common precursor cell responsible for both delayed hypersensitivity and antibody formation? *Immunology* 15: 159.
11. Baldwin, R. W., Embleton, M. J., Jones, J. S., and Langman, M. J. 1973. Cell-mediated and humoral immune reactions to human tumors. *Int. J. Cancer* 12: 73.
12. Baldwin, R. W., Price, M. R., and Robins, R. A. 1972. Blocking of lymphocyte-mediated cytotoxicity for rat hepatoma cells by tumor-specific antigen-antibody complexes. *Nature* 238: 185.
13. Bansal, S. C., Hargraeves, R., and Sjögren, H. O. 1972. Facilitation of polyoma tumor growth in rats by blocking sera and tumor eluates. *Int. J. Cancer* 9: 97.
14. Bansal, S. C., and Sjögren, H. O. 1971. Unblocking serum activity *in vitro* in the Polyoma system may correlate with antitumor effect of antiserum *in vivo*. *Nature* 233: 76.
15. Bansal, S. C., and Sjögren, H. O. 1973. Regression of Polyoma tumor metastases by combined unblocking and BCG treatment correlation with induced alterations in tumor immunity status. *Int. J. Cancer* 12: 179.
16. Bartlett, G. L. 1972. Effect of host immunity on antigenic strength of primary tumors. *J. Natl. Cancer Inst.* 49: 493.
17. Batchelor, J. R., and Silverman, M. S. 1962. Further studies on interactions between sessile and humoral antibodies in homograft reactions, *in CIBA Foundation Symposium on Transplantation*, p. 216. CIBA, London.

18. Bennett, M., and Steeves, R. A. 1970. Immunocompetent cell function in mice infected with Friend leukemia virus. *J. Natl. Cancer Inst.* 44: 1107.

19. Bernstein, I. D., Thor, D. E., Zbar, B. et al. 1971. Tumor immunity: Suppression in vivo initiated by soluble products of specifically stimulated lymphocytes. *Science* 172: 729.

20. Biberfeld, P., and Perlman, P. 1970. Morphological observations on the cytotoxicity of human blood lymphocytes for antibody-coated chicken erythrocytes. *Exp. Cell Res.* 62: 433.

21. Billingham, R. E., Brent, L., and Medawar, P. B. 1954. Quantitative studies on tissue transplantation immunity. II. The origin, strength, and duration of activity and adoptively acquired immunity. *Proc. Roy. Soc. S. B.* 143: 58.

22. Biozzi, G., Asofsky, R., Liberman, R., et al. 1970. Serum concentrations and allotypes of immunoglobulins in two lines of mice genetically retested for "High" or "Low" antibody synthesis. *J. Exp. Med.* 132: 752.

23. Blair, P., Kripke, M., Lappe, M., Benhag, R., and Young, L. 1971. Immunologic deficiency associated with mammary tumor virus (MTV) infection in mice: Hemeagglutinating response and allograft survival. *J. Immunol.* 106: 364.

24. Blomgren, H., and Jacobsson, H. 1974. Interaction between thymocytes and lymph node cells in the graft-versus-host response: Evidence for a syngeneic and an antagonistic activity mediated by mouse thymocytes. *Cell. Immunol.* 12: 296.

25. Bloom, E. T., and Hildemann, W. H. 1970. Mechanisms of tumor-specific enhancement versus resistance towards a methylcholanthrene-induced murine sarcoma. *Transplantation* 10: 321.

26. Borsos, T., and Rapp, H. 1965. Hemolysin titration based on fixation of the activated first component of complement. Evidence that one molecule of hemolysin suffices to sensitize an erythrocyte. *J. Immunol.* 95: 559.

27. Bosmann, H. B., Bieber, G., Brown, A., et al. 1972. Biochemical parameters correlated with tumor. *Proc. Natl. Acad. Sci. U.S.A.* 69: 485.

28. Boyse, E. A., Old, L. J., and Stockert, E. 1962. Immunological enhancement of a leukemia. *Nature* 194: 1142.

29. Boyse, E., Stockert, E., and Old, L. 1968. Isoantigens of the H2 and Tla loci of the mouse. *J. Exp. Med.* 128: 85.

30. Bretscher, P. 1972. The control of humoral and associative antibody synthesis. *Transplant. Rev.* 11: 217.

31. Broder, S., and Whitehouse, F. 1968. Immunologic enhancement of tumor xenografts by pepsin-degraded immunoglobulin. *Science.* 162: 1494.

32. Brown, R. J. 1971. In vitro desensitization of sensitized murine lymphocytes by a serum factor (soluble antigen?). *Proc. Natl. Acad. Sci. U.S.A.* 68: 1634.

33. Bubenik, J., Jakou-Kova, J., Krakora, P., et al. 1971. Cellular immunity to renal carcinomas in man. *Int. J. Cancer* 8: 503.

34. Bubenik, J., Perlman, P., Helmstein, K., and Marberger, B. 1970. Cellular and humoral immune responses to human bladder carcinomas. *Int. J. Cancer* 5: 310.

35. Bubenik, J., and Turano, A. 1968. Enhancing effect on tumor growth of humoral antibodies against tumor-specific transplantation antigens in tumors induced by murine sarcoma virus (Harvey). *Nature* 220: 928.

36. Buck, C. A., Glick, M. C., and Warren, L. 1971. Glycopeptides from the surface of control and virus-transformed cells. *Science* 172: 169.

37. Casey, A. E. 1941. Experiments with a material from the Brown Pearce tumor. *Cancer Res.* 1: 134.

38. Celada, D. 1968. Cancer and aging, *in* A. Engel and T. Larson (eds.), *Thule International Symposium*, p. 97.

39. Ceppellini, R., Bigliani, S., Curtani, E. S., and Lerghed, G. 1969. Experimental allotransplantation in man. II. The role of A1, A2, and B antigens. III. Enhancement by circulating antibody. *Transplant. Proc.* 1: 39.

40. Cerilli, J., and Hattan, D. 1974. Immunosuppression and oncogenesis. *Amer. J. Clin. Pathol.* 62: 218.

41. Chantler, S. M. 1967. Characteristics of the cellular response in pretreated recipients exhibiting enhanced tumor growth. *Transplantation* 5: 1400.

42. Chantler, S. M., and Batchelor, J. R. 1964. Changes in the host response following treatment with lyophilized tissue. *Transplantation* 2: 75.

43. Chard, T. 1968. Immunological enhancement by mouse isoantibodies. The importance of complement fraction. *Immunology* 14: 583.

44. Charney, J. 1968. Production of self-directed antigens by tumor cells. *Nature* 220: 504.

45. Chutna, V. 1971. The mechanism of immunological enhancement of H-2 incompatible skin grafts in mice. *Transplantation* 12: 28.

46. Cikes, M., and Klein, G. 1972. Effects of inhibitors of protein and nucleic acid synthesis on the expression of H-2 and Moloney leukemia virus-determined cell surface antigens on cultured murine lymphoma cells. *J. Natl. Cancer Inst.* 48: 509.

47. Cohen, I. R., and Wekerle, H. 1973. Regulation of autosensitization. The immune activation and specific inhibition of self-recognizing thymus-derived lymphocytes. *J. Exp. Med.* 137: 224.

48. Cohen, J., Stringer, S., and Lloyd, W. 1974. Abrogation of cell-mediated immunity by hyperimmune alloantiserum: Mechanism and correlation with allograft enhancement. *Int. J. Cancer* 13: 463.

49. Cohen, S. 1968. The requirement for the association of two adjacent rabbit γG molecules in the fraction of complement by immune complexes. *J. Immunol.* 100: 407.

50. Cohen, S., and Milstein, C. 1967. Structure and biological properties of immunoglobulins. *Adv. Immunol.* 7:1.

51. Coman, D. R. 1953. Mechanism responsible for the origin and distribution of blood-borne tumor metastases. A review. *Cancer Res.* 13: 397.

52. Coman, D. R. 1961. Adhesiveness and stickiness. Two independent properties of cell surfaces. *Cancer Res.* 21: 1436.

53. Cremer, N. E., Taylor, D. O. N., and Hagens, S. J. 1966. Antibody formation, latency and leukemia; infection with Moloney virus. *J. Immunol.* 96: 495.

54. Cruse, J. M., Germany, W. W., and Dulaney, A. D. 1965. Effects of immune serum and spleen cells on C3Hf/He tumor graft survival in Tennessee Swiss mice. *Lab. Invest.* 14: 1554.

55. Dauphinee, M. J., Talal, N., and Witz, I. P. 1974. Generation of noncom-

plement fixing, blocking factors by lysozomal extract treatment of cytotoxic antitumor antibodies. *J. Immunol.* 113: 948.

56. Dent, P. B. 1972. Immunodepression by oncogenic viruses. *Progr. Med. Virol.* 14: 1.

57. Diehl, V., Jereb, B., Stjernsword, J., et al. 1971. Cellular immunity to nephroblastoma. *Int. J. Cancer* 7: 277.

58. Diener, E., and Armstrong, W. P. 1967. Induction of antibody formation and tolerance in vitro to a purified protein antigen. *Lancet* 2: 1281.

59 Dupuy, J. M., and Good, R. A. 1970. Passive transfer of delayed hypersensitivity in guinea pigs: Role of conventional antibody and antigen. *J. Immunol.* 106: 528.

60. Dupuy, J. M., Perey, D. Y., and Good, R. A. 1969. Passive transfer with plasma of delayed allergy in guinea pigs. *Lancet* 1: 551.

61. Dupuy, J. M., Perez, D. Y., and Good, R. A. 1970. Transfer of skin homograft immunity with a plasma factor. *J. Immunol.* 104: 1523.

62. Evans, R., and Alexander, P. 1972. Mechanisms of immunologically specific killing of tumor cells by macrophages. *Nature* 236: 167.

63. Fass, L., Herbermann, R. B., and Ziegler, J. L. 1970. Cutaneous hypersensitivity reactions to autologous extracts of malignant melanoma cells. *Lancet* 1: 116.

64. Fass, L., Herbermann, R. B., and Ziegler, J. L. 1970. Delayed cutaneous hypersensitivity reactions to autologous extracts of Burkitt's lymphoma cells. *N.E.J.M.* 28: 776.

65. Feldman, J. D. 1972. Immunological enhancement. A study of blocking antibodies. *Adv. Immunol.* 15: 167.

66. Feldman, M. 1973. Induction of B cell tolerance by antigen-specific T cell factor. *Nature* 242: 84.

67. Feldman, M. 1974. T cell suppression in vitro. II. Nature of specific suppressive factor. *Eur. J. Immunol.* 4: 667.

68. Feldman, M., and Basten, A. 1972. Specific collaboration between T and B lymphocytes across a cell-impermeable membrane in vitro. *Nature* 237: 13.

69. Feldman, M., and Diener, E. 1970. Antibody-mediated suppression of the immune response in vitro. I. Evidence for a control effect. *J. Exp. Med.* 131: 247.

70. Fenyo, E. M., Klein, E., and Klein, G. 1968. Selection of an immunoresistant Moloney lymphoma subline with decreased concentration of tumor-specific surface antigens. *J. Natl. Cancer Inst.* 40: 69.

71. Ferrer, J. F., and Gibbs, F. A., Jr. 1969. Concomitant loss of specific cell surface antigen and demonstrable type C virus particles in lymphomas induced by radiation leukemia virus. *J. Natl. Cancer Inst.* 43: 1317.

72. Ferrer, J. F., and Mihich, E. 1968. Effect of splenectomy on the regression of transplantable tumors. *Cancer Res.* 28: 1116.

73. Ferrer, J. F., and Mihich, E. 1968. Prevention of therapeutically induced regression of sarcoma 180 by immunologic enhancement. *Cancer Res.* 28: 245.

74. Folkman, J. 1972. Anti-angiogenesis: New concept for therapy of solid tumors. *Ann. Surg.* 175: 409.

75. Fox, T. O., Sheppard, J. R., and Burger, M. M. 1971. Cyclic membrane

charges in animal cells: Transformed cells permanently display a surface architecture detected in normal cells only during mitosis. *Proc. Natl. Acad. Sci. U.S.A.* 68: 244.

76. Fridman, W. H., and Kourilsky, F. M. 1969. Stimulation of lymphocytes by autologous leukaemic cells in acute leukaemia. *Nature* 224: 277.

77. Fujimoto, S., Greene, M., and Sehon, A. H. 1975. Immunosuppressor T cells in tumor-bearing hosts. *Immunol. Commun.* 4: 201.

78. Galti, R. A., and Good, R. A. 1971. Occurrence of malignancy in immunodeficiency diseases. *Cancer* 28: 89.

79. Gershon, R. K. 1974. T cell control of antibody production. *Contemp. Top. Immunobiol.* 3: 1.

80. Gershon, R. K., Carter, R. L., and Lane, N. J. 1967. Studies on homotransplantable lymphoma in hamsters. IV. Observation of macrophages in the expression of tumor immunity. *Amer. J. Pathol.* 31: 1117.

81. Gledhill, A. W. 1961. Enhancement of the pathogenicity of mouse hepatitis virus (MHV) by prior infection of mice with certain leukemia agents. *Brit. J. Cancer* 15: 531.

82. Gorczynski, R. M. 1974. Immunity to murine sarcoma virus-induced tumors. II. Suppression of T cell-mediated immunity by cells from progressor animals. *J. Immunol.* 112: 1826.

83. Gorer, P. A. 1958. Some reactions of H-2 antibodies *in vitro* and *in vivo*. *Ann. N.Y. Acad. Sci.* 73: 707.

84. Gorer, P. A., and Kaliss, N. 1959. The effect of isoantibodies *in vivo* on three different transplantable neoplasms in mice. *Cancer Res.* 19: 824.

85. Ha, T. Y., and Waksman, B. H. 1973. Role of thymus in tolerance. X. Suppressor activity of antigen-stimulated rat thymocytes transferred to normal recipients. *J. Immunol.* 110: 1290.

86. Halasz, N. A., and Orloff, M. J. 1965. The passive transfer of enhancement as applied to skin homografts. *J. Immunol.* 95: 253.

87. Halliday, W. J. 1971. Blocking effect of serum from tumor-bearing animals on macrophage migration inhibition with tumor antigens. *J. Immunol.* 106: 855.

88. Halliday, W. J. 1972. Macrophage migration inhibition with mouse tumor antigen. Properties of serum and peritoneal cells during tumor growth and after tumor loss. *Cell. Immunol.* 3: 113.

89. Hayami, M., Hellström, I., and Hellström, K. E. 1973. Serum effect of cell-mediated destruction of Rous sarcomas. *Int. J. Cancer* 12: 667.

90. Haywood, G. R., and McKhann, C. F. 1971. Antigenic specificities on murine sarcoma cells. Reciprocal relationship between normal transplantation antigens (H-2) and tumor-specific immunogenicity. *J. Exp. Med.* 133: 1171.

91. Hellström, I. 1967. A colony inhibition (CI) technique for demonstration of tumor cell destruction by lymphoid cells *in vitro*. *Int. J. Cancer* 2: 65.

92. Hellström, I., Evans, C. A., and Hellström, K. E. 1969. Cellular immunity and its serum-mediated inhibition in shope virus-induced rabbit pappilomas. *Int. J. Cancer* 4: 601.

93. Hellström, I., and Hellström, K. E. 1969. Studies on cellular immunity

and its serum-mediated inhibition in Moloney virus-induced mouse sarcomas. *Int. J. Cancer* 4: 587.

94. Hellström, I., and Hellström, K. E. 1970. Colony inhibition study on blocking and nonblocking serum effects on cellular immunity to Moloney sarcomas. *Int. J. Cancer* 5: 195.

95. Hellström, I., and Hellström, K. E. 1972. Can "blocking" serum factors protect against autoimmunity? *Nature* 230: 49.

96. Hellström, I., and Hellström, K. E. 1972. Can "blocking" serum factors protect against autoimmunity? *Nature* 230: 49.

97. Hellström, I., Hellström, K. E., and Trontin, J. J. 1973. Cellular immunity and blocking serum activity in chimeric mice. *Cell. Immunol.* 7: 73.

98. Hellström, I., Hellström, K. E., Pierce, G. E., and Fefer, A. 1969. Studies on immunity to autochthonous mouse tumors. *Transplant. Proc.* 1: 90.

99. Hellström, I., Hellström, K. E., and Shepard, T. H. 1970. Cell-mediated immunity against antigens common to human colonic carcinomas and fetal gut epithelium. *Int. J. Cancer* 6: 346.

100. Hellström, I., Hellström, K. E., and Sjögren, H. O. 1970. Serum-mediated inhibition of cellular immunity to methylcholanthrene-induced murine sarcomas. *Cell. Immunol.* 1: 18.

101. Hellström, I., Hellström, K., and Warner, G. 1973. Increase of lymphocyte-mediated tumor cell destruction by certain patient sera. *Int. J. Cancer* 12: 348.

102. Hellström, I., Hellström, K. E., Sjögren, H. O., and Warner, G. A. 1971. Demonstration of cell-mediated immunity to human neoplasm of various histological types. *Int. J. Cancer* 7: 1.

103. Hellström, I., Hellström, K. E., Sjögren, H. O., and Warner, G. A. 1971. Serum factors in tumor-free patients cancelling the blocking of cell-mediated tumor immunity. *Int. J. Cancer* 8: 185.

104. Hellström, K. E., and Hellström, I. 1970. Immunological enhancement as studied by cell culture techniques. *Ann. Rev. Microbiol.* 24: 373.

105. Hellström, K. E., and Hellström, I. 1974. Lymphocyte-mediated cytotoxicity and blocking serum activity to tumor antigens. *Adv. Immunol.* 18: 209.

106. Heiniger, H. J., Meier, H., Kaliss, N., et al. 1974. Hereditary immunodeficiency and leukemogenesis in HRS/J mice. *Cancer Res.* 34: 201.

107. Heppner, G. H. 1970. Neonatal thymectomy and mouse mammary tumorigenesis, in L. Seversi (ed.), *Immunity and Tolerance in Oncogenesis*, p. 503. Division of Cancer Research, Perugia, Italy.

108. Heppner, G. H. 1972. Blocking antibodies and enhancement. *Ser. Haematol.* 5: 41.

109. Heppner, G. H., Griswold, D. E., Di Lorenzo, J., et al. 1974. Selective immunosuppression by drugs in balanced immune responses. *Fed. Proc.* 33: 1882.

110. Hirsch, M. S., and Murphy, F. A. 1968. Effects of antilymphoid sera on viral infections. *Lancet* 2: 37.

111. Hirsch, M. S., and Murphy, F. A. 1968. Effects of antilymphocyte serum on Rauscher virus infection in mice. *Nature* 218: 478.

112. Haughton, G., and Nash, D. 1969. Specific immunosuppression by minute doses of passive antibody. *Transplant. Proc.* 1: 616.

113. Howard, R. J., Mergenhage, S. E., Natkins, A. L., and Dougherty, S. F. 1969. Inhibition of cellular immunity and enhancement of humoral antibody formation in mice infected with lactic dehydrogenase virus. *Transplant. Proc.* 1: 586.

114. Hsu, C. C. S., and Cooperband, S. R. 1971. *In vitro* responses of lymphocytes from cancer-bearing patients to autochthonous tumor tissues. *Soc. Exp. Biol. Med.* 136: 446.

115. Hughes, L. E., and Lytton, B. 1964. Antigenic properties of human tumors: Delayed cutaneous hypersensitivity reactions. *Brit. Med. J.* 1: 209.

116. Hutchin, P., Amos, D. B., and Prioleau, W. H. 1967. Interactions of humoral antibodies and immune lymphocytes. *Transplantation* 5: 68.

117. Irvin, G. L., and Eustace, T. C. 1970. The enhancement and rejection of tumor allografts by immune lymph node cells. *Transplantation* 10: 555.

118. Irvin, G. L., and Eustace, J. C. 1971. A study of tumor allografts sensitized lymph nodes in mice. I. Biologic activities of transferred cells and antibody titers of donor and recipient mice. *J. Immunol.* 106: 956.

119. Irvin, G. L., Eustace, J. C., and Fahey, J. L. 1967. Enhancement activity of mouse immunoglobulin classes. *J. Immunol.* 99: 1085.

120. Jones, J. M., and Feldman, J. D. 1971. Reactions *in vitro* with target cells and subcellular fractions of enriched rat alloantibodies with enhancing sera. *Transplantation* 12: 114.

121. Jones, J. M., Peter, H., and Feldman, J. 1972. Binding *in vivo* of enhancing antibodies to skin allografts and specific allogeneic tissues. *J. Immunol.* 108: 301.

122. Jose, D. G., and Seshadri, R. 1974. Circulating immune complexes in human neuroblastoma-direct assay and role in blocking specific cellular immunity. *Int. J. Cancer* 13: 824.

123. Jose, D. G., and Skvaril, F. 1974. Serum inhibition of cellular immunity in human neuroblastoma. IgG subclass of blocking activity. *Int. J. Cancer* 13: 824.

124. Judd, K. P., Stephens, K., and Trentin, J. T. 1971. Effects of heterologous antilymphocyte antibody on the development of spontaneous and transplanted lymphoma in AKR mice. *Cancer Res.* 27: 1161.

125. Kaliss, N. 1958. Immunological enhancement of tumor homografts in mice, a review. *Cancer Res.* 18: 992.

126. Kaliss, N. 1966. Immunological enhancement. Conditions for its expression and its relevance for grafts of normal tissues. *Ann. N.Y. Acad. Sci.* 192: 155.

127. Kaliss, N. 1970. Dynamics of immunological enhancement. *Transplant. Proc.* 2: 59.

128. Kaliss, N., and Molomut, N. 1952. The effect of prior injections of tissue antiserums on the survival of cancer homografts in mice. *Cancer Res.* 12: 110.

129. Kaliss, N., and Suter, R. B. 1968. Altered survival times of murin skin allografts from cancer-bearing donors. *Transplant.* 6: 844.

130. Kantiarinen, S., and Mitchison, N. A. 1975. Blocking antigen-antibody complexes on the T lymphocyte surface identified with defined protein antigens. II. Lymphocyte activation during *in vitro* incubation before adoptive transfer. *Immunology* 28: 523.

131. Kateley, J. R., Kamo, I., Kaplan, G., et al. 1974. Suppressive effect of leukemia virus-infected lymphoid cells on in vitro immunization of normal splenocytes. J. Natl. Cancer Inst. 53: 1371.

132. Katz, D., and Benacerraf, B. 1972. Regulating influences of activated T cells on B cell responses to antigens. Advan. Immunol. 15: 1.

133. Kirkwood, J. M., and Gershon, R. K. 1974. A role for suppressor T cells in immunological enhancement to tumor growth. Progr. Exp. Tumor Res. 19: 157.

134. Klein, G., Sjögren, H. O., Klein, E., and Hellström, K. E. 1960. Demonstration of resistance against methylcholanthrene-induced sarcomas in the primary autochthonous host. Cancer Res. 20: 1561.

135. Konda, S., Napao, Y., and Smith, R. T. 1973. The stimulatory effect of tumor bearing upon the T and B cell subpopulations of the mouse spleen. Cancer Res. 37: 2247.

136. Kouri, R. E., and Whitmire, C. E. 1974. Genetic control of susceptibility to cancers induced by 3-methylcholanthrene (MCA). Proc. 11th Cancer Congr. 2: 77.

137. Kourilsky, F. M., Silvestre, D., Levy, J. P., et al. 1971. Immunoferritin study of the distribution of HL-A antigens on human blood cells. J. Immunol. 106: 454.

138. Lagrange, P. H., Mackanes, G. B., and Miller, T. E. 1974. Potentiation of T cell-mediated immunity by selective suppression of antibody formation with cyclophosphamide. J. Exp. Med. 139: 1529.

139. Lance, E., Cooper, S., and Boyse, E. 1971. Antigenic change and cell maturation in murine thymocytes. Cell. Immunol. 1: 536.

140. Law, L. N., Ting, R. C., and Allison, A. C. 1968. Effects of antilymphocyte serum on the induction of tumors and leukaemia by murine sarcoma virus. Nature 220: 611.

141. Lerner, K. G., Glick, B., and McDuffie, F. C. 1971. Role of the bursa of Fabricius in IgG and IgM production in the chicken. Evidence for the role of nonbursal site in the development of humoral immunity. J. Immunol. 107: 493.

142. Levey, R. H., Trainin, N., Law, L., et al. Lymphocytic choriomeningitis infection in neonatally thymectomized mice bearing diffusion chambers containing thymus. Science 142: 483.

143. Levinthal, J. D., Buffet, R. F., and Furth, J. 1959. Prevention of viral lymphoid leukemia of mice by thymectomy. Proc. Soc. Exp. Biol. Med. 100: 610.

144. Levy, H. B., Law, L. W., and Robson, A. S. 1969. Inhibition of tumor growth by polyinosinic-polycytidilic acid. Proc. Natl. Acad. Sci. U.S.A. 62: 357.

145. Lian, M. C., Hunt, J. B., Smith, D. W., et al. 1973. Inhibition of transfer and ribosomal RNA methylases by polyinosinate. Cancer Res. 33: 323.

146. Lilly, F. 1970. Fv-2: Identification and location of a second gene governing the spleen focus response to Friend leukemia virus in mice. J. Natl. Cancer Inst. 45: 163.

147. Lilly, F., and Pincus, T. 1973. Genetic control of murine viral leukemogenesis. Adv. Cancer Res. 17: 231.

148. Linscott, W. D. 1970. Effect of cell surface antigen density on immunological enhancement. Nature 228: 824.

149. McCoy, J. L., Fefer, A., and Glynn, J. P. 1968. Inhibition and enhance-

ment of syngeneic Friend virus-induced lymphoma cells by passively transferred anti-Friend serum. *Exp. Hematol.* 16: 24.

150. McDevitt, H., and Benacerraf, B. 1969. Genetic control of specific immune responses. *Advan. Immunol.* 11: 31.

151. McDevitt, H., and Chinitz, A. 1969. Genetic control of the antibody response: Relationship between immune response and histocompatability (H-2) type. *Science* 163: 1207.

152. McErdy, D. P., Boon, M. C., and Furth, J. 1944. On the role of thymus, spleen, gonads in the development of leukemia in a high-leukemia incidence stock. *Cancer Res.* 4: 377.

153. McKenzie, I., Koene, R., and Winn, H. 1971. Mechanism of skin graft enhancement in the mouse. *Transplant. Proc.* 3: 711.

154. McKhann, C. F., and Jagarlamoody, S. M. 1971. Evidence for immune reactivity against neoplasms. *Transplant. Rev.* 7: 55.

155. MacLennan, I., Laurel, G., and Howard, A. 1969. A human serum immunoglobulin with specificity for certain homologous target cells which induced target cell damage by normal human lymphocytes. *Immunology* 17: 897.

156. Martin, M. C., Magnusson, S., Goscienski, P. J., et al. 1961. Common human viruses as carcinogen vectors. *Science* 134: 1985.

157. Martinez, C. 1964. Effect of early thymectomy on development of mammary tumors in mice. *Nature* 203: 1188.

158. Matsuoka, K., Hozumi, M., Koyowa, T., et al. 1964. Tumor toxohormone unrelated to bacterial contamination. *Gann* 55: 411.

159. Medina, A., and Heppner, G. 1973. Cell-mediated immunostimulation induced by mammary tumor virus-free Balble mice. *Nature* 242: 329.

160. Miller, J. F. A. P. 1960. Studies on mouse leukemia: The role of thymus leukemogenesis by cell-free leukemic filtrates. *Brit. J. Cancer* 14: 93.

161. Mitchell, M. S. 1972. Central inhibition of cellular immunity to leukemia L1210 by isoantibody. *Cancer Res.* 32: 825.

162. Mitchell, M. S., and Mokry, M. B. 1972. Specific inhibition of receptors for cytophilic antibody on macrophages by isoantibody. *Cancer Res.* 32: 832.

163. Mitchison, N. A. 1954. Passive transfer of transplantation immunity. *Proc. Roy. Soc. S. B.* 142: 72.

164. Mitchison, N. A. 1955. Studies on the immunological response to foreign tumor transplants in the mouse. I. The role of lymph node cells in conferring immunity by adoptive transfer. *J. Exp. Med.* 102: 157.

165. Mitchison, N. A. 1971. The carrier effect in the secondary response to hapten-protein conjugates. II. Cellular cooperation. *Eur. J. Immunol.* 1: 18.

166. Möller, E. 1965. Antagonistic effects of humoral isoantibodies on the *in vitro* cytotoxicity of immune lymphoid cells. *J. Exp. Med.* 122: 11.

167. Moller, E. 1963. Quantitative studies on the differentiation of isoantigens in newborn mice. *Transplantation* 1: 165.

168. Moller, G. 1964. Prolonged survival of allogeneic (homologous) normal tissue in antiserum-treated recipients. *Transplantation* 2: 281.

169. Moller, G. 1966. Biologic properties of 19S and 7S mouse isoantibodies directed against H-2 isoantigens. *J. Immunol.* 96.

170. Nakakera, W., and Fukuoka, A. 1949. Toxohormone: A characteristic

toxic substance produced by cancer tissue. *Gann* 40: 45.

171. Nandi, S., and Helmick, C. 1974. Genetical analysis of vertical transmission of mammary tumor virus (MTV) by female G. R. mice. *Proc. 11th Int. Cancer Cong.* 2: 75.

172. Nelson, D. S. 1969. The role of macrophages in transplantation immunity and tumor immunity, *in* A. Neuberger and E. L. Tatum (eds.), *Macrophages and Immunity*, Vol. II, p. 211. North Holland Research Monographs, Frontiers of Biology.

173. Nelson, K., Pollack, S. B., and Hellström, K. E. 1975. Specific antitumor responses by cultured immune spleen cells. I. *In vitro* culture method and initial characterization of factors which block immune cell-mediated cytotoxicity *in vitro*. *Int. J. Cancer* 15: 806.

174. Nowotny, A., Groshman, J., Abdelmoor, A., *et al.* 1974. Escape of TA3 tumors from allogeneic immune rejection: Theory and Experiments. *Eur. J. Immunol.* 4: 73.

175. Old, L. J., Stockert, E., Boyse, E., and Kimm, J. H. 1968. Antigenic modulation: Loss of TL antigen from cells exposed to TL antibody. Study of phenomena *in vitro*. *J. Exp. Med.* 127: 523.

176. Oldstone, M. B. A., and Dixon, F. J. 1971. Virus-antiviral antibody complexes, *in* B. Amos (ed.), *Progress in Immunology* (First International Congress of Immunology). Academic Press, New York.

177. Oren, M. E., and Herbermann, R. B. 1971. Delayed cutaneous hypersensitivity reactions to membrane extract of human tumor cells. *Clin. Exp. Immunol.* 9: 45.

178. Parsekevas, F., Orr, K. B., Anderson, E. P., Lee, S. T., and Israels, L. G. 1972. The biological significance of Fc reception on mouse B lymphocytes. *J. Immunol.* 108: 1729.

179. Penn, I., Helgrinson, C. G., and Starzl, T. E. 1971. De novo malignant tumors in organ transplant recipients. *Transplant. Proc.* 3: 773.

180. Perlman, P., and Holm, G. 1969. Cytotoxic effects of lymphoid cells *in vitro in* F. J. Dixon, Jr., and H. G. Kunkel (eds.), *Advances in Immunology* 11: 117.

181. Perlman, P., Perlman, H., Wasserman, J., and Packalen, T. 1970. Lysis of chicken erythrocytes sensitized with PPD by lymphoid cells from guinea pigs immunized with tubercle bacilli. *Int. Arch. Allergy* 38: 204.

182. Peter, H., and Feldman, J. 1972. Cell-mediated cytotoxicity during rejection and enhancement of allogeneic skin grafts in rats. *J. Exp. Med.* 135: 1301.

183. Peterson, D. A. R., Hendrickson, R., and Good, R. A. 1963. Reduced antibody-forming capacity during incubation period of passage A leukemia in C3H mice. *Proc. Soc. Exp. Biol. Med.* 114: 517.

184. Polak, L., and Turk, J. L. 1974. Reversal of immunological tolerance by cyclophosphamide through inhibition of suppressor cell activity. *Nature* 249: 654.

185. Pollack, S. 1973. Specific arming of normal lymph node cells by sera from tumor-bearing mice. *Int. J. Cancer* 11: 138.

186. Pollack, S., Heppner, G., Brown, J., and Nelson, K. 1972. Specific killing of tumor cells *in vitro* in the presence of normal lymphoid cells and sera from hosts immune to the tumor antigens. *Int. J. Cancer*. 9: 316.

187. Poulter, L. W., and Turk, J. L. 1972. Proportional increase in the *theta-*

carrying lymphocytes in peripheral lymphoid tissue following treatment with cyclophosphamide. *Nature* 238: 17.

188. Prehn, R. T. 1972. The immune reaction as a stimulator of tumor growth. *Science* 176: 170.

189. Reif, A., and Allen, J. 1966. Mouse thymic isoantigens. *Nature* 209: 521.

190. Ron, M., and Witz, I. 1970. Tumor-associated immunoglobulins. The elution of IgG2 from mouse tumors. *Int. J. Cancer.* 6: 361.

191. Ron, M., and Witz, I. 1972. Tumor-associated immunoglobulins. Enhancement of syngeneic tumors by IgG2 containing tumor eluates. *Int. J. Cancer.* 9: 242.

192. Rosenau, W., and Morton, D. L. 1966. Tumor-specific inhibition of growth of methylcholanthrene-induced sarcoma *in vivo* and *in vitro* by sensitized isologous lymphoid cells. *J. Natl. Cancer Inst.* 36: 825.

193. Rotter, V., and Trainin, N. 1975. Inhibition of tumor growth in syngeneic chimeric mice mediated by depletion of suppressor cells. *Transplantation* 20: 65.

194. Rubin, H., Fanshier, L., Cornelius, A., et al. 1962. Tolerance and immunity in chickens after congenital and contact infections with an avian leukosis virus. *Virology* 17: 143.

195. Salaman, M. H. 1968. The effect of some leukemogenic viruses on immune reactions. *Bibl. Haematol.* 31: 92.

196. Sanford, B. 1967. An alteration in tumor histocompatability induced by neuraminidase. *Transplantation* 5: 1273.

197. Savel, H. 1969. Effect of autologous tumor extracts on cultured human peripheral blood lymphocytes. *Cancer* 24: 56.

198. Schempl, A., and Wecher, E. 1972. Replacement of T cell function by a T cell product. *Nature* 237: 15.

199. Sinkovics, J. G., Di Saia, P. J., and Rutledge, F. 1970. Tumor immunology and evolution of the placenta. *Lancet* 2: 1190.

200. Sjöberg, O. H., Anderson, J., and Moller, G. 1972. Reconstitution of the antibody response *in vitro* of T cell-derived spleen cells by supernatants from spleen cell cultures. *J. Immunol.* 109: 1379.

201. Sjögren, H. O., Hellström, I., Bansal, S. C., and Hellström, K. E. 1971. Suggestive evidence that the blocking antibodies of tumor-bearing individuals may be antigen-antibody complexes. *Proc. Natl. Acad. Sci. (Wash.)* 68: 1375.

202. Sjögren, H. O., Hellström, I., Bansal, S., Warner, G., and Hellström, K. E. 1972. Elution of blocking factors from human tumors capable of abrogating tumor cell destruction by specifically immune lymphocytes. *Int. J. Cancer* 9: 274.

203. Smith, R. T. 1968. Tumor-specific mechanisms. *N.E.J.M.* 278: 1268.

204. Smith, R. T. 1972. Possibilities and problems of immunologic interventions in cancer. *N.E.J.M.* 287: 439.

205. Snell, G. D. 1954. The enhancing effect (or actively acquired tolerance) and the histocompatability 2 locus in the mouse. *J. Natl. Cancer Inst.* 15: 665.

206. Snell, G. D. 1956. The suppression of the enhancing effect in mice by addition of donor lymph nodes to the tumor inoculum. *Transplant. Bull.* 3: 83.

207. Snell, G. D., and Stimpfling, J. H. 1966. Genetics of tissue transplantations, in E. L. Green (ed.), *Biology of the Laboratory Mouse*, p. 457. McGraw Hill, New York.

208. Squartini, F., Olivi, M., and Bolis, G. B. 1970. Mouse strain and breeding stimulation as factors influencing the effect of thymectomy on mammary tumorigenesis. *Cancer Res.* 30: 2069.

209. Steeves, R. A., Mirand, E. A., Thomson, S., *et al.* 1969. Enhancement of spleen focus formation and virus replication in Friend virus-infected mice. *Cancer Res.* 29: 1111.

210. Steinmuller, D. 1969. Allograft immunity produced with skin isografts from immunologically tolerant mice. *Transplant. Proc.* 1: 593.

211. Takassugi, M., and Haldemann, W. H. 1969. Regulation of immunity toward allogeneic tumors in mice. I. Effect of antiserum fractions on tumor growth. *J. Natl. Cancer Inst.* 43: 843.

212. Takassugi, M., and Haldemann, W. H. 1969. Regulation of immunity toward allogeneic tumors in mice. II. Effect of antiserum and antiserum fractions on cellular and humoral responses. *J. Natl. Cancer Inst.* 43: 857.

213. Taskvaklides, E., Smith, C., Kersey, J. H., *et al.* 1974. Transplantation antigens (H-2) on virally and chemically transformed Balb/3T3 fibroblasts in culture. *J. Natl. Cancer Inst.* 52: 1499.

214. Taylor, H. E., and Culling, C. F. 1968. Production of complement by spleen cells *in vitro* and its possible role in an allograft rejection model. *Nature* 220: 506.

215. Treves, A. J., Carnaud, C., Trainin, N., *et al.* 1974. Enhancing T lymphocytes from tumor-bearing mice suppress host resistance to a syngeneic tumor. *Eur. J. Immunol.* 4: 722.

216. Tubergen, D. G., and Feldman, J. D. 1971. The role of thymus and bone marrow cells in delayed hypersensitivity. *J. Exp. Med.* 134: 1144.

217. Uhr, J. W., and Möller, G. 1968. Regulatory effect of antibody on the immune response. *Adv. Immunol.* 8: 81.

218. Umiel, T., and Trainin, N. 1974. Immunological enhancement of tumor growth by syngeneic thymus-derived lymphocytes. *Transplantation* 18: 244.

219. Vaage, J. 1974. Circulating tumor antigens versus immune serum factors in depressed concomitant immunity. *Cancer Res.* 34: 2979.

220. Voisin, G., Kinsky, R., Jansen, F., and Bernard, C. 1969. Biological properties of antibody classes in transplantation immune sera. *Transplantation* 8: 618.

221. Voisin, G. A. 1971. Nature of enhancing-facilitation antibodies. *Transplant. Proc.* 3: 1229.

222. Volkert, M., and Hannover, Larsen, J. 1965. Immunological tolerance to viruses. *Prog. Med. Virol.* 7: 160.

223. Volkman, A., and Collins, F. M. 1971. The restorative effect of peritoneal macrophages on delayed hypersensitivity following ionizing radiation. *Cell. Immunol.* 2: 552.

224. Waldmann, H., and Munro, A. J. 1974. T cell dependence of B cell unresponsiveness *in vitro*. *Eur. J. Immunol.* 4: 410.

225. Watkins, E., Ogata, Y., Anderson, L., and Waters, M. 1971. Activation of host lymphocytes cultured with cancer cells treated with neuraminidase. *Nature* 231: 83.

226. Weston, B. J., Carter, R. L., Easty, G. C., *et al.* 1974. The growth and metastses of an allograft lymphoma in normal, deprived and reconstituted mice.

Int. J. Cancer 14: 176.

227. Wegmann, T. G., Hellström, I., and Hellström, K. E. 1971. Immunological tolerance: "Forbidden clones" allowed in tetraparental mice. *Proc. Natl. Acad. Sci. U.S.A.* 68: 1644.

228. Winn, J. H. 1970. Humoral antibody in allograft reactions. *Transplant. Proc.* 2: 83.

229. Yoshida, T. O., and Southam, C. M. 1963. Attempts to find cell-associated immune reaction against autochthonous tumors. *Japan. J. Exp. Med.* 33: 369.

230. Zarling, J. M., and Terethia, S. S. 1973. Transplantation immunity to simian virus 40-transformed cells in tumor-bearing mice. I. Development of cellular immunity to simian virus 40 tumor-specific transplantation antigens during tumorigenesis by transplanted cells. *J. Natl. Cancer Inst.* 40: 137.

231. Zarling, J. M., and Tevethia, S. S. 1973. Transplantation immunity to simian virus 40-transformed cells in tumor-bearing mice. II. Evidence for macrophage participation at the effector level of tumor cell rejection. *J. Natl. Cancer Inst.* 50: 149.

232. Zbar, B., Wepsic, H. T., borsos, T., *et al.* 1970. Tumor graft rejection in syngeneic guinea pigs. Evidence for a two-step mechanism. *J. Natl. Cancer Inst.* 44: 473.

233. Zbar, B., Wepsic, A., Rapp, H., *et al.* 1970. Two-step mechanism of tumor graft rejection in syngeneic guinea pigs. II. Initiation of reaction by a cell fraction containing lymphocytes and neutraphils. *J. Natl. Cancer Inst.* 44: 701.

234. Zimmerman, B., and Feldman, J. 1969. Bioassay of enhancement. *J. Immunol.* 102: 507.

235. Zimmerman, B., and Feldman, J. 1970. Enhancing antibody. III. Site of activity. *J. Immunol.* 104: 626.

CHAPTER 10

TUMOR-SPECIFIC ANTIGENS ASSOCIATED WITH HUMAN OVARIAN CYSTADENO-CARCINOMA

Malaya Bhattacharya
and Joseph J. Barlow

Department of Gynecology
Roswell Park Memorial Institute
Buffalo, New York 14263

Evidence has been reviewed for at least one tumor-associated antigen in human cystadenocarcinoma of the ovary which is apparently absent in normal ovaries and other histologically similar normal organs, ovarian carcinomas other than serous and mucinous cystadenocarcinomas, and other cancers thus far tested. The antigenic determinant of this ovarian cystadenocarcinoma-associated glycoprotein is immunologically unrelated to blood group substances, nonspecific serum and tissue antigens, carcinoembryonic antigen, alphafetoprotein, histocompatibility antigens, and human fibrin. It consists of about 50% protein and 30 to 40% carbohydrate. High levels of this glycoprotein antigen have been detected in the sera of ovarian cancer patients with advanced disease, and the level of circulating antigen appears to correlate with the tumor volume of the patient.

1. Introduction

During recent years increasing evidence has accumulated indicating that some human cancers are associated with demonstrable protein, glycoprotein or glycolipid antigens that are either newly acquired during the process of neoplastic transformation or reflect an augmentation of certain, usually undetectable, normal cell antigens.

Sensitive serologic techniques have revealed the presence of both humoral and cell-mediated immunity in many human cancers suggesting that some of these, like animal tumors, possess tumor-specific (associated) antigens. Among human tumors reported to possess tumor-associated antigens are colonic adenocarcinoma (38), primary liver hepatoma (37), leukemia (27), Burkitt's lymphoma (20), melanoma (28), neuroblastoma (18), osteosarcoma (29), Hodgkin's disease (30), and many others. The demonstration of these tumor-associated antigens has spurred a great deal of research directed toward the development of immunodiagnostic and immunotherapeutic methods for human cancers. Extensive studies have been published on the detection of circulating carcinoembryonic antigen (CEA), which was originally derived from human colonic cancer (38), and circulating alpha-fetoprotein (α-fp), which was derived from primary liver hepatoma (37). Although cross-reactivity with other tumors has been reported for CEA and α-fp (24–26, 33, 35, 39), they continue to be useful tumor-markers as aids in diagnosis, in following response to therapy, and in detecting early tumor recurrence. CEA and α-fp have also been detected in the plasma and tumors of patients with female genital cancers (17, 19, 24, 40, 41). However, the plasma assays of these two fetal antigens have been only of limited use in screening for female genital cancers and monitoring ovarian malignancy (24, 33, 41). It is obvious that an immunologic test based on the antigen isolated from ovarian tumor is needed to improve the specificity and clinical application in the diagnosis and detection of ovarian cancer.

The presence of tumor-associated antigens in ovarian cancers has been suggested by work in our laboratory (1–5) as well as by other investigators (9, 13, 16, 21, 23, 32). We have reported evidence for at least two common tumor-associated antigens or antigenic determinants in human cystadenocarcinomas of the ovary which are apparently absent in normal ovaries and other histologically similar normal organs. These antigenic determinants are immunologically unrelated to blood group substances, nonspecific serum and tissue antigens, CEA, α-fp, histocompatibility antigens, and human fibrin (2).

One of these two antigens appears to be specific for cystadenocarcinomas of the ovary in that it does not cross-react with any other ovarian carcinomas except serous and mucinous types, other gynecologic malignancies or nongynecologic malignancies thus far tested (1, 3). We have termed this antigen(s) as ovarian cystadenocarcinoma-associated antigen (OCAA). Interestingly, OCAA has not been detected in benign ovarian cystadenomas despite the similarities in histological appearance and tissue of origin between the benign serous and mucinous cystadenomas and their malignant counterparts. OCAA is present in both the solid and cyst fluid components of cystadenocarcinomas (3).

In this review we will attempt to summarize our work concerning the isolation, purification, and immunochemical characterization of tumor-specific antigens associated with cystadenocarcinomas of the ovary, the most common types of ovarian cancer, and their clinical application.

2. Sources for Cystadenocarcinoma-Associated Antigens

Three types of tumor materials are available as starting material for the isolation of the antigens: (a) solid ovarian tumors obtained from laparotomies performed for diagnosis and treatment of patients with ovarian cancer; (b) tumor cells in ascites fluids obtained from ovarian cancer patients who require multiple paracenteses; and (c) cyst fluids. Large quantities of cyst fluids may be obtained from a single patient from cystic areas of cystadenocarcinomas. This is a potential source for isolation of the tumor-associated antigens in large quantities.

3. Production of Heteroantisera for the Demonstration of Ovarian Tumor-Associated Antigens

Antisera were produced in rabbits against individual or pooled surgical specimens of serous or mucinous cystadenocarcinomas buffered saline extracts. The same results have been achieved using solid areas or the cyst fluids from these tumors. The anti-cystadenocarcinoma sera obtained were serially absorbed with pooled human sera and red cells representing all the major blood groups, with homogenates of pooled normal ovaries and other normal reproductive organs, and with sediments of human liver and kidney (2). These absorptions were designed to remove antibodies against blood group substances, normal reproductive organ components, nonspecific serum components, tissue antigens and fibrin. Absorbed antiserum was then used to perform the assays for tumor-associated antigenic reactivity. Ouchterlony double diffusion and immunoelectrophoretic studies were done with normal ovarian and tumor tissue extracts and the antitumor antiserum before and after absorptions (2). Numerous precipitin bands appeared against both antigenic mixtures prior to absorption, but at least two precipitin bands remained after absorption, and only between the tumor extract and the absorbed antitumor antiserum. Only prior absorption of the antitumor antiserum with extracts of cystadenocarcinoma-inhibited precipitin band formation between the tumor extract and the antitumor antiserum. In most specimens tested serous cystadenocarcinomas and mucinous cystadenocarcinomas of the ovary were immunologically indistinguishable. Each contained at least two tumor-associated antigens (1, 3). Similar findings for a close antigenic relationship between serous and mucinous ovarian carcinomas have been also presented by other investigators (9, 13, 21). Chen and colleagues (11) observed cross-inhibition of cellular hypersensitivity to tumor antigen(s) with both serous and mucinous cystadenocarcinomas.

In analyzing large numbers of serous and mucinous cystadenocarcinomas, there were some samples that gave rise to the formation of as many as four precipitin lines instead of two lines seen in most instances. Figure 1 illustrates immunoelectrophoresis patterns developed between absorbed antitumor serum and one such tumor extract. All the four precipitin bands had β-electrophoretic mobility and the two innermost bands and the two outermost bands tended to superimpose each other. Figure 2 shows the Ouchterlony double diffusion patterns developed between ab-

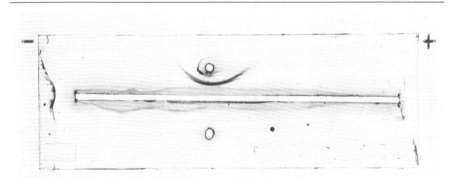

Fig. 1. Examples of immunoelectrophoresis patterns with normal ovary and tumor antigens against absorbed antitumor sera. Upper well: cystadenocarcinoma extract; lower well: normal ovary extract; trough: absorbed antisera against pooled cystadenocarcinoma extract.

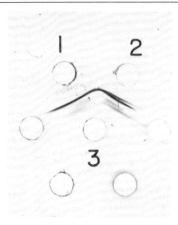

Fig. 2. Examples of immunodiffusion patterns developed between absorbed antitumor sera and two cystadenocarcinoma extracts. Well No. 1: cystadenocarcinoma extract. Well No. 2: another cystadenocarcinoma extract. Well No. 3: absorbed antisera against pooled cystadenocarcinoma extract.

sorbed antitumor serum and two cystadenocarcinoma extracts 1 and 2, one of which forms two lines and the other four. A complete reaction of identity was obtained between the two tumor extracts. The outer band of extract 1, which was closer to the antigen well, fused completely with the two outer bands of extract 2. Similarly, the broad diffuse inner band of extract 1, which was closer to the antisera well, fused with the two inner bands of extract 2. Evidence that these two tumor extracts were antigenically similar also came from precipitin-inhibition studies. Further absorption of the antitumor sera with either of these two extracts abolished precipitin band formation between the tumor extracts and the antisera. These observations indicate that ovarian cystadenocarcinomas contain two distinct antigenic systems each consisting of more than one similar antigenic components. Depending on physicochemical properties, polydispersity, charge, etc. the antigenically similar molecules sometimes form different lines and sometimes fail to do so either due to coincidence of the lines or to a genuine common line.

These two antigenic systems of ovarian cystadenocarcinomas did not cross-react with CEA, α-fp, or histocompatability antigens by radioimmunoassay inhibition technique (2). They appeared to be of cytoplasmic origin by immunofluorescent studies (2). They were also unrelated to ferritin, another tumor-associated antigen of Hodgkin's disease reported to be present in ovarian carcinomas (31).

4. Distribution of Cystadenocarcinoma-Associated Antigens

An immunologic comparison was made between cystadenocarcinoma of the ovary and other human gynecologic and nongynecologic tumors and sera by immunodiffusion and precipitin-inhibition techniques (3). Figure 3 shows the Ouchterlony patterns developed between absorbed antitumor serum and various representative gynecological tumor extracts. Two major precipitin bands formed between serous and mucinous cystadenocarcinomas, whereas only one precipitin band formed between other gynecologic tumor extracts and the absorbed antitumor antisera. The inner precipitin band of serous and mucinous cystadenocarcinomas, which did not cross-react with other gynecologic cancer extracts, showed a pattern of nonidentity with the outer precipitin band.

Precipitin-inhibition experiments indicated that complete inhibition was achieved when mucinous and serous cystadenocarcinoma extracts were mixed with absorbed antiserum, whereas treatment of the absorbed antiserum with other gynecologic tumor extracts eliminated only the outer cross-reacting band. The inner antigenic band is referred to as OCAA which does not cross-react with other tumors thus far tested. Next the absorbed anticystadenocarcinoma serum was tested against two specimens of primary colon and breast cancers (1, 5). Neither of these two antigenic systems were demonstrable in these tumors. But when we tested

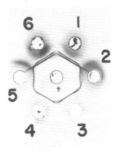

Fig. 3 (Ref. 1, 5). Examples of immunodiffusion patterns developed between absorbed anti-cystadenocarcinoma sera and various gynecologic tumor extracts. Center well: absorbed antitumor sera, peripheral wells: (1) mucinous cystadenocarcinoma extract, (2) endometrioid carcinoma of ovary extract, (3) squamous cell carcinoma of the cervix extract, (4) carcinosarcoma of the uterus extract, (5) granulosa cell tumor of ovary extract, and (6) serous cystadenocarcinoma extract.

a large number of primary breast cancer specimens, 7 out of 26 primary breast tumor extracts showed the presence of the cross-reacting outer precipitin band of cystadenocarcinomas. They were all negative for OCAA. Hence the second antigenic system of cystadenocarcinomas was not restricted within gynecologic tumors as was originally thought. The frequency distribution of this antigen in gynecologic tumors was however, much greater (about 90%) compared to nongynecologic tumors.

Both the antigenic systems of cystadenocarcinomas were apparently absent in normal ovary and other normal reproductive organs such as uterus, cervix, endometrium and fallopian tubes (1, 3). The presence of the second cross-reacting antigenic system was, however, indicated in one apparently normal autopsy specimen of kidney obtained from a patient who died of malignant disease. One out of 15 different apparently normal uterine cervices obtained from cancer patients at surgery also showed the presence of the second antigenic system.

We tested sera from ovarian cancer patients and from normal healthy age-matched controls for the presence of the two antigenic systems of cystadenocarcinomas by Ouchterlony double diffusion technique. None of the control sera showed the presence of any of these two antigens. All ovarian cancer patients' sera were negative for OCAA by immunodiffusion technique. But about 80% of the preoperative and pretreatment ovarian cancer patients' sera were positive for the second antigen. When sera were collected from these same patients after surgery or chemo- or radiation therapy, the immunodiffusion technique was unable to demonstrate the presence of the second antigen anymore. All these data indicate that the second antigenic system of cystadenocarcinomas is more abundant than OCAA. One human umbilical cord serum was also positive for the second antigen, whereas pregnancy sera obtained at the third trimester was negative for both OCAA and the second antigen of cystadenocarcinomas.

Table 1 lists the distribution of these two antigenic systems in different normal and neoplastic tissues and sera we have examined so far by immunodiffusion technique. A wide variety of other cancerous and noncancerous diseased tissue and sera will, however, have to be screened by more sensitive detection methods to ascertain whether OCAA is solely associated with ovarian cystadenocarcinomas or it may be present in other histologic types of cancer or disease also.

5. Isolation and Purification of OCAA

The starting point for the purification procedure was the clear 20,000 g supernatant from sonicated, buffered saline tumor extracts.

Table 1. Distribution of ovarian cystadenocarcinoma-associated antigens in different normal and neoplastic specimens and sera

Specimen Extracts	Double Diffusion Test	
	OCAA Positive	Second Antigen Positive
Serous cystadenocarcinoma	26/37	30/37
Mucinous cystadenocarcinoma	7/7	5/7
Serous cystadenocarcinoma cyst fluid	2/3	3/3
Mucinous cystadenocarcinoma cyst fluid	3/3	2/3
Serous cystadenoma tissue and cyst fluid	0/2	0/2
Mucinous cystadenoma tissue and cyst fluid	0/3	0/3
Endometrioid ovarian carcinoma	0/3	3/3
Granulosa cell cancer of ovary	0/5	4/5
Malignant teratoma of ovary	0/3	2/3
Squamous cell carcinoma of cervix	0/8	8/8
Carcinosarcoma of uterus	0/2	2/2
Adenocarcinoma of uterine corpus	0/7	5/7
Carcinoma of the vulva	0/1	1/1
Primary colon cancer	0/2	0/2
Metastatic colon cancer to ovary	0/5	2/5
Primary breast cancer	0/26	7/26
Metastatic breast cancer to ovary	0/6	2/6
Metastatic pancreatic cancer to ovary	0/2	1/2
Normal ovary	0/60	0/60
Normal cervix	0/15	1/15
Normal fallopian tube	0/2	0/2
Normal endometrium	0/2	0/2
Normal colon	0/2	0/2
Normal age-matched women's sera	0/54	0/54
Ovarian cancer patient's sera, preoperative or pretreatment	0/22	17/22
Ovarian cancer patient's sera, postoperative or posttreatment	0/14	0/14
Human umbilical cord serum	0/1	1/1
Pregnancy sera at third trimester	0/3	0/3

Source: Ouchterlony.

These were first chromatographed on a Sephadex G-200 column in which the antigenic activity came off in the void volume of the column. Treatment of this excluded peak with an equal volume of 1.2 M perchloric acid solubilized the OCAA whereas the second antigenic system was inactivated. The perchloric acid soluble material was then subjected to two further gel filtration columns, a Sepharose 4B column followed by another Sephadex G-200 column, which finally gave a single major peak. The details of these purification procedures have been published in detail elsewhere (5). The material from the final column formed a single precipitin arc in the electrophoretic region for β-globulins in immunoelectrophoresis against both absorbed and unabsorbed anticystadenocarcinoma serum. These results are shown in Figure 4 which also shows the results of reaction between unabsorbed and absorbed antitumor serum before purification of the antigen (1, 5).

Purification of OCAA by the classical gel filtration technique is a long and laborious procedure and the yield is low. Recently, we have employed the antibody-precipitation method (8) for the isolation of the antigen. Antisera were prepared in rabbits by injection of OCAA purified by the gel filtration technique. The antisera were carefully absorbed with perchloric acid extracted, pooled normal human sera and normal ovary to

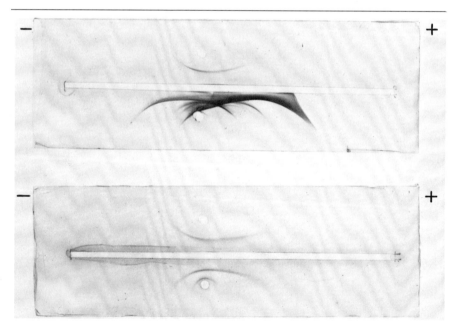

Fig. 4 (Ref. 1, 5). Examples of immunoelectrophoresis patterns with purified tumor antigen and crude tumor extract against antitumor sera before and after absorptions. **A.** Upper well: purified tumor antigen, lower well: crude tumor extract, trough: anti-cystadenocarcinoma sera unabsorbed. **B.** Upper well: purified tumor antigen, lower well: crude tumor extract, trough: absorbed anti-cystadenocarcinoma sera.

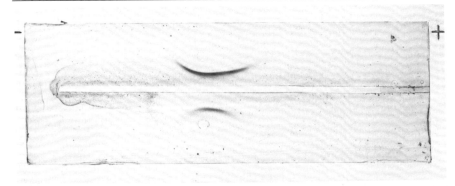

Fig. 5. Examples of immunoelectrophoresis patterns developed between purified tumor antigen and anti-tumor sera. Upper well: OCAA purified by the gel filtration technique, lower well: OCAA purified by the antibody precipitation technique, trough: anti-cystadenocarcinoma sera, unabsorbed.

render it operationally monospecific. A given volume of the absorbed antisera was then mixed with concentrated, soluble buffered saline extracts of ovarian cystadenocarcinomas and the immunoprecipitate formed was then dissociated with low pH buffer. Antigen was extracted with an equal volume of 1.2 M perchloric acid which denatured the antibody in the mixture. The perchloric acid soluble antigen was then dialyzed thoroughly against deionized water and lyophilized. OCAA isolated by this technique was found to be identical with OCAA isolated by gel filtration technique in double diffusion test. In immunoelectrophoresis their precipitin lines had the same β-electrophoretic mobility and shape as has been shown in Figure 5.

The purity of OCAA was further checked by analytical disc electrophoresis (5). In the presence of 6M urea, OCAA traveled as a single broad diffused band at both basic and acidic pH and was stained by both periodic acid-Schiff reagent and amido black, indicating that the antigen is a glycoprotein (Fig. 6).

6. Chemical Composition and Nature of Antigenic Determinants of OCAA

OCAA consists (based on dry weight) of about 50–60% protein and 30–40% carbohydrate. The ratio of protein to carbohydrate varies from sample to sample to some extent. Table 2 shows the amino acid and carbohydrate composition of OCAA (1, 5). The amino acid composition is characterized by a high percentage of threonine, serine, proline and val-

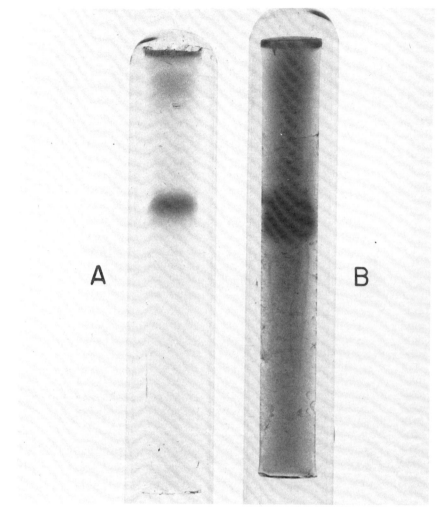

Fig. 6. Analytic disc electrophoresis patterns with purified tumor antigen in basic condition (Tris-glycine, pH 8.3). **A.** Stained with periodic acid-Schiff reagent (PAS). **B.** Stained with amido black.

ine. Galactose and N-acetylglucosamine are the principle carbohydrate constituents.

The chemical nature of the antigenic determinant of OCAA was studied by incubating the pure antigen with various degradative enzymes (1, 5). Antigenicity, as measured by the intensity of the precipitin band of

Table 2. Amino acid and carbohydrate composition of OCAA

Component	μmoles/100 mg dry weight of antigen	Component	μmoles/100 mg dry weight of antigen
Amino acid		*Amino acid* (continued)	
Aspartic acid	9.1	Lysine	6.1
Threonine	21.0	Histidine	3.8
Serine	22.0	Arginine	6.7
Glutamic acid	13.0		
Proline	16.0	*Carbohydrate:*	
Glycine	13.0	L-Fucose	8.4
Alanine	14.0	D-Mannose	27.0
Valine	48.0	D-Galactose	36.4
½ Cystine	7.8	N-acetyl-D-	
Isoleucine	4.0	glucosamine	52.6
Leucine	9.0	N-acetyl-D-	
Tyrosine	4.7	galactosamine	4.3
Phenylalanine	6.1	Sialic acid	9.2

Source: Refs. 1, 5.

OCAA against unabsorbed anti-OCAA serum, was not affected by treatment with deoxyribonuclease, ribonuclease, trypsin, or insoluble protease. Nor was antigenicity altered by treatment with neuraminidase, suggesting that terminal sialic acid probably does not have any role in its antigenicity. The intensity of the precipitin band of OCAA against unabsorbed anti-OCAA serum was, however, reduced as compared to the control sample, after periodate oxidation (Fig. 7), which indicates that at least part of the antigenicity of the OCAA molecule resides in the carbohydrate moiety.

7. OCAA and Blood Group Antigens

The purified preparation of OCAA isolated from tumor materials obtained from patients belonging to all major blood groups (ABO system) was tested for content of blood group antigens by hemagglutination inhibition technique and was found to have no blood group specificity. This, however, does not exclude the possibility of the presence of any blood group antigenic determinants in OCAA molecule. The hemagglutination inhibition technique is highly sensitive for authentic blood group substances but may be inadequate to detect the presence of low density blood

Periodate Oxidation

Fig. 7.   Effect of periodate oxidation on antigenicity of OCAA. Upper well: OCAA (control), middle well: anti-OCAA serum, unabsorbed, and lower well: periodate-treated OCAA.

group determinants associated with the OCAA molecule. We plan to do sensitive radiolabeled antigen binding studies with anti-blood group antisera in the future. The chemical composition of OCAA is, however, quite different from blood group substances, which have high carbohydrate content.

8. Utilization of OCAA as a Tumor Marker

Taking advantage of the lack of OCAA in nongynecologic cancers, we have utilized testing for the presence of OCAA as an aid in determining the primary site of origin in widely metastasizing intraabdominal tumors. Since the ovaries are a frequent metastatic site for gastrointestinal and breast carcinomas, it is sometimes difficult, especially when the ovaries are extensively involved, to determine by laparotomy and even histopathology the primary site of tumor origin. By simultaneously setting up immunodiffusion reactions between absorbed anti-cystadenocarcinoma serum, anti-CEA serum, and extracts of tumor biopsy specimens, we have been able, with apparent success, to distinguish between primary ovarian malignancies and various gastrointestinal and breast primaries metastatic to the ovaries. In 29 of 31 attempts, the correct primary site diagnosis was indicated by this technique. Two cases of apparent primary ovarian cancer gave false-negative reactions.

The ultimate goal of our work with OCAA has been to develop an immunodiagnostic serologic screening test for early ovarian cancer. Using the Farr technique as modified by Kupchik et al. (22) we have developed a radioimmunoassay for the detection of circulating OCAA in ovarian cancer patients.

Antisera were produced in rabbits against the purified OCAA. Although the preparation of OCAA appeared to be pure, when the anti-OCAA serum was tested against OCAA and a highly concentrated extract of perchloric acid extracted pooled normal human serum or normal ovarian glycoprotein by immunodiffusion technique, a typical reaction of partial identity was obtained. OCAA appeared to share a common antigenic determinant with a normal serum or normal ovarian glycoprotein and, at the same time, had its unique antigenic determinant which gave spur formation. After absorptions of the antisera with perchloric acid extract of pooled normal human sera and normal ovarian glycoprotein, only reaction against OCAA remained. We iodinated OCAA and did binding studies with the antisera. The standard radioimmunoassay inhibition curve obtained with these reagents had a relatively flat slope. When the sera of patients with serous and mucinous cystadenocarcinomas of the ovary were tested, the radioimmunoassay did indeed indicate circulating OCAA in the sera of these patients. However, the sensitivity of the assay was inadequate at low levels of antigen.

We have followed 15 patients with advanced-stage ovarian cancer with serial determinations over a long period of time. High levels of circulating OCAA were detected in preoperative and pretreatment sera of these patients. Serial measurements of circulating OCAA appeared to correlate with tumor volume as well as the clinical status of the patient. The OCAA antigen assay appears very promising for the followup surveillance of ovarian cancer patients but is currently inadequate for early immunodiagnosis or for detecting small tumor burdens. Present studies are underway to improve the sensitivity and specificity of the present radioimmunoassay so that it can be successfully used for early immunodiagnostic purposes.

9. Immunogenicity of Ovarian Cystadenocarcinoma-Associated Antigens to the Host

Both humoral and cell-mediated immunity have been demonstrated in ovarian cancer patients against their tumors (11, 12, 14, 23). Dorsett *et al.* have isolated tumor-specific antibodies from peritoneal effusions of patients with ovarian cancer (14). Levi (23) reported evidence for the presence of circulating antibodies in advanced ovarian cancer patients to a tumor-associated antigen of ovarian cystadenocarcinoma by immunodiffusion studies. Utilizing both immunodiffusion and tanned cell hemagglutination technique, we have been unable to detect circulating antibodies to autologous crude, soluble tumor extracts in 20 patients with ovarian cancer (6). All these patients had advanced stage ovarian cancer, but several had relatively small tumor burdens in that they had known small amounts of residual tumor when they were tested. We plan to renew our search for circulating antibodies using purified antigen and more sensitive detection methods in patients with early stage disease.

Cell-mediated immunity to autologous tumor in patients with ovarian carcinoma has been demonstrated by leukocyte migration inhibition technique (11). Also, cytotoxicity by peripheral lymphocytes from ovarian cancer patients has been shown. However, the target cells in these studies were homologous tumor cells in tissue culture (12).

In order to detect cell-mediated immunity in ovarian cancer patients we tested the *in vitro* lymphocyte blastogenic response to phytohemagglutinin (PHA) and various concentrations of autologous tumor extracts (10). To evaluate immunocompetence *in vivo*, the same group of ovarian cancer patients was studied for delayed cutaneous hypersensitivity reactions against a battery of recall antigens and against their own tumor extracts (10).

None of the peripheral lymphocytes from ovarian cancer patients or control normal age-matched individuals were significantly stimulated in the presence of tumor extracts as measured by thymidine incorporation. In parallel experiments stimulation with PHA was observed indicating no inherent defect in the T-lymphocyte system of ovarian cancer patients. The tumor extracts tested did not have any cytotoxic effect on autologous or on homologous normal healthy lymphocytes. Hence, with this test system, no evidence for cell-mediated immunity to autologous tumor in ovarian cancer patients was observed. However, the possibility exists that *in vitro* lymphocyte blastogenic transformation is an inappropriate assay method with the tumor antigen under consideration. Under some circumstances lymphocyte transformation may be negative, while macrophage migration inhibition as an index of cell-mediated immunity is positive

(36). The exposure of presensitized lymphocytes to specific antigen may not necessarily induce activation leading to blast transformation. Instead, activation leading to the production of soluble factors which subsequently influence various cell types may occur. So, an attempt will be made to develop a macrophage migration inhibition test with purified tumor antigen to check the cell-mediated immunity of ovarian cancer patients.

Only a few of the ovarian cancer patients, when tested for delayed hypersensitivity reaction against a battery of recall antigens and Keyhole limpet haemocyanin, were completely anergic. None of the patients responded when skin tested with their own tumor extracts. It will be interesting to employ the purified tumor antigen for skin testing in the future.

10. Discussion

Evidence has been reviewed for the presence of a specific tumor-associated antigen for serous and mucinous cystadenocarcinomas of the ovary. Since serous and mucinous cystadenocarcinomas comprise 60–70% of all ovarian cancers, the potential applicability of OCAA as a tumor marker in the diagnosis and surveillance of women with ovarian cancer is extremely important. Ovarian cancer is an insidious disease in a deep seated organ which usually does not produce symptoms until the advanced stages of the disease. There is no reliable means of early diagnosis. It is also a cancer that has a high cure rate if treated in its early stages, but a very poor cure rate when treated in the advanced stages when, unfortunately, most patients are diagnosed. If a reliable immunodiagnostic screening test based on OCAA could be developed, most of the 10,000 women dying annually from ovarian cancer might be saved. Also, a reliable tumor marker for ovarian cancer would, as in the case of hCG in choriocarcinoma, be of enormous help in evaluating patients with regard to the need for additional or alternative therapy as well as determining the effect of present therapy.

The radioimmunoassay results indicate circulating OCAA in patients with advanced stage serous and mucinous cystadenocarcinomas of the ovary. However, cross-reactivity of OCAA with a normal serum and normal ovarian glycoprotein renders the current assay relatively insensitive. Our data suggest the feasibility of the detection of OCAA as an immunodiagnostic technique for early ovarian cancer if the sensitivity and specificity of this test can be improved.

In addition to OCAA, it will be important to search for a variety of other markers that may occur in cancer cells and some of which may correlate positively with ovarian cancer. Embryonic proteins that have been examined in ovarian cancers include Regan isoenzymes (15), hormones such as hCG (15), placental lactogen (34), CEA (40, 41), and α-fp (24, 42). Björklund (7) isolated from human placenta a tumor polypeptide antigen present in fifty percent of ovarian cancer patients' sera.

When sufficient data have been accumulated on ovarian cancers, they may reveal the presence of only a few distinct antigenic systems for this disease so a patient's urine, serum, or other tissue samples could be rapidly assayed for these known tumor antigen systems if panels of specific immunological reagents become available. The application of tumor-associated antigen assays in the management of patients with ovarian malignancy also offers a very promising area in the near future.

REFERENCES

1. Barlow, J. J., and Bhattacharya, M. 1975. Tumor markers in ovarian cancer: Tumor-associated antigens. *Seminars Oncol.* 2: 203–209.

2. Bhattacharya, M., and Barlow, J. J. 1973. Immunologic studies of human serous cystadenocarcinoma of ovary. Demonstration of tumor-associated antigens. *Cancer* 31: 588–595.

3. Bhattacharya, M., and Barlow, J. J. 1973. An immunologic comparison between serous cystadenocarcinoma of the ovary and other human gynecologic tumors. *Amer. J. Obstet. Gynecol.* 117: 849–853.

4. Bhattacharya, M., Barlow, J. J., Chu, T. M., and Piver, M. S. 1974. Tumor-associated antigen(s) from granulosa cell carcinomas of the ovary. *Cancer Res.* 34: 818–822.

5. Bhattacharya, M., and Barlow, J. J. 1975. A tumor-associated antigen for cystadenocarcinomas of the ovary. *Natl. Cancer Inst. Monogr.* 42: 25–32.

6. Bhattacharya, M., and Barlow, J. J. 1974. Tumor-associated antigen(s) from human cystadenocarcinoma of the ovary. *XI International Cancer Congress (Abstr.)* 2: 105.

7. Björklund, B. 1972. Immunological techniques for the detection of cancer, in B. Björklund (ed.), *Proc. Folksam Symp.* 1972. Stockholm, Sweden.

8. Burtin, P., and Chavanel, G. 1973. A new and fast method of preparation of CEA. *Ann. Immunol. (Inst. Pasteur).* 124C: 583–587.

9. Burton, R. M., Hope, N. J., Lubbers, L. M. 1976. A thermostable antigen associated with ovarian cancer. *Amer. J. Obstet. Gynecol.* 125: 472–477.

10. Chatterjee (Bhattacharya), M., Barlow, J. J., Allen, H. J., Chung, W. S., and Piver, M. S. 1975. Lymphocyte response to autologous tumor antigen(s) and phytohemagglutinin in ovarian cancer patients. *Cancer* 36: 956–962.

11. Chen, S. Y., Koffler, K., Cohen, C. J. 1973. Cell-mediated immunity in patients with ovarian carcinomas. *Amer. J. Obstet. Gynecol.* 115: 467–470.

12. DiSaia, P. J., Rutledge, F. N., Smith, J. P., and Sinkovics, J. G. 1971. Cell-mediated immune reaction to two gynecologic malignant tumors. *Cancer* 28: 1129–1137.

13. Dorsett, B. H., Ioachim, H. L. 1973. Common antigenic component in ovarian carcinomas: Demonstration by double diffusion and immunofluorescence techniques. *Immunol. Commun.* 2: 173–184.

14. Dorsett, B. H., Ioachim, H. L., Stolbach, L., Walker, J., and Barber, H. R. K. 1975. Isolation of tumor-specific antibodies from effusions of ovarian carcinomas. *Int. J. Cancer* 16: 779–786.

15. Fishman, W. H., Inglis, N. R., Vaitukaitis, J. L., and Stolbach, L. L. 1975. Regan isoenzyme and human chorionic gonadotropin in ovarian cancer. *Natl. Cancer Inst. Monogr.* 42: 63–73.

16. Gall, S. A., Walling, J., Pearl, J. 1973. Demonstration of tumor-associated antigens in human gynecologic malignancies. *Amer. J. Obstet. Gynecol.* 115: 387–393.

17. Goldenberg, D. M., Pletsch, Q. A., VanNagell, J. R. 1976. Characterization and localization of carcinoembryonic antigen in a squamous cell carcinoma of the cervix. *Gynecol. Oncol.* 4: 204–211.

18. Hellström, I., Hellström, K. E., Pierce, G. E., and Bill, A. H. 1968. Demonstration of cell-bound and humoral immunity against neuroblastoma cells. *Proc. Natl. Acad. Sci. U.S.A.* 60: 1231–1238.

19. Khoo, S. K. 1974. Radioimmunoassay for carcinoembryonic antigen: Its application to diagnosis and post-treatment follow-up of human cancer. *Med. J. Aust.* 1: 1025–1029.

20. Klein, G., Clifford, P., Klein, E., Smith, R. T., Minowarda, J., Kourilsky, F. M., and Burchenal, J. H. 1967. Membrane immunofluorescence reaction of Burkitt's lymphoma cells from biopsy specimens and tissue cultures. *J. Natl. Cancer Inst.* 39: 1027–1044.

21. Knauf, S., Urbach, G. I. 1974. Ovarian tumor-specific antigens. *Amer. J. Obstet. Gynecol.* 119: 966–970.

22. Kupchik, H. Z., Zamcheck, N., and Saravis, C. A. 1973. Immunochemical studies of carcinoembryonic antigens: Methodologic considerations and some clinical implications. *J. Natl. Cancer Inst.* 51: 1741–1749.

23. Levi, M. M. 1971. Antigenicity of ovarian and cervical malignancies with a view toward possible immunodiagnosis. *Amer. J. Obstet. Gynecol.* 109: 689–698.

24. Masopust, J., Kithier, K., Radl, J., Kouteck, Y. G., and Kotal, L. 1968. Occurrence of fetoprotein in patients with neoplastic and non-neoplastic diseases. *Int. J. Cancer* 3: 364–373.

25. Meeker, W. R., Kashmiri, R., Hunter, L., Clapp, W., Griffen, W. O. 1973. Clinical evaluation of carcinoembryonic antigen test. *Arch. Surg.* 107: 266–274.

26. Mehlman, D. J., Bulkley, B. H., Wiernik, P. H. 1971. Serum alpha-1-fetoglobulin with gastric and prostatic carcinomas. *N. Engl. J. Med.* 285: 1061–1960.

27. Metzgar, R. S., Mohankumar, T., Miller, D. S. 1972. Antigens specific for human lymphocytic and myeloid leukemia cells: Detection by nonhuman primate antiserums. *Science* 178: 986–988.

28. Morton, D. L., Malmgren, R. A., Holmes, E. C., and Ketcham, A. S. 1968. Demonstration of antibodies against human malignant melanoma by immunofluorescence. *Surgery* 65: 233–240.

29. Morton, D. L., and Malmgren, R. A. 1968. Human osteosarcomas: Immunologic evidence suggesting an associated infectious agent. *Science* 162: 1278.

30. Order, S. E., Chism, S., Hellman, S. 1973. Hodgkin's disease-associated antigens: Studies on segregation and specificities. *Natl. Cancer Inst. Monogr.* 36: 239–245.

31. Order, S. E., Thurston, J., and Knapp, R. 1975. Ovarian tumor antigens: A new potential for therapy. *Natl. Cancer Inst. Monogr.* 42: 33–43.

32. Pecora, P. F., Miroff, G., Li, M. C. 1974. Chemical and physical properties of a specific marker from mucinous cystadenocarcinoma of the human ovary. *XI. Int. Cancer Congress (Abstr.)* 1: 357.

33. Reynoso, G., Chu, T. M., Holyoke, D., Cohen, E., Nemoto, T., Wang, J. J., Chung, J., Guinan, P., and Murphy, G. P. 1972. Carcinoembryonic antigen in patients with different cancers. *J. Amer. Med. Assoc.* 220: 361–365.

34. Rosen, S. E., Weintraub, B. D., Vaitukaitis, J. L. 1975. Placental proteins and their subunits as tumor markers. *Ann. Int. Med.* 82: 71–83.

35. Smith, J. B. 1970. Alpha-fetoprotein. Occurrence in certain malignant diseases and review of clinical applications. *Med. Clin. North Amer.* 54: 797–803.

36. Spitler, L., Benjamini, E., Young, J. D., Kaplan, H., and Fudenberg, H. H. 1970. Studies on the immune response to a characterized antigenic determinant of the tobacco mosaic virus protein. *J. Exp. Med.* 131: 133–148.

37. Tatarinov, J. S. 1964. Presence of embryonal α-globulin in the serum of patients with primary hepatocellular carcinoma. *Vopr. Med. Khim.* 10: 90–91.

38. Thomson, D. M. P., Krupey, J., Freedman, S. O., and Gold, P. 1969. The radioimmunoassay of circulating carcinoembryonic antigen of the human digestive system. *Proc. Natl. Acad. Sci. U.S.A.* 54: 161–167.

39. VanKleist, S. 1973. Substances immunologically related to CEA. *Ann. Immunol. (Inst. Pasteur).* 124C: 589–593.

40. VanNagell, J. R., Meeker, W. R., Parker, J. C., and Harralson, J. D. 1975. Carcinoembryonic antigen in patients with gynecologic malignancy. *Cancer Res.* 35: 1372–1376.

41. VanNagell, J. R., Pletsch, Q. A., and Goldenberg, D. M. 1975. A study of cyst fluid and plasma carcinoembryonic antigen in patients with cystic ovarian neoplasms. *Cancer Res.* 35: 1433–1437.

42. Wilkinson, E., Frederick, E. G., Hosty, T. A. 1973. Alpha-fetoprotein and endodermal sinus of the ovary. *Amer. J. Obstet. Gynecol.* 116: 711–714.

CHAPTER 11

ROLE OF T CELLS, B CELLS AND MACROPHAGES IN IMMUNITY TO TESTICULAR TERATOCARCINOMAS OF THE MOUSE

Abdallam M. Isa

Departments of Microbiology and Ophthalmology
School of Medicine
Meharry Medical College
Nashville, Tennessee 37208

The role of T, B lymphocytes and macrophages in the immunity to teratocarcinoma 402 AX of the mouse has been studied. The effector cell type appears to have macrophage properties, while neither T nor B lymphocytes exhibit effector activity. The T lymphocyte appears to act as a suppressor cell, thus suppressing effector activity of the macrophage. Some soluble suppressor factor(s) are present in the ascitic fluid of tumor-bearing animals, and some of these factors are cytotoxic to normal lymphocytes and tumor cells.

I. INTRODUCTION

Teratocarcinomas, as other tumors, arise from normal stem cells. Confirmation of this was brought about by the discovery of Stevens (13) that embryonal carcinoma cells originate in the primordial germ cells of strain 129/J mice. These embryonic carcinomas may differentiate into embryonic tissue giving rise to a benign teratoma or to a malignant teratocarcinoma. When embryonic carcinoma cells differentiate into embryonic tissue the resulting tumors consist of derivatives of the three germ layers namely, the ectoderm, mesoderm, and endoderm (11).

II. DEFINITIONS AND PROPERTIES

Mouse testicular teratomas may arise spontaneously from cells of the testes or experimentally by the implantation of male fetal genital ridges into adult testes or presomitic embryos to extrauterine sites (13).

Mouse teratomas consist of ectodermal, mesodermal, and endodermal tissues. Teratomas originate from primordial germ cells and consist of multipotential cells which are capable of differentiating into different tissues. Based on their cell composition gonadal tumors were classified by Stevens and Pierce (15) as follows:

a. Embryonal carcinoma cells: These cells resemble embryonic cells, contain multipotential cells and are malignant. They can invade and metastasize.
b. Teratocarcinoma cells: Tumors containing embryonal carcinoma cells, ectodermal, mesodermal, and endodermal germ cells.
c. Teratoma cells: Are tumor cells in which the embryonal cells differentiate and the tumor stops growing.
d. Parietal yolk sac tumors: Are tumors of extra embryonic fetal membranes arising from embryonal carcinoma cells and consisting of distal endodermal cells that secrete Reichert's membrane.
e. Parietal yolk sac carcinoma: Are malignant parietal yolk sac tumors.

III. EMBRYO-TERATOMA RELATIONSHIP

Embryos develop following the fertilization of an ovum by a sperm cell. Primordial germ cells developing in the seminiferous tubules of the mouse fetus during the 12th day of gestation give rise to testicular teratomas (13). Ovarian teratomas arise from the parthenogenetic activation of eggs of female mice that are over one month of age.

In mature mice both testicular and ovarian teratomas have a variety of tissue types. In the early developmental stages however, cells resembling cleaving eggs appear in the ovarian but not in the testicular teratomas. Further, in the early stages of development unlike ovarian teratomas, testicular teratomas do not form trophoblastic cells. One exception to this was found in a spontaneous testicular teratocarcinoma in mice which contained trophoblastic giant cells. Normal embryos, ovarian and testicular teratomas are derived from germ cells and in the early stages of development, cells equivalent to the inner mass of normal blastocysts and the primary ectoderm of a 6-day embryo are present in the three of them.

IV. GROWTH PATTERNS OF TERATOMAS

A. In Vivo

We have been working with mouse testicular teratocarcinoma 402AX. This teratocarcinoma is an embryo-like tumor cell line originally derived from strain 129/J. Teratocarcinoma 402AX cells appear to consist of a mixture of cell types including cartilage, muscle and embryonal cells of various degrees of maturity (13).

In our experience teratocarcinoma 402AX cells grew much faster in the male than in the female. Development of the tumor started by the appearance of a nodule at the site of injection following the inoculation of the host a few days following tumor implantation (Fig. 1). This nodule represented a solid tumor growth which was then followed by an ascitis growth (Fig. 2), which led to death of the animal. The time of appearance of the tumor and death of the host was proportional to the tumor dose used. These data are depicted in Tables 1 and 2.

From the above data it would appear that male mice are more susceptible to infection by and death due to teratocarcinoma 402AX than female mice. This observation suggests that hormonal factors play a role in the growth and dissemination of this tumor, by possibly modifying the immune system of the host.

Enhancement of teratocarcinoma 402AX growth in the female as well as in the male however, was achieved by impairing the function of host macrophages (5). Tumor recipients were infused with a rabbit antiserum that was prepared specifically against mouse macrophages one day prior to, at the time of and one day post tumor implantation. Antimacrophage serum treatment of the host resulted in a significant reduction in the time of appearance of tumor growth and also in the time of death of both male

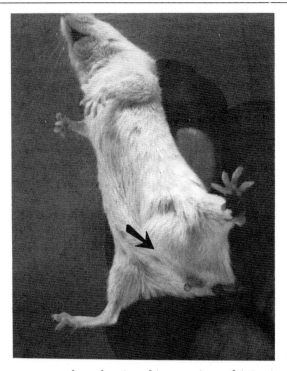

Fig. 1.   Solid tumor growth at the site of intraperitoneal injection (arrow).

and female mice, over that observed in recipients receiving normal rabbit sera.

Pluripotent embryonal carcinomas can be isolated from solid tumor growth. These solid tumors, in addition to containing embryonal carcinoma cells, they also contain a variety of differentiated cells. When grown in the ascitis form the cells aggregate forming embryoid bodies of two different types:

1.   Simple embryoid bodies consisting of inner cores of embryonal carcinoma cells and outer layers of endodermal cells.
2.   Cystic embryoid bodies consisting of embryoid carcinoma cells and variety of differentiated tissue and a cyst (10).

B. In Vitro

Several teratocarcinoma tumor cell lines have been isolated from mouse strain 129 tumors. These isolated clonal cell lines have been

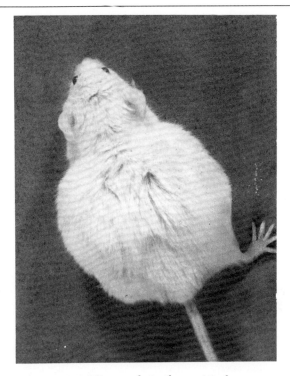

Fig. 2. Teratocarcinoma 402AX growth in the ascitis form.

shown to be multipotent since injection into syngeneic hosts resulted in tumors containing ectodermal, mesodermal and endodermal germ layer cells. Some of these clones require the help of feeder cultures to survive (9) others requires gelatin-coated substrate (8) and yet others do not require any help at all.

Table 1. Time of appearance of tumor and of death of Balb/c male mice following Teratocarcinoma 402AX cell implantation into the peritoneal cavity

Tumor Dose (cells)	Tumor Appearance (days)	Death of Host (days)
10^5	14 ± 2	29 ± 3
10^6	14 ± 2	28 ± 2
10^7	12 ± 3	26 ± 2
10^8	7 ± 2	14 ± 3

Table 2. Time of appearance of tumor growth and death of Balb/c female mice following teratocarcinoma 402AX cells implantation into the peritoneal cavity

Tumor Dose (cells)	Tumor Appearance (days)	Death of Host (days)
10^5	20 ± 1	44 ± 3
10^6	18 ± 2	39 ± 2
10^7	16 ± 2	36 ± 2
10^8	15 ± 2	30 ± 1

V. SURFACE ANTIGENS ON TERATOMAS

A. Histocompatibility Antigens

The ability of teratocarcinoma 402AX cells to grow in various strains of mice differing at the H-2 locus, in our laboratory, suggested to us that this tumor did not carry any of the major H-2 antigens (5). We have examined teratocarcinoma 402AX cells for H-2 antigens by immuno-fluorescence and by dye-exclusion cytotoxicity studies using anti-H-2 alloantisera. These alloantibodies were obtained through the courtesy of Dr. John G. Ray (Transplantation and Immunology Branch, National Institute of Allergy and Infectious Diseases, National Institutes of Health, Bethesda, Maryland).

1. Dye-Exclusion Cytotoxicity Assay.   Spleen cells from various strains were used as controls for the cytotoxicity assay. Spleen as well as 402AX teratocarcinoma cells were mixed with alloantisera of known H-2 specificity and incubated at 37°C for 30 minutes, in the presence of guinea pig complement. Following incubation, cells were washed three times with buffer containing both Ca^{++} and Mg^{++}. Trypan blue solution was added to each tube and the number of viable/dead cells counted. Spleen cells lysed in the presence of homologous allo-antiserum but in no instance we were able to demonstrate lysis of teratocarcinoma 402AX cells with any of the mouse anti-H-2 alloantisera in the presence of guinea pig or rabbit complement. Furthermore, when the anti-H-2 alloantisera were absorbed with teratocarcinoma 402AX cells the anti-H-2 activity in these allo-antisera was not changed thus suggesting that no H-2 antigenic specificities could be demonstrated on the surface of these teratocarcinoma 402AX cells (4).

2. Direct Immunofluorescence Assays. Anti-H-2 mouse al-loantisera were labeled with fluorescein-iso-thiocyanate according to the method of Cebra and Goldstein (3). Teratocarcinoma 402AX cells as well as spleen cell controls were treated with the fluorescein-labeled alloantis-era, mixed and incubated at 37°C for 30 minutes. Cells were washed three times with buffer and the cells were then spread on microscope slides, allowed to dry and then fixed in 95% ethanol. Cells treated in this manner were examined under ultraviolet light using a Zeiss fluorescence micro-scope illuminated with an Osram HBO-200 watt vapor lamp. A minimum of 200 cells were counted by two independent observers who did not know the identity of the cells. Cells showing fluorescence were recorded as positive. Spleen cells tested against homologous anti-H-2 alloan-tiserum were the only cells showing fluorescence. In no instance were we able to demonstrate fluorescence on teratocarcinoma 402AX cells. This observation indicated to us that the tumor cells were devoid of any dem-onstrable H-2 antigens. Indirect immunofluorescence assays could not be carried out on such ascites tumor cells because the cells were coated with anti-tumor antibodies. However, when the antibodies were eluted from the surface of tumor cells and then the cells treated with unlabeled anti-H-2 mouse alloantisera followed by treatment with fluorescein-labeled goat antimouse immunoglobulin, none of the cells showed any fluores-cence thus indicating that the tumor cells lacked any detectable H-2 anti-gens on their surface (4). The finding that teratocarcinoma 402AX cells lack any detectable H-2 antigens confirms the findings of Artzt and Jacob (2), who were unable to show the presence of H-2 antigens by reporting that antisera and complement were ineffective in causing lysis of F9 cells maintained *in vitro*.

3. ^{3}H-thymidine Cytotoxicity Assay. Tumor or spleen cells were labeled with ^{3}H-thymidine according to the method of Jagarlamoody et al. (7). Twenty million target cells were labeled with 40 microCurie of ^{3}H-thymidine provided as the methyl-^{3}H form from New England Nuclear. The cells were incubated with the label in a 5% CO_2-95% air and saturated humidity atmosphere at 37°C for 20–24 hours. the spe-cific activity of ^{3}H-thymidine used is 53.1 Ci/millimole. After incubation, the cells were washed in medium RPMI 1640 containing 10% fetal calf serum, and supplemented with penicillin, streptomycin and glutamine. Prior to the cytotoxicity assay, labeled target cells were suspended to contain one million cells per sample. Effector cells (macrophages, T lym-phocytes, or B lymphocytes) were added at an effector to target cell ratio of 10:1. The effector target cell mixture was incubated for 24 hours, and then the cells washed and resuspended in scintillation liquid and read for

Table 3. Percent cytotoxicity of ³H-thymidine-labeled 402AX cells when treated with effector cells

Effector Cell	Treatment	% Cytotoxicity
Spleen Cells	none	36
	anti-φ serum	88
Spleen Cells	none	30
	anti-kappa, lambda	35
Macrophage	none	65

radioactivity in a Beckman scintillation counter. Soluble suppressor factors (obtained from the fractionation of peritoneal exudate fluid on Sephadex G-200 or Bio-Gel A1.5m) was added in lieu of the effector cells at the ratio of 0.1 ml of the fraction to each 1 million labeled target cells. Per cent cytotoxicity was calculated according to the following formula:

$$\% \text{ Cytotoxicity} = 100 - \frac{\text{Sample Count} - \text{Background}}{\text{Control Count} - \text{Background}} \times 100$$

The results of these experiments are depicted in Table 3.

B. Tumor-Specific Antigens

A cell surface antigen that is shared by primitive teratocarcinoma cell lines is also demonstrable on the surface of morulae and spermatozoa as reported by Artzt et al. (1). This embryonic antigen was demonstrated by hyperimmunizing strain 129 male mice with primitive carcinoma cells. This antigen is expressed on all cells even after they differentiate into trophoblast and inner mass cells.

In our work (5) we have found teratocarcinoma 402AX cells to be immunogenic even in the original host, mouse strain 129. This immunogenicity was evidenced by the presence of antibodies coating the tumor cell surface (Fig. 3). These antibodies appear to be produced by the host in response to antigens present on the surface of tumor cells but absent from host tissues. Of course, this antigen is not a histocompatibility antigen since the mouse strain in which the tumor originated reacted by the production of antibodies specific to this antigen and also all attempts to demonstrate such H-2 antigens on the surface of 402AX tumor cells were unsuccessful. On the other hand, it is possible that this antigen might be a weak histocompatibility antigen which could not be detected by the reagents we used that are highly specific to the H-2 antigens.

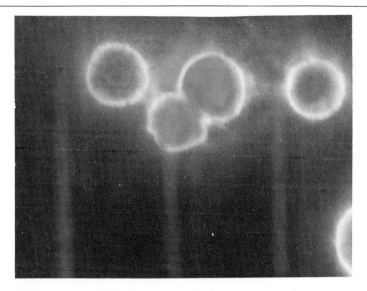

Fig. 3.   Ascitis 402AX cells coated with antibody.

We have attempted to produce tumor-specific antibodies in the rabbit by immunizing white New Zealand rabbits with suspensions of teratocarcinoma 402AX. Each animal received a total of 3×10^8 tumor cells via the intraperitoneal route over a period of six weeks. The first injection was given in complete Freund's adjuvants and the subsequent doses in normal saline. One week after the last injection, rabbits were bled and the serum separated, inactivated, and assayed for antibody activity by immuno-fluorescence and cytotoxicity assays. Since the ascitis 402AX tumor cells were used as the immunizing antigen, and although antibodies were eluted from the surface of these cells, rabbit anti-402AX antisera were repeatedly absorbed with mouse serum in order to remove any antibodies that might have been produced in response to mouse immunoglobulin and to insure that all the antibody activity in the rabbit serum is directed against 402AX specific antigens. In our experience, 402AX injected into mice via the subcutaneous route resulted in the production of solid tumor growth. Cells obtained from such solid tumors were consistently devoid of any antibody on their surfaces. Cells from solid 402AX growth were therefore used as the test antigen in immunofluorescence assays utilizing rabbit anti-402AX antisera. The presence of tumor-specific antibodies in the serum of rabbits was ascertained by the visible fluorescence observed on the surface of solid tumor cells following treatment with rabbit antiserum. Further absorption of the rabbit serum with mouse globulins did not remove antibody activity, but absorption with ascites or solid tumor cells rendered the rabbit antiserum devoid of any antibody activity against tumor cells. These findings indicate very strongly that rabbits reacted by the production of antibodies specific to 402AX specific antigens.

VI. TERATOMA-HOST INTERACTION

A. Humoral Immune Response

Almost invariably all 402AX tumor-bearing mice including syngeneic strain 129 responded by the production of antibodies to the tumor. In no instance were we able to demonstrate antitumor antibodies in the serum, but rather—almost invariably—these antibodies were found to be coating the ascitis tumor cells. Tumor cells from solid growth were always devoid of antibody on their surface. The antibodies that coat the surface of ascitis tumor cells were not limited to any one class of immunoglobulin. Using immunofluorescence assays, we were able to demonstrate antibodies of the IgM, IgA, IgG1, IgG2a, and IgG2b classes of immunoglobulins (5).

B. Cellular Immune Response

The findings in our laboratory that antibodies are produced in response to tumor-specific antigens and that these antibodies are coating the surface of the tumor cell, and the tumor is never rejected, but rather proliferates and kills the host regardless of its H-2 specificity suggested to us that immunity to this form of tumor is not mediated by antibody but rather might be mediated by a cellular immune mechanism.

Evidence implicating the macrophage as the possible effector cell type in immunity to 402AX came from studies with anti-macrophage serum. In these studies (5) we have produced an acceleration of the time of appearance and time of death of the host following impairment of the macrophage function by the injection of anti-macrophage serum. This effect was reproduced in both males and females irrespective of their histocompatibility antigenic specificity.

In order to unequivocally identify the effector cell type, we have to deal with 'purified' cell preparations of macrophages, thymus-dependent (T) lymphocytes and thymus-independent (B) lymphocytes. Effector cells were prepared from the spleen, thymus, lymph nodes, and peritoneal cavity from normal and from tumor-bearing animals at various times following tumor implantation in the following manner:

T Lymphocytes. Thymus-dependent (T) lymphocytes were prepared by teasing the cells from the lymphoid organs and preparation of single cell suspensions was achieved by passaging of the cells through various gauge needles. To eliminate macrophage contamination of the T cell population, the cells were incubated for 4–24 hours at 37°C in an atmosphere of 5% CO_2-95% air and saturated humidity. The adherent cells (macrophages) were discarded and the resulting cell suspension was treated with anti-macrophage serum and complement to remove any other macrophages not sticking to the solid surface, and also treated with anti-κ and anti-lambda antiserum and complement to remove any contaminating B lymphocytes. The resulting cells obtained in this manner were examined by immunofluorescence using fluorescein-labeled anti-θ alloantiserum, and also with fluorescein-labeled anti-κ and lambda antiserum. This cell population consisted of cells having the properties of T lymphocytes (about 95% and less than 1% B lymphocytes. The 'purified' T lymphocyte cell population prepared in this manner was then examined for its effector activity against 402AX target tumor cells, by the dye-exclusion and ^{3}H-thymidine cytoxicity assays. Cytotoxicity due to T lymphocytes was not higher than background levels.

B Lymphocytes. Thymus-independent B lymphocytes were prepared by the selective elimination of T lymphocytes and macrophages from the lymphoid cell population. T lymphocytes were eliminated by treating the cell population with anti-θ antiserum and complement and macrophages by incubation for 4–24 hours at 37 C in an atmosphere of 5% CO_2-95% air and saturated humidity and also by the addition of anti-macrophage serum and complement. B lymphocytes obtained following this treatment were examined for immunoglobulin content by immunofluorescence using fluorescein-labeled goat antimouse globulin or anti-κ and lambda antisera. The B cell population consisted of about 95% cells having the properties of B lymphocytes by virtue of their content of immunoglobulin. Examination of the effector activity of B lymphocytes on 402AX cells by dye exclusion and ^{3}H-thymidine cytotoxicity assays showed little activity that can be attributed to B lymphocytes.

Macrophages. Animals were stimulated for the production of macrophages by the injection of irradiated teratocarcinoma 402AX tumor cells, viable tumor cells or thioglycollate fluid medium. Four days after stimulation the peritoneal exudate was aspirated from the cavity and the peritoneal exudate was incubated at 37 C in an atmosphere of 5% CO_2-95% air and saturated humidity for 24–48 hours. The adherent cell population was then treated with anti-κ and lambda and anti-θ antisera and complement to remove any B cell and T cell contamination respectively.

After washing the macrophage monolayers, these macrophages were tested for their effector activity against teratocarcinoma 402AX target tumor cells by ^{3}H-thymidine and dye exclusion cytotoxicity assays. Effector cell activity was clearly demonstrated in the macrophage cell population (6).

C. Suppressor Activity

T-lymphocytes. "Purified" populations of T lymphocytes were prepared as described above. When the T lymphocyte cell population is used as an effector cell no demonstrable cytotoxic activity can be seen. If however, the ϕ-bearing lymphocytes are removed from this population there is an increase in the cytotoxic activity. Cytotoxic activity can be shown in the whole unfractionated lymphoid cell population, but highly significant increase in the cytotoxic activity is evidenced by the massive release of ^{3}H-thymidine from labeled target tumor cells by the selective removal of ϕ-bearing lymphocytes, by addition of anti-ϕ antiserum and complement. This effect was observed only when the effector cell population came from tumor-bearing animals. This 'suppressor activity' by T lymphocytes reached peak levels in C^{57}B1/6 mice at one week and in C^{3}H/HeJ mice at two weeks following tumor implantation. This effect was abolished and the cytotoxic activity declined to background levels by the third week following tumor implantation (6).

B Lymphocytes. Populations of B lymphocytes were prepared by the selective elimination of T lymphocytes and macrophages as described above. The ability of B lymphocytes to act as suppressor cells was assayed by cytotoxicity studies employing ^{3}H-thymidine tagged teratocarcinoma 402AX target tumor cells. The rationale for these studies was that if a cell type is behaving as a suppressor cell type then elimination of this cell type should show an increase in cytotoxic activity. B lymphocytes therefore, were treated with anti-κ and anti-lambda antisera in the presence of complement to eliminate any possible B lymphocyte contamination from lymphoid cell populations, and the resulting cell population was tested for its cytotoxic activity against ^{3}H-thymidine labeled teratocarcinoma 402AX cells. Our preliminary data indicate that the B lymphocyte population does not show any increase in the cytotoxic activity, indicating that B lymphocytes are not acting as suppressor cells.

Macrophages. Our studies indicate that the effector cell type against 402AX tumor cells whether in vivo by impairment of the macrophage function or in vitro by cytotoxicity studies is a cell having the characteristic of the macrophage. Removal of the macrophages by treatment with antimacrophage serum and complement or by incubation did not show an enhanced cytotoxic effect of the lymphoid cell population in the ^{3}H-thymidine cytotoxicity assay. We interpreted this effect to indicate that the macrophage does not appear to have any suppressor activity.

D. Soluble Suppressor Factors

Ascitis fluid was obtained from tumor-bearing animals prior to their death. Survival of the animals was prolonged following removal of the peritoneal exudate containing the tumor and the ascitis fluid. This ascitis fluid was separated by Gel filtration on Sephadex G-200 or on Bio-Gel A-1.5m columns. Using either separation method we were able to get 7 fractions, although the fractions on Bio-Gel were more distinct than those obtained on Sephadex G-200. Each fraction was pooled separately and concentrated to one fifth of the original fluid volume, and examined for its content of immunoglobulin by gel diffusion. Whereas fractions 1–3 had immunoglobulins, fractions 4–7 were either completely devoid of it or had very small amounts. We examined the fractions that did not contain any immunoglobulin by cytotoxicity assay on spleen cells from normal as well as from tumor-bearing animals and also on 402AX tumor

Table 4.   Percent viability of normal spleen cells after treatment with teratocarcinoma 402AX ascitis fluid fractions

Dilution	Fraction Number			
	IV	V	VI	VII
0	78	70	70	70
1/4	30	22	30	30
1/8	28	40	30	30
1/16	28	40	30	30
1/32	28	30	30	50
1/64	28	50	30	50
1/128	28	50	30	40
1/256	28	50	30	55
1/512	52	50	50	60
1/1024	56	73	50	60
1/2048	58	73	70	60

Table 5. Percent viability of teratocarcinoma 402AX cells folllowing
treatment with ascitis fluid fractions

Dilution	Fraction Number			
0	62	42	27	24
1/4	22	20	20	20
1/8	30	20	20	30
1/16	43	37	30	30
1/32	50	60	60	30
1/64	50	60	60	70
1/128	58	90	70	70
1/256	58	95	82	92
1/512	95	100	100	100
1/1024	100	100	100	100
1/2048	100	100	100	100

cells. We used a ratio of one-tenth milliliter of fraction for each one million cells and cytotoxicity was estimated by the dye-exclusion assay which was performed as follows:

Spleen or tumor cells were incubated with dilutions of the ascitis fluid fractions for one hour at 37 C. At the end of the incubation period the cells were washed three times in RPMI 1640 containing 10% fetal calf serum and to each tube was added 0.05 ml of freshly prepared trypan blue solution. The tubes were mixed and allowed to stand in an ice bath for 15 minutes and then the viability estimated. Results of a sample experiment are presented in Tables 4 and 5.

VII. CONCLUSIONS

From the foregoing discussion it would appear that immunity to teratocarcinoma 402AX in the mouse is mediated by a cellular immune mechanism, and not by antibodies. It does not appear that the cell-mediated immune reactions in this tumor system are antibody dependent since repeated studies with complement did not cause an enhancement of tumor cell killing in the presence of the effector cell or antibody, but on the contrary we showed that complement was protective against cell killing in many instances.

In attempting to identify the nature of the effector cell type, by selective elimination of one cell type at a time, we were able to show that the cell type capable of destroying tumor cells, whether by the dye exclusion cytotoxicity assay or by the ³H-thymidine cytotoxicity assay, to have macrophage properties.

Neither T lymphocytes nor B lymphocytes were capable of acting as effector cells. On the contrary, T lymphocytes acted as suppressor cells by somehow inhibiting cytotoxicity by other cells, but removal of T lymphocytes from the cell suspension led to an enhanced cytotoxic response sometimes exceeding 100% enhancement.

In an attempt to identify the suppressor factors, we were able to fractionate ascitis fluid from tumor bearing animals and found that several fractions had the ability to kill normal spleen cells in addition to killing tumor cells. In all instances spleen cell killing was more pronounced than tumor cell killing.

It does not seem inappropriate to speculate that the soluble factor(s) present in ascitis fluid of tumor-bearing animals have some resemblance to lymphokines; some of these are capable of killing spleen cells while others kill tumor target cells. It may follow that the killing of some spleen cells which might have acted as effector cells pave the way for the tumor to proliferate unabated. This might explain the invasiveness of this tumor which is never rejected, until death of the host.

REFERENCES

1. Artzt, K., Kobois, P., Babinet, D., Condamine, H., Babinet, C., and Jacob, F. 1973. Surface antigens common to mouse cleavage embryos and primitive teratocarcinoma cells in culture. Proc. Natl. Acad. Sci. (U.S.A.) 70: 2988.

2. Artzt, K., and Jacob, F. 1974. Absence of serologically detectable H-2 antigens on primitive teratocarcinoma cells in culture. Transplantation 17: 632.

3. Cebra, J. J., and Goldstein, G. 1965. Chromatographic purification of tetramethylrhodamice immune globulin conjugates and their use in the cellular localization of rabbit gamma-globulin polypeptide chains. J. Immunol. 95: 230.

4. Isa, A. M. 1976. Lack of demonstrable H-2 antigens on the surface of teratocarcinoma 402AX of the mouse maintained in vivo. Transplantation 21: 195–198.

5. Isa, A. M., and Sanders, B. R. 1975. Enhancement of tumor growth in allogeneic mice following impairment of macrophage function. Transplantation 20: 296–302.

6. Isa, A. M., and Sanders, B. R. 1976. Identification of suppressor cells in tumor immunity, in Ray G. Crispen (ed.), Neoplasm Immunity: Mechanism. 39, ITR, Chicago.

7. Jagarlamoody, S. M., Aust, J. C., Tew, R. H., and McKhann. 1971. In vitro detection of cytotoxic cellular immunity against tumor-specific antigens by a radioisotopic technique. Proc. Natl. Acad. Sci. (U.S.A.) 68: 1346.

8. Jami, J., and Ritz, E. 1974. Multipotentiality of single cells of transplantable teratocarcinomas derived from mouse embryo grafts. J. Natl. Cancer Inst. 52: 1547.

9. Kahan, B. W., and Ephrussi, B. 1970. Development potentialities of clonal *in vitro* cultures of mouse testicular teratomas. *J. Natl. Cancer Inst.* 44: 1015.

10. Martin, G. R., and Evans, M. J. 1975. The formation of embryoid bodies *in vitro* by homogeneous embryonal carcinoma cell cultures derived from isolated single cells, *in* M. I. Sherman and D. Solter (ed.), *Teratomas and Differentiation*, p. 169. Academic Press, Inc., New York.

11. Pierce, G. B. 1975. Teratomas: Introduction and Perspectives, *in* M. I. Sherman and D. Solter (ed.), *Teratomas and Differentiation*, p. 3. Academic Press, Inc., New York.

12. Stevens, L. C. 1958. Studies on transplantable testicular teratomas of strain 129 mice. *J. Natl. Cancer Inst.* 20: 1257.

13. Stevens, L. C. 1964. Experimental production of testicular teratomas in mice. *Proc. Natl. Acad. Sci. (U.S.A.)* 52: 654.

14. Stevens, L. C. 1968. The development of teratomas from intratesticular grafts of tubal mouse eggs. *J. Embryol. Exp. Morph.* 20: 329.

15. Stevens, L. C. 1975. Comperative development of normal and parthenogenetic mouse embryos and embryoid bodies, *in* M. I. Sherman and D. Solter (ed.), *Teratomas and Differentiation*, p. 17. Academic Press, Inc., New York.

16. Stevens, L. C., and Pierce, G. B. 1975. Definitions and Terminology, *in* M. I. Sherman and D. Solter (ed.), *Teratomas and Differentiation*, p. 13. Academic Press, Inc., New York.

CHAPTER 12

SECRETORY IMMUNOGLOBULINS AND CANCER

Rama Ganguly
and Robert H. Waldman

Departments of Internal Medicine
and Microbiology
West Virginia University
School of Medicine
Morgantown, West Virginia 26506

Studies of humoral immunity in patients with cancers have provided variable results. Immunoglobulin concentrations in serum and secretions have been found to be elevated, normal or decreased, reflecting various stages and types of malignancy, as well as amount and kind of therapy these patients received prior to evaluation. Correlation has been made between these levels and disease states for the purpose of screening and prognosis. Application of fluorescence microscopy for the detection of secretory component in mammary carcinoma tumor cells has been suggested for detecting metastatic breast cancer. Lack of an IgA antibody response to herpes virus type II in cervicovaginal secretions in women with carcinoma of the cervix has been reported and its implication in the development of this neoplasm is discussed.

Besredka, more than 50 years ago, proposed that there was an independent immune system resident on mucosal surfaces (4). For more than 30 years, it has been known that external secretions, such as those of the respiratory and gastrointestinal tracts, contain antibodies to various foreign substances, including viral and bacterial antigens (59, 15). Despite these and other observations, the vast majority of immunologists felt that antibody in external secretions were the result of transudation of serum antibody into the secretions. This "spill-over" concept was put to rest with the discovery by Hanson and Tomasi (20, 50) that the predominant immunoglobulin in external secretions is IgA, a relatively minor immunoglobulin in serum. This was strengthened by the observation that this IgA in secretions is of a slightly different structure than that found in serum, serum IgA being monomeric, 7S, with a molecular weight of about 170,000 daltons, while IgA in secretions is predominantly dimeric, 11S with a molecular weight of about 400,000. In addition, secretory IgA, as the IgA in secretions is called, contains a unique polypeptide attached to the heavy chains of the molecule, called secretory component, and also J chain, a polypeptide associated with polymeric immunoglobulins. Over the past 15 years, data have accumulated showing that secretory IgA is locally produced by plasma cells beneath the epithelium of mucosal surfaces, that local application of antigen is more efficient in stimulating the production of this antibody than is systemic immunization, and that antibody in secretions is important in protection against several infections of secretory surfaces (reviewed in Ref. 55).

The vast majority of infections occur either entirely on mucosal surfaces, or enter the body through mucosal surfaces. In fact, it is easier to think of exceptions to this, rather than to give examples of mucosal infections, the exceptions being infectious diseases which enter the body through breaks in the skin, such as hepatitis B (in many cases), malaria (through the bite of the mosquitoe), and so on. Because of this, most of the work concerning the secretory immune system has been in relationship to infectious diseases. However, as with infectious diseases, the vast majority of life-threatening malignancies also occur on secretory surfaces (42). Thus, the most common fatal malignancies are those of the respiratory, gastrointestinal, and genital tract. Therefore, it certainly seems reasonable to consider the relationship of the secretory immune system and cancer.

In addition to the fact that most fatal malignancies occur on mucosal surfaces, another reason for being concerned with the secretory immune system and cancer is the interesting relationship between IgA production and the thymus (49, 47, 54). Thymectomy in animal models has been commonly associated with subsequent IgA deficiency, and patients with IgA deficiency very commonly have defects in their cell-mediated immunity. This association of defects in IgA production and T cells may be of importance because of the strong association of cell-mediated immunity and protection against neoplasia (23, 43).

In considering the secretory immune system and its relationship to malignancies, there is not an overwhelming amount of data available. Therefore, in evaluating the situation, we must consider data that indirectly tell us something about the status of mucosal immunity, i.e., measurements of serum IgA levels. This is not ideal, but is not useless information either, since, with very few exceptions, patients who are deficient in serum IgA are also deficient in secretory IgA, and vice versa. There may be unrecognized exceptions to this generalization, however, and data are not available to delineate whether patients with slightly elevated or slightly depressed serum IgA levels also have correspondingly slightly elevated or depressed secretory IgA levels. Another unanswered question is whether there are patients with normal serum and secretory IgA levels who have a deficiency in antibody production, i.e., patients who have quantitatively normal levels of immunoglobulin, but qualitatively a deficiency in antibody production.

Secretory Immunoglobulins and Cancer

As stated above, IgA is the predominant immunoglobulin class secreted onto the mucosal surfaces of the lacrimal, respiratory, gastrointestinal, and genitourinary tracts and into saliva and colostrum (10, 48). The predominant antibody in all human secretions, including milk and colostrum, is IgA, and is synthesized in the submucosal plasma cells and linked with secretory component in the epithelial cells. External secretions contain immunoglobulins in concentrations different from those in serum, indicating the presence of a distinct secretory immune system (47, 49, 54). These secretory antibodies have been shown to be involved in protection against viral and bacterial diseases (7, 18, 55). Experimentally, local immunoglobulin production is greatly enhanced by local antigenic stimulation, e.g., by antigen injected into the lactating mammary gland or ingested so as to reach the intestinal mucosa (14, 17, 19, 32). Data suggest that complete development of the IgA system depends on a functioning thymus (9, 35, 36). This might explain the increased incidence of neoplasia, especially pulmonary and gastrointestinal malignancies, and autoimmune disorders in patients with IgA deficiency (58).

Most fatal neoplasms occur at contact points where we meet our external environment (42). In other words, these life-threatening disorders develop along the mucosal or secretory surfaces of the gastrointestinal, respiratory or genitourinary tracts and are epithelial in nature. Most of the reported studies have centered around measuring immunoglobulin levels in secretions and sera of cancer patients and studied their variations with the clinical course of the disease. While these data are helpful, the cause and/or effect relationship to the neoplastic disease remains speculative.

Serum IgA Levels

Studies of humoral immunity in patients with malignancies have provided variable results. Immunoglobulin concentrations in serum have been found to be elevated, normal or decreased, and this is also the case with secretory immunoglobulin levels. One possible explanation for this variability is that these data reflect various types and stages of malignancy, as well as amount and kind of therapy the patients received prior to evaluation.

Increased levels of IgA in the serum and whole saliva of patients with neoplastic disease have been reported. Hughes et al. (25) (Table 1) studied serum concentrations of IgG, IgA, and IgM immunoglobulins in patients with carcinoma, melanoma, and sarcoma. They observed that patients with carcinoma of the skin and lung had significantly increased IgG and

Table 1. IgG immunoglobulin concentrations in sera from normal controls and some patients with cancer

Group	Number	Range	Mean (mg/100 ml)	SD	P [b]
Normal controls					
Male	106	672–1984	1148	224	
Female	150	577–2257	1157	271	
Skin[a]					
Male	32	787–2200	1344	357	0.01 > p > .001
Female	19	820–1620	1150	241	
Lung					
Male	89	598–3300	1403	417	0.001 > p
Female	9	880–2120	1534	359	10.001 > p

a. Consists of squamous cell carcinoma of skin, vulva, sweat glands adenoma, penis.
b. P values on basis of student's t test.

Source: Modified from Hughes et al. (25).

IgA levels. IgA was significantly increased in patients with cancer of the mouth, gut, and uterus. Serum IgM concentrations were significantly increased in male patients with sarcoma and in female patients with melanoma. Patients with primary ovarian cancer had a significantly lower than normal IgM concentration. The authors suggested that cancer of such tissues as the lung, mouth and gastrointestinal tract could result in an increased infection rate and therefore an enhanced local antigenic stimulus of those sites, thus inducing higher levels of local immunoglobulin synthesis. Since most of serum IgA comes from synthesis in the mucosae, it would be expected that IgA levels in sera would be elevated. It is interesting to note that in patients with lung cancer and carcinoma of the skin, a concomitant rise in serum IgG levels was also noticed, resulting in no change in the IgA/IgG ratio. This is in contrast to the exclusive IgA rise in patients with carcinoma of the orogastric tract. Levels of immunoglobulins in secretions were not studied in these patients.

The malignant tissues involved in the patients described above, those with increased IgA and/or IgG levels, are those continually exposed to the external environment, i.e., skin, mouth, lung, and gut. The authors observed that since IgA and IgG levels in most remaining patients with cancers of organs less directly exposed to infection were within normal range, the most likely explanation of the increased immunoglobulin levels is that they are a response to microbial invasion through the malignant epithelium.

Elevated IgA levels in patients with cancer of epithelial secretory organs such as the prostate, uterus, and lung have also been reported (1, 53, 56) (Table 2). Others have reported elevated levels of IgG and IgA with the stage of tumor progress (24, 60, 63). Zeromski et al. (62) studied the behavior of local and systemic immunoglobulins in patients with lung cancer. They observed that in the vicinity of the primary lung cancer and in the regional lymph nodes, intensive immunoglobulin synthesis in plasma cells with a predominance of the IgA and IgG classes was taking place. There were significantly elevated serum immunoglobulin levels with a predominance of IgA and IgG. Inoperable patients showed higher immunoglobulin concentrations than those who underwent surgery.

Wara et al. (60, 61) suggested that serum IgA levels may be of value as a screening test for nasopharyngeal carcinoma in a high risk population, i.e., Chinese with recurrent otitis media. They evaluated serum immunoglobulin levels, antibody responses and cell-mediated immunity (CMI) in patients with carcinoma of the nasopharynx. They noted elevated levels of serum IgA in patients with nasopharyngeal carcinoma and paranasal sinus carcinoma prior to radiation therapy. After treatment, the IgA levels were lower in the nasopharyngeal carcinoma patients. Elevated IgA levels were also noticed in patients with recurrent disease. Seven out of fourteen

Table 2. IgA immunoglobulin concentrations in sera from normal controls and some patients with cancer

Group	Number	Range	Mean (mg/100 ml)	SD	P[a]
Normal controls					
Male	106	60–528	201	89	
Female	150	17–395	174	80	
Skin					
Male	32	141–471	273	105	0.001 > P
Female	19	87–530	204	97	
Lung					
Male	89	70–792	280	144	0.001 > P
Female	8	84–265	164	63	

a. P values on basis of Student's *t* test as in Table 1.
Source: Modified from data of Hughes *et al.* (25).

patients demonstrated depressed CMI as measured by delayed hypersensitivity skin testing, total lymphocyte count, *in vitro* blastogenic response to PHA and T-cell-rosette formation. The authors suggested, therefore, that in the high risk population, in the absence of any lesions in the nasopharynx but an elevated serum IgA level, a biopsy may be indicated. The differential diagnosis of recurrent tumor or radionecrosis following therapy for nasopharyngeal carcinoma is relatively common. In these patients, an elevated serum IgA indicated recurrent tumor, prompting a new biopsy of the nasopharynx and additional therapy. As association between EBV and tumor has been demonstrated (24, 63), the elevated IgA levels could be due to specific antibody formation against EBV antigen or against a complex of EBV and tumor cells. In their study, Wara *et al.* (60) isolated and partially characterized the serum IgA from patients with nasopharyngeal carcinoma. Preliminary studies utilizing direct fluorescent microscopy indicate that IgA surrounds nasopharyngeal carcinoma cells, indicating IgA specificity against a unique tumor antigen. In addition, these patients had elevated serum IgA antibody titers to EBV.

In contrast to the above study, Meyer *et al.* (33) found no correlation in patients with breast cancer, who had not been irradiated, between IgA levels and recurrence. They studied IgA levels and total lymphocyte counts in 42 women with axillary node metastases at mastectomy. Recurrence after irradiation was, however, found to correlate significantly with an IgA level of less than 200 mg/100 ml and a lymphocyte count of less than 1500/cu mm. The irradiated group with high IgA levels remained tumor-free. From these results it was concluded that postmastectomy ir-radiation is detrimental to patients with a low IgA concentration, and may improve survival in women with a high preoperative IgA level.

Secretory Component

Harris et al. (21) recently studied localization of secretory compo-nent (SC) in human mammary carcinoma. It is known that SC is a distinct antigenic glycoprotein component of the whole secretory IgA molecule. It is synthesized by the epithelial cells. The dimeric IgA molecule (devoid of SC) is synthesized by the plasma cells (8, 51) of the lamina propria, and on its passage through epithelial cells combines with the SC. This complex is then secreted from the luminal side of the cells as intact secretory IgA (S-IgA). Harris and co-workers determined whether SC, which is a normal glandular epithelial product, could be demonstrated in an epithelial cancer by employing immunofluorescence microscopy (21). Ten cases of normal breast tissue showed fluorescent epithelial cells confined to nor-mal ducts. This was found to be in marked contrast to invasive mammary carcinomas (20 cases), which showed intense staining of tumor cells and stromal cells in addition to the normal ductular epithelium. Intense fluorescence for secretory component was observed in axillary lymph nodes with metastases (2 cases) whereas axillary lymph nodes without metastases (2 cases) showed no fluorescence. In both normal and tumor tissue, antisera to IgA stained only ducts and subepithelial plasma cells. Preliminary studies of colon, lung and bladder carcinoma also revealed similar findings of tumor cells with cytoplasmic fluorescence for SC. In contrast, they observed that tumor cells in two cases of sarcoma did not show fluorescence for SC. It is difficult to determine from these data if the fluorescence seen is the result of the local production of SC by the tumor cells or the result of absorption onto the tumor cells after SC has been synthesized by the normal ductular epithelial cells. However, since there are no normal ductular epithelial cells in lymph node metastases, it is strongly suggestive of synthesis of SC by the neoplastic cells themselves. Since the normal axillary lymph nodes from two patients with mammary carcinoma did not show fluorescing cells, it appeared that drainage of the involved area is not sufficient to give the fluorescent cellular pattern but the presence of tumor cells in the section was required. They also ob-served that cells in the adjacent normal lymph node structure of cancer-ous nodes had fluorescence. They postulated that the SC was produced in nearby tumor cells and subsequently was absorbed onto these apparently normal cells. This probably also explained the stromal fluorescence seen in the primary lesions. Tumor cells did not show fluorescence with anti-

IgA sera, indicating that the SC seen in tumor cells was not part of an intact S-IgA molecule or host response to tumor. They also pointed out that SC in the tumor cells from a variety of cancers may have potential significance in understanding regulation of the immune response to these neoplasms. An obvious clinical application of this finding and one that needs to be evaluated is the use of immunofluorescence microscopy to examine suspected metastases of epithelial cancers for the presence of SC, which also may be a more sensitive technique compared to light-microscopic examination for tiny foci of tumor cells. Further work is needed in this area to characterize and confirm the endogenous production of SC by neoplastic cells. Surface immunoglobulin positive lymphocytes in human breast cancer tissue and lymph nodes have been reported in several studies (38, 39, 52).

IgA Levels in Secretions

Mandel et al. (30, 31) investigated salivary immunoglobulins in patients (Table 3) with oropharyngeal and bronchopulmonary carcinoma. These workers observed that oropharyngeal cancers are found almost exclusively in patients with histories of smoking and/or alcoholism (26, 37). They determined the relationship between these habits, the secretion of local immunoglobulins, and cancer. IgA was found to be the predominant, often exclusive immunoglobulin in the secretion. Also, they noted that the highest salivary immunoglobulin levels were present in patients

Table 3. Salivary IgA titers in patients with cancer

	Mean Titers (mg)/15 min Collection		
	Smoker	Smokers and Drinkers	Total
Oropharyngeal carcinoma	1,97 (20) (SD ± 0.46)	2.37 (14) (SD ± 0.70)	2.15 (35)[a] (SD ± 0.65)
Bronchogenic carcinoma	1.98 (11) (SD ± 0.31)	2.14 (23) (SD ± 0.52)	2.11 (35)[b] (SD ± 0.49)

a. Includes one non-smoker and non-drinker with oropharyngeal carcinoma having titer 2.90 mg/15 min collection.

b. Includes bronchogenic carcinoma patient with non-smoker and non-drinker whose titer was 2.55 mg/15 min collection.

Source: Modified from data of Mandel et al. (31).

with oropharyngeal and bronchopulmonary carcinomas. Furthermore, smoking and alcoholism resulted in markedly elevated salivary immunoglobulin secretion. The workers postulated that drinking and smoking affect salivary IgA production, acting as chronic irritants like nonspecific secretagogues (13) or as antigenic stimuli (22).

The effects of nonrelated cancer and oral inflammation on salivary IgA was also studied. Patients with cancer of the genitourinary tract who neither smoked nor drank had normal IgA titers. Patients with oropharyngeal neoplasms had consistently higher titers of salivary IgA than did groups of age-controlled normal patients. This might represent the body's attempt to eliminate neoplastic clones. Since spontaneous regression of tumor was not observed in any patient, this response was obviously ineffective. This salivary IgA could be enhancing type antibody (2, 34) helping in inducing or maintaining neoplastic growth, with a net deleterious effect on the host. Another possibility is that these high levels of IgA result from serum transudation through inflamed capillary networks or that under these disease conditions, changes in secretory dynamics occur, resulting in an alteration in the relative proportions of immunoglobulin-producing cells in the oropharyngeal tract. Patients with oral inflammatory conditions were found to have comparable IgA titers with the chronic smokers, but qualitatively the relative proportions of 7S and 11S IgA were quite different. These data suggest that the processes responsible for the elevated titers in the chronic smokers and oral inflammatory group of patients are mediated through different mechanisms.

Brown et al. (5, 6) more recently studied the correlation of the secretory immunoglobulins in the saliva of patients with progress of their neoplastic disease. They observed that oral and laryngeal cancer patients had a two-fold increase of serum and salivary IgA compared to controls. Recurrent cancer patients had an even greater elevation of salivary IgA. Cured patients exhibited a persistent elevation of serum, but a return to normal of salivary IgA. A follow up study of 26 patients confirmed this pattern of a drop in whole salivary IgA with cure and a spike with recurrence. In this study IgG in saliva of patients also was detected, indicating probable serum leakage or exudation (45). However, the salivary IgA of these patients did not correlate with their elevated albumin or IgG levels, indicating IgA production occurred predominantly locally in these individuals. These authors suggested, based on their data, that salivary IgA levels may prove to be useful in distinguishing patients with possible recurrent diseases.

The above data refute the contention that higher serum immunoglobulin levels in patients with cancer of epithelial secretory organs are due to reabsorption of salivary contents back into the serum due to widespread inflammation of the epithelial surfaces (46). Other reports suggest that damage due to chronic respiratory infection in lung disease is, in fact, associated with unchanged or depressed serum IgA levels (56, 44). Similar observations of unchanged levels of serum and salivary immunoglobulins were made by Lehner with regard to patients with oral aphthous stomatitis (28).

Levy et al. (29) studied gastric IgA levels in patients with carcinoma of the stomach. Secretory IgA levels were found to be significantly higher in patients with gastric malignancies than in patients with benign lesions of the stomach. Patients in whom the cancer was locally confined to the stomach and not metastatic or massively invading the entire gastric wall, IgA levels were found to be significantly elevated. As the tumor progressed, the secretory IgA levels seemed to decline, as a result of either direct invasion of the tumor into the wall of the stomach with loss of secretory cell mass, overwhelming antigen excess, or immunologic exhaustion of the comitted cell clones. They also suggested that locally produced immunoglobulin titers may be of value when used in conjunction with other diagnostic modalities in determining the nature of gastrointestinal lesions.

Dent and Bienenstock (11) observed that cervicovaginal secretions of 57 patients with carcinoma of the cervix and 28 normal women contained no IgA antibodies to herpes virus type II. Approximately one-third of both groups possessed IgA antibodies to another local pathogen, Candida albicans. There was higher frequency of serum IgA anti-herpes antibodies in these patients studied. They also observed that total IgA immunoglobulin levels in serum and secretions were significantly higher in the patient group.

It is noteworthy in this regard that herpes virus type II (HSV II) has been implicated in the etiology of carcinoma of the cervix on the basis of a considerable accumulation of indirect evidence (3, 16, 60, 61). The absence of a local IgA antibody response to HSV II in both patients and controls is of interest with regard to the nature of the immunologic response this particular pathogen elicits. It is possible that the secretory IgA response to this pathogen is of short duration in the absence of repeated exposure. Dent and Bienenstock speculated that the absence of an IgA antibody response to HSV II could play a critical role in determining the oncogenic potential of this pathogen.

Secretory IgA Levels in Serum

Secretory IgA was thought not to be found in serum until its presence was demonstrated in the serum of normal individuals and, in increased frequency, in the serum of patients with chronic inflammatory

Table 4.   Secretory IgA levels in sera of patients with various diagnoses

Diagnosis	Serum S IgA	≥0.10/Total[a]
Liver diseases		
Laennec's cirrhosis	0.10	6/10
Hepatitis	0.07	1/5
Lymphoma-leukemia involving liver	0.15	3/4
Carcinoma metastatic to liver	0.10	3/4
Hepatoma	0.31	1/1
Pulmonary diseases		
Carcinoma	0.07	2/5
Chronic bronchitis	0.04	0/4
Pulmonary embolus	0.04	0/4
Other	0.05	1/5
Renal diseases	0.04	0/12
Hematologic diseases		
Lymphoma	0.09	2/4
Leukemia	0.11	3/6
Myeloma	0.11	1/2
Endocrinologic diseases		
Thyroid	0.06	0/4
Diabetes mellitus	0.06	1/13
Cardiovascular diseases		
Myocardial infarction	0.05	1/8
Hypertension	0.04	0/10
Cerebrovascular	0.08	1/5
Neurologic diseases	0.05	3/20
Psychiatric disorders	0.05	3/11
Cancer	0.06	4/14
Metastatic	0.07	3/9
Not metastatic	0.04	1/5
Metastatic to liver	0.10	3/4
Metastatic, not to liver	0.06	0/5
Allergic conditions	0.02	0/5
Infectious diseases	0.04	3/21

a. Number of specimens with levels ≥0.10 per total number examined.
Source: Modified from Waldman et al. (57).

diseases of the bowel (57). This observation was extended in a study which described a more sensitive and quantitative technique for measuring serum S IgA levels (28). In that study it was shown that S IgA was present in small quantities (average of 0.03 mg per ml) in nearly all normal individuals, and in increased amounts in a variety of conditions, including cancers, lactating females, and, in particularly high levels, in a patient with primary hepatoma (Table 4).

When patients with neoplasms were divided into those with no metastases, metastases elsewhere than to the liver, and those with hepatic metastases, there was no significant difference between the patients with no metastases and those with metastases to non-hepatic foci; however, significantly elevated levels were found in patients with hepatic involvement. Measurement of S IgA levels in serum might be useful in identifying patients with neoplasms with hepatic involvement.

REFERENCES

1. Ablin, R. J., Gorden, M. J., and Soane, W. A. 1972. Levels of immunoglobulin in the sera of patients with carcinoma of the prostate. Neoplasma 19: 57–60.

2. Amos, D. B., Cohen, I., and Klein, W. J. 1970. Mechanisms of immunological enhancement. Transplant. Proc. 2: 68–75.

3. Aurelian, L., Strandberg, J. D., Melendez, L. V., and Johnson, L. A. 1971. Herpes virus type 2 isolated from cervical tumor cells grown in tissue culture. Science 174: 704–707.

4. Besredka, A. 1927. Local Immunizations, p. 181. Williams and Wilkins, Baltimore.

5. Brown, A. M., Lally, E. T., Frankel, A., Harwick, R., Davis, L. W., and Rominger, C. J. 1975. The association of the IgA levels of serum and whole saliva with the progression of oral cancer. Cancer 35: 1154–1162.

6. Brown, A. M., Lally, E. T., and Frankel, A. 1975. IgA and IgG content of the saliva and serum of oral cancer patients. Arch. Oral Biol. 20: 395–398.

7. Burrows, W., Deupree, N. G., and Moore, D. E. 1950. The effect of x-radiation on fecal and urinary antibody response. J. Inf. Dis. 87: 169–193.

8. Cebra, J. J., and Small,P. A. 1967. Polypeptide chain structure of rabbit immunoglobulins. III. Secretory gamma A immunoglobulins from colostrum. Biochemistry 6: 503–512.

9. Clough, J. D., Mims, L. H., and Strober, W. J. 1971. Deficient IgA antibody responses to arsanilic acid bovine serum albumin (BSA) in neonatally thymectomised rabbits. J. Immunol. 106:1624–1629.

10. Dayton, D. H. (ed.) 1971. Conference on the secretory immunologic system, Vero Beach, FL, 1969, Bethesda, MD; National Institute of Child Health and Human Development.

11. Dent, P. B., and Bienenstock, J. 1974. Absence of IgA antibody to Herpes virus in cervicovaginal secretions of patients with carcinoma of the cervix. Clin. Immunol. Immunopath. 3: 171–177.

12. Dostalova, O., Schol, E., Wagnerova, M., Jelinek, J., and Wagner, V. 1976. Serum immunoglobulin levels in cancer patients. II. Serum immunoglobulins and stage of tumor progress. Neoplasma 23: 95–102.

13. Falk, H. L., Kotin, P., and Rowlette, W. 1967. The response of mucus secreting epithelium and mucus to irritants. Ann. N.Y. Acad. Sci. 106: 583–608.

14. Felsenfeld, O. 1968. Proteins and related subjects: Immunoglobulin production and secretion into the intestinal tract of primates under the influence of some antigenic stimuli, in H. Peters (od.), Protides of the Biological Fluids, Vol. 16, p. 469. Pergamon Press, Oxford.

15. Francis, T., Jr. 1941–42. Factors conditioning resistance to epidemic influenza. Harvey Lectures 37: 69.

16. Frenkel, N., Roizman, B., Cassai, E., and Nahmias, A. 1972. A DNA fragment of herpes simplex 2 and its transcription in human cervical cancer tissue. Proc. Natl. Acad. Sci. 69: 3784–3789.

17. Ganguly, R., Clem, L. W., Bencic, Z., Sinha, R., Sakazaki, R., Waldman, R. H. 1975. Antibody response in the intestinal secretions of volunteers immunized with various cholera vaccines. Bull. Wld. Hlth. Org. 52: 323–330.

18. Ganguly, R., Ogra, P. L., Regas, S., Waldman, R. H. 1973. Rubella immunization of volunteers via the respiratory tract. Inf. Immun. 8: 497–502.

19. Genco, R. J., Taubman, M. A. 1969. Secretory gamma A antibodies induced by local immunization. Nature 221: 679–687.

20. Hanson, L. A. 1961. Comparative immunological studies of the immunoglobulins of human milk and blood serum. Int. Arch. Allergy Appl. Immunol. 18: 241–267.

21. Harris, J. P., Caleb, M. H., and South, M. A. 1975. Secretory component in human mammary carcinoma. Cancer Res. 35: 1861–1864.

22. Hattler, B., and Amos, B. 1966. The immunobiology of cancer. Tumor antigens and the responsiveness of the host. Monogr. Surg. Sci. 3: 1–34.

23. Hellström, I., Hellström, K. E., Sjögren, H. O., and Warner, G. A. 1971. Demonstration of cell-mediated immunity to neoplasms of various types. Int. J. Cancer 7: 1–6.

24. Henle, W., Henle, G., Ho, G. C., Burtin, P., Cachin, Y., Clifford, P., Schryver, A., De-The, G., Diehl, and Klein, G. 1970. Antibodies to Epstein Barr virus in nasopharyngeal carcinoma, other head and neck neoplasms and control groups. J. Natl. Cancer Inst. 44: 225–231.

25. Hughes, N. G. 1971. Serum concentrations of IgG, IgA and IgM immunoglobulins in patients with carcinoma, melanoma and sarcoma. J. Natl. Cancer Inst. 46: 1015–1027.

26. Keller, A. Z. 1967. Cirrhosis of the liver, alcoholism and heavy smoking associated with cancer of the mouth and pharynx. Cancer 20: 1015–1022.

27. Krant, M. J., Manskopf, G., Brandrup, C. S., Madoff, M. A. 1968. Immunologic alterations in bronchogenic cancer. Cancer 21: 623–631.

28. Lehner, T. 1969. Immunoglobulin estimation of blood and saliva in human recurrent oral ulceration. Arch. Oral Biol. 14: 351–364.

29. Levy, M., Petreshock, P., Mandell, C., Deysine, M., Katzka, I., and Aufses, A. H. 1974. Response of gastric IgA in patients with gastric malignant neoplasms. Surg. Forum 25: 91–93.

30. Mandel, M. A., Dvorak, K., and DeCosse, J. J. 1972. Secretory immunoglobulin levels in cancer patients. Surg. Forum 23: 512–514.

31. Mandel, M. A., Dvorak, K., DeCosse, J. J. 1973. Salivary immunoglobulins in patients with oropharyngeal and bronchopulmonary carcinoma. Cancer 31: 1408–1413.

32. McDowell, G. H., and Lascelles, A. K. 1969. Local production of antibody of ovine mammary glands infused with Salmonella flagellar antigens. Aust. J. Exp. Biol. Med. Sci. 47: 669–678.

33. Meyer, K. K., Mackler, G. L., and Beck, W. C. 1973. Increased IgA in women free of recurrence after mastectomy and radiation. Arch. Surg. 107: 159–161.

34. Mollar, G. 1963. Studies on the mechanism of immunological enhancement of tumor homografts. II. Effect of isoantibodies on various tumor cells. J. Natl. Cancer Inst. 30: 1153–1226.

35. Perey, D. T. E., and Bienenstock, J. J. 1976. Effects of bursectomy and thymectomy on ontogeny of fowl IgA, IgG and IgM. J. Immunol. 111: 633–637.

36. Perey, D. Y. E., Frommel, D., Hog, R., and Good, R. A. 1970. The mammalian homologue of the avian bursa of Fabricius: II. Extirpation, lethal X-irradiation and reconstitution in rabbits: Effects on humoral immune responses, immunoglobulins, and lymphoid tissue. Lab. Invest. 22: 212–227.

37. PHS Publication No. 1696. 1968. The Health Consequences of Smoking. United States Department of Health, Education and Welfare.

38. Richters, A., and Kaspersky, C. J. 1974. Human breast cancer and lymph node lymphocyte surface immunoglobulins. Fed. Proc. 33: 610.

39. Richters, A., and Kaspersky, C. L. 1975. Surface immunoglobulin positive lymphocytes in human breast cancer tissue and homolateral axillary lymph nodes. Cancer 35: 129–133.

40. Rowinska-Zakrewska, E., Lazar, P., and Burtin, P. 1970. Serum immunoglobulin levels in malignant disease. Ann. Inst. Pasteur Paris 119: 621–625.

41. Royston, I., and Aurelian, L. 1969. Immunofluorescent detection of herpes virus antigens in exfoliatic cells from human cervical carcinoma. Proc. Natl. Acad. Sci. 67: 204–212.

42. Silverberg, E., and Holleb, A. I. 1971. Cancer statistics, 1971. Can. J. Clin. 21: 12–31.

43. Smith, R. T., and Landy, M. 1970. Immune Surveillance. Academic Press, New York.

44. South, M. A., Cooper, J., Wooheim, F. A., and Good, R. 1968. The IgA system II. The clinical significance of IgA deficiency. Amer. J. Med. 44: 168–198.

45. Strober, W., Blaese, R. M., and Waldman, T. A. 1970. The origin of salivary IgA. J. Lab. Clin. Med. 75: 856–862.

46. Thompson, R. A., and Asquith, P. 1970. Quantitation of exocrine IgA in human serum in health and disease. Clin. Exp. Immunol. 7: 491–500.

47. Tomasi, T. B. 1972. Secretory immunoglobulins. N. Engl. J. Med. 287: 500–506.

48. Tomasi, T. B., and Grey, H. M. 1972. Structure and function of immunoglobulin A. Prog. Allergy 16: 87–213.

49. Tomasi, T. B., Jr., Tan, E. M., Solomon, A., Prendergast, R. A. 1965. Characteristics of an immune system common to certain external secretions. *J. Exp. Med.* 121: 101–124.

50. Tomasi, T. B. Jr., Zigelbeaum, S. D. 1963. The selective occurrence of γ1 A globulins in certain body fluids. *J. Clin. Invest.* 42: 1552–1560.

51. Tourville, D. R., Adler, R. H., Bienenstock, J., and Tomasi, T. B. 1969. The human secretory immunoglobulin system: Immunohistological localization of gamma A₁ secretory "piece" and lactoferrin in normal human tissues. *J. Exp. Med.* 129: 411–429.

52. Tsakraklides, E., Tsakraklides, V., and Good, R. A. 1974. T and B cells in the axillary lymph nodes of patients with operable breast carcinoma. *Fed. Proc.* 33: 610.

53. Vasudevan, D. M., Balakrishnan, K., and Talwars, G. P. 1971. Immunoglobulins in carcinoma of the cervix. *Ind. J. Med. Res.* 59: 1653–1659.

54. Waldman, R. H., Bencic, Z., Sinha, R., Deb, B. C., Sakazaki, R., Tamura, K., Mukerjee, S., and Ganguly, R. 1972. Cholera Immunology II Serum and intestinal secretion antibody response after naturally occurring cholera. *J. Inf. Dis.* 126: 401–407.

55. Waldman, R. H., and Ganguly, R. 1974. Immunity to infections on secretory surfaces. *J. Inf. Dis.* 130: 419–440.

56. Waldman, R. H., Mach, J. P., Stella, M. M., and Rowe, D. S. 1970. Secretory IgA in human serum. *J. Immunol.* 105: 43–47.

57. Waldman, R. H., Rowe, D. S., and Mach, J. P. 1973. Secretory IgA levels in serum of patients with various disorders. *Clin. Med.* 80: 11–13.

58. Waldman, T. A. 1972. Immunodeficiency disease and malignancy. *Ann. Intern. Med.* 77: 605–628.

59. Walsh, T. E., Cannon, P. R. 1938. Immunization of the respiratory tract: a comparative study of the antibody content of the respiratory and other tissues following active, passive and regional immunization. *J. Immunol.* 35: 31–46.

60. Wara, W. M., Ammann, A. J., Wara, D. W., and Phillips, T. L. 1975. Serum IgA in the diagnosis of nasopharyngeal and paranasal sinus carcinoma. *Radiology* 116: 409–411.

61. Wara, W. B., Wara, D. W., Phillips, T. L., and Ammann, A. J. 1975. Elevated IgA in carcinoma of the nasopharynx. *Cancer* 35: 1313–1315.

62. Zermoski, J., Gorny, M. K., Wruck, M., and Sapula, J. 1975. Behavior of local and systemic immunoglobulins in patients with lung cancer. *Int. Arch. Allergy Appl. Immunol.* 49: 548–563.

63. Zur Hausen, H., Schulte-Holthausen, H., Klein, G., Henle, W., Henle, G., Clifford, P., and Santesson, L. 1970. EBV DNA in biopsies of the Burkett tumors and anaplastic carcinomas of the nasopharynx. *Nature* 228: 1056–1058.

INDEX